NEUROLOGICAL FOUNDATIONS OF COGNITIVE NEUROSCIENCE

NEUROLOGICAL FOUNDATIONS OF COGNITIVE NEUROSCIENCE

edited by
Mark D'Esposito

A Bradford Book
The MIT Press
Cambridge, Massachusetts
London, England

This book was set in Times Roman by SNP Best-set Typesetter Ltd., Hong Kong and was printed and bound in the United States of America.

Library of Congress Cataloging-in-Publication Data

Neurological foundations of cognitive neuroscience / edited by Mark D'Esposito.
     p.   cm.—(Issues in clinical and cognitive neuropsychology)
  "A Bradford book."
  Includes bibliographical references and index.
  ISBN 0-262-04209-6 (hc. : alk. paper)
  1. Cognition disorders. 2. Cognitive neuroscience. I. D'Esposito, Mark. II. Series.

RC533.C64 N475 2002
616.8—dc21   2002021912

10 9 8 7 6 5 4 3 2 1

To Judy, Zoe, and Zack

Contents

Preface

It is an exciting time for the discipline of cognitive neuroscience. In the past 10 years we have witnessed an explosion in the development and advancement of methods that allow us to precisely examine the neural mechanisms underlying cognitive processes. Functional magnetic resonance imaging, for example, has provided markedly improved spatial and temporal resolution of brain structure and function, which has led to answers to new questions, and the reexamination of old questions. However, in my opinion, the explosive impact that functional neuroimaging has had on cognitive neuroscience may in some ways be responsible for moving us away from our roots—the study of patients with brain damage as a window into the functioning of the normal brain. Thus, my motivation for creating this book was to provide a collection of chapters that would highlight the interface between the study of patients with cognitive deficits and the study of cognition in normal individuals. It is my hope that reading these chapters will remind us as students of cognitive neuroscience that research aimed at understanding the function of the normal brain can be guided by studying the abnormal brain. The incredible insight derived from patients with neurological and psychiatric disorders provided the foundation for the discipline of cognitive neuroscience and should continue to be an important methodological tool in future studies.

Each chapter in this book was written by a neurologist who also practices cognitive neuroscience. Each chapter begins with a description of a case report, often a patient seen by the author, and describes the symptoms seen in this patient, laying the foundation for the cognitive processes to be explored. After the clinical description, the authors have provided a historical background about what we have learned about these particular neurobehavioral syndromes through clinical observation and neuropsychological investigation. Each chapter then explores investigations using a variety of methods—single-unit electrophysiological recording in awake-behaving monkeys, behavioral studies of normal healthy subjects, event-related potential

and functional neuroimaging studies of both normal individuals and neurological patients—aimed at understanding the neural mechanisms underlying the cognitive functions affected in each particular clinical syndrome. In many chapters, there are conflicting data derived from different methodologies, and the authors have tried to reconcile these differences. Often these attempts at understanding how these data may be convergent, rather than divergent, has shed new light on the cognitive mechanisms being explored.

The goal of preparing this book was not to simply describe clinical neurobehavioral syndromes. Such descriptions can be found in many excellent textbooks of behavioral and cognitive neurology. Nor was the goal to provide a primer in cognitive neuroscience. The goal of this book is to consider normal cognitive processes in the context of patients with cognitive deficits. Each of the clinical syndromes in this book is markedly heterogeneous and the range of symptoms varies widely across patients. As Anjan Chatterjee aptly states in his chapter on the neglect syndrome: "This heterogeneity would be cause for alarm if the goal of neglect research was to establish a unified and comprehensive theory of the clinical syndrome. However, when neglect is used to understand the organization of spatial attention and representation, then the behavioral heterogeneity is actually critical to its use as an investigative tool." These words capture perfectly my intent for this book.

Many neurologists in training and in practice lack exposure to cognitive neuroscience. Similarly, many newly trained cognitive neuroscientists lack exposure to the rich history of investigations of brain–behavior relationships in neurological patients. I am optimistic that this book will serve both groups well. It is a privilege to have assembled an outstanding group of neurologists and cognitive neuroscientists to present their unique perspective on the physical basis of the human mind.

NEUROLOGICAL FOUNDATIONS OF COGNITIVE NEUROSCIENCE

1 Neglect: A Disorder of Spatial Attention

Anjan Chatterjee

Unilateral spatial neglect is a fascinating clinical syndrome in which patients are unaware of entire sectors of space on the side opposite to their lesion. These patients may neglect parts of their own body, parts of their environment, and even parts of scenes in their imagination. This clinical syndrome is produced by a lateralized disruption of spatial attention and representation and raises several questions of interest to cognitive neuroscientsts. How do humans represent space? How do humans direct spatial attention? How is attention related to perception? How is attention related to action?

Spatial attention and representation can also be studied in humans with functional neuroimaging and with animal lesion and single-cell neurophysiological studies. Despite the unique methods and approaches of these different disciplines, there is considerable convergence in our understanding of how the brain organizes and represents space. In this chapter, I begin by describing the clinical syndrome of neglect. Following this description, I outline the major theoretical approaches and biological correlates of the clinical phenomena. I then turn to prominent issues in recent neglect research and to relevant data from human functional neuroimaging and animal studies. Finally, I conclude with several issues that in my view warrant further consideration.

As a prelude, it should be clear that neglect is a heterogeneous disorder. Its manifestations vary considerably across patients (Chatterjee, 1998; Halligan & Marshall, 1992, 1998). This heterogeneity would be cause for alarm if the goal of neglect research were to establish a unified and comprehensive theory of the clinical syndrome. However, when neglect is used to understand the organization of spatial attention and representation, then the behavioral heterogeneity is actually critical to its use as an investigative tool.

Distributed neuronal networks clearly mediate spatial attention, representation, and movement. Focal damage to parts of these networks can produce subtle differences in deficits of these complex functions. These differences themselves are of interest. A careful study of spatial attention and representations through the syndrome of neglect is possible precisely because neglect is heterogeneous (Chatterjee, 1998).

Case Report

Neglect is more common and more severe with right than with left brain damage. I will refer mostly to left-sided neglect following right brain damage, although similar deficits are seen sometimes following left brain damage.

A 65-year-old woman presented to the hospital because of left-sided weakness. She was lethargic for 2 days after admission. She tended to lie in bed at an angle, oriented to her right, and ignored the left side of her body. When her left hand was held in front of her eyes, she suggested that the limb belonged to the examiner. As her level of arousal improved, she continued to orient to her right, even when approached and spoken to from her left. She ate only the food on the right side of her hospital tray. Food sometimes collected in the left side of her mouth.

Her speech was mildly dysarthric. She answered questions correctly, but in a flat tone. Although her conversation was superficially appropriate, she seemed unconcerned about her condition or even about being in the hospital. When asked why she was hospitalized, she reported feeling weak generally, but denied any specific problems. When referring to her general weakness, she would look at and lift her right arm. Over several days, after hearing from her physicians that she had had a stroke and having repeatedly been asked by her physical therapist to move her left side, she acknowledged her left-sided weakness. However, her insight into the practical restrictions imposed by her weakness was limited. Her therapists noted that she was pleasant and engaging for short periods, but not particularly motivated during therapy sessions and fatigued easily.

Three months after her initial stroke, obvious signs of left neglect abated. Her left-sided weakness also improved. She had slightly diminished somatosensory sensation on the left, but after about 6 months she also experienced uncomfortable sensations both on the skin and "inside" her left arm. The patient continued to fatigue

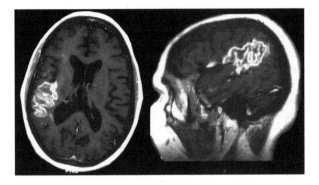

Figure 1.1
Contrast-enhanced magnetic resonance image showing lesion in the posterior division of the right middle cerebral artery, involving the inferior parietal lobule and the posterior superior temporal gyrus.

easily and remained at home much of the time. Her magnetic resonance imaging (MRI) scan showed an ischemic stroke in the posterior division of the right middle cerebral artery (figure 1.1). Her lesion involved the posterior inferior parietal lobule, Brodmann areas (BA) 39 and 40 and the posterior part of the superior temporal gyrus, BA 22.

Clinical Examination of Neglect

Bedside tests for neglect are designed to assess patients' awareness of the contralesional parts of their own body (personal neglect), contralesional sectors of space (extrapersonal neglect), and contralesional stimuli when presented simultaneously with competing ipsilesional stimuli (extinction).

Personal Neglect

Personal neglect refers to neglect of contralesional parts of one's own body. Observing whether patients groom themselves contralesionally provides a rough indication of personal neglect. Patients who ignore the left side of their body might not use a comb or makeup, or might not shave the left side of their face (Beschin & Robertson, 1997). To assess personal neglect, patients are asked about their left arm after this limb is brought into their

view. Patients with left personal neglect do not acknowledge ownership of the limb. When asked to touch their left arm with their right hand, these patients fail to reach over and touch their left side (Bisiach, Perani, Vallar, & Berti, 1986).

A phenomenon called anosognosia for hemiplegia can also be thought of as a disorder of personal awareness. In this condition, patients are aware of their contralesional limb, but are not aware of its paralysis (Bisiach, 1993). Anosognosia for hemiplegia is not an all-or-none phenomenon, and patients may have partial awareness of their contralesional weakness (Chatterjee & Mennemeier, 1996). Misoplegia is a rare disorder in which patients are aware of their own limb, but develop an intense dislike for it (Critchley, 1974).

Extrapersonal Neglect

Extrapersonal neglect can be assessed using bedside tasks such as line bisection, cancellation, drawing, and reading. Line bisection tasks assess a patient's ability to estimate the center of a simple stimulus. Patients are asked to place a mark at the midpoint of lines (usually horizontal). The task is generally administered without restricting head or eye movements and without time limitations. Patients with left-sided neglect typically place their mark to the right of the true midposition (Schenkenberg, Bradford, & Ajax, 1980). Patients make larger errors with longer lines (Chatterjee, Dajani, & Gage, 1994a). If stimuli are placed in space contralateral to their lesion, patients frequently make larger errors (Heilman & Valenstein, 1979). Thus, using long lines (generally greater than 20 cm) placed to the left of the patient's trunk increases the sensitivity of detecting extrapersonal neglect using line bisection tasks.

Cancellation tasks assess how well a patient explores the contralesional side of extrapersonal space (figure 1.2). Patients are presented with arrays of targets which they are asked to "cancel." Cancellation tasks are also administered without restricting head or eye movements and without time limitations. Patients typically start at the top right of the display and often search in a vertical pattern (Chatterjee, Mennemeier, & Heilman, 1992a). They neglect left-sided targets (Albert, 1973) and often targets close to their body, so that a target in the left lower quadrant is most likely to be ignored (Chatterjee, Thompson, & Ricci, 1999; Mark & Heilman, 1997). Sometimes patients cancel right-sided targets repeatedly. Increasing the number of targets may uncover neglect that is not evident on arrays with fewer targets (Chatterjee, Mennemeier, & Heilman, 1992b; Chatterjee et al., 1999). The use

of arrays in which targets are difficult to discriminate from distracter stimuli (Rapcsak, Verfaellie, Fleet, & Heilman, 1989) may increase the sensitivity of cancellation tasks. Thus, using arrays with a large number of stimuli (generally more than fifty) and with distracters that are difficult to discriminate from the targets increases the sensitivity of cancellation tasks in detecting extrapersonal neglect.

In drawing tasks, patients are asked to either copy drawings presented to them or to draw objects and scenes from memory (figures 1.3 and 1.4). When asked to copy drawings with multiple objects, or complex objects with multiple parts, patients may omit left-sided objects in the array and/or omit the left side of individual objects, regardless of where they appear in the array (Marshall & Halligan, 1993; Seki & Ishiai, 1996). Occasionally, patients may draw left-sided features of target items with less detail or even misplace left-sided details to the right side of their drawings (Halligan, Marshall, & Wade, 1992).

Reading tasks can be given by having patients read text or by having them read single words. Patients with left-sided neglect may have trouble bringing their gaze to the left margin of the page when reading text. As a consequence, they may read lines starting in the middle of the page and produce sequences of words or sentences that do not make sense. When reading single words, they may either omit left-sided letters or substitute confabulated letters (Chatterjee, 1995). Thus the word "walnut" might be read as either "nut" or "peanut." This reading disorder is called "neglect dyslexia" (Kinsbourne & Warrington, 1962).

Extinction to Double Simultaneous Stimulation

Patients who are aware of single left-sided stimuli may neglect or "extinguish" these stimuli when left-sided stimuli are presented simultaneously with right-sided stimuli (Bender & Furlow, 1945). Extinction may occur for visual, auditory, or tactile stimuli (Heilman, Pandya, & Geschwind, 1970). Visual extinction can be assessed by asking patients to count fingers or to report finger movements

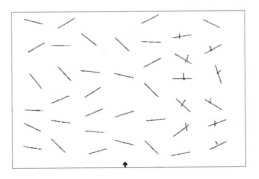

Figure 1.2
Example of a cancellation task showing left neglect. That task is given without time constraints and without restricting eye or head movements.

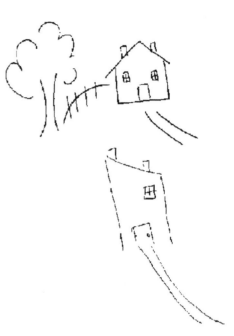

Figure 1.4
Example of a drawing copied by a patient with left neglect.

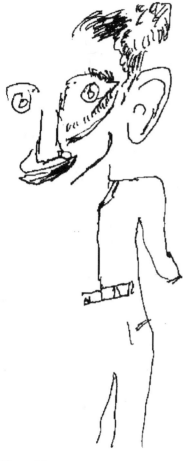

Figure 1.3
Example of a spontaneous drawing by a patient with left neglect.

presented to both visual fields compared with single visual fields. Auditory extinction can be assessed by asking them to report which ear hears a noise made by snapped fingers or two coins rubbed together at one or both ears. Tactile extinction can be assessed by lightly touching patients either unilaterally or bilaterally and asking them to report where they were touched. Patients' eyes should be closed when tactile extinction is being assessed since their direc-

tion of gaze can modulate extinction (Vaishnavi, Calhoun, & Chatterjee, 1999).

Extinction may even be elicited by having patients judge relative weights placed in their hands simultaneously (Chatterjee & Thompson, 1998). Patients with extinction may dramatically underestimate left-sided weights when a weight is also placed on their right hand. Finally, extinction may also be observed with multiple stimuli in ipsilesional space (Feinberg, Haber, & Stacy, 1990; Rapcsak, Watson, & Heilman, 1987).

General Theories of Neglect

General theories emphasize behaviors common to patients with neglect and try to isolate the core deficit, which produces the clinical syndrome. These theories include attentional and representational theories.

Attentional Theories

Attentional theories are based on the idea that neglect is a disorder of spatial attention. Spatial attention is the process by which objects in certain spatial locations are selected for processing over objects in other locations. The processing may involve selection for perception or for actions. The idea that objects in spatial locations are selected for action has given rise to the notion of "intentional neglect," in which patients are disinclined to act in or toward contralesional space. (Intentional neglect is discussed more fully later in this chapter.)

Attention is generally considered effortful and usually operates serially. Normally, the nervous system processes visual information in stages. Visual elements, such as color, movement, and form, are extracted initially from the visual scene. These elements are segregated or grouped together "preattentively," to parse the visual scene before attention is engaged. Preattentive processing is generally considered automatic and often operates in parallel across different spatial locations. Brain damage can produce selective deficits at this preattentive level with relatively normal spatial attention (Ricci, Vaishnavi, & Chatterjee, 1999; Vecera & Behrmann, 1997). By contrast, patients with neglect often have relatively preserved preattentive vision, as evidenced by their ability to separate figure from ground and their susceptibility to visual illusions (Driver, Baylis, & Rafal, 1992; Mattingley, Davis, & Driver, 1997; Ricci, Calhoun, & Chatterjee, 2000; Vallar, Daini, & Antonucci, 2000).

In neglect, attention is directed ipsilesionally, and therefore patients are aware of stimuli only in this sector of space. A major concern of general attentional theories is to understand why neglect is more common and severe after right than after left brain damage. Kinsbourne postulates that each hemisphere generates a vector of spatial attention directed toward contralateral space, and these attentional vectors are inhibited by the opposite hemisphere (Kinsbourne, 1970, 1987). The left hemisphere's vector of spatial attention is strongly biased, while the right hemisphere produces only a weak vector. Therefore, after right brain damage, the left hemisphere's unfettered vector of attention is powerfully oriented to the right. Since the right hemisphere's intrinsic vector of attention is only weakly directed after left brain damage, there is not a similar orientation bias to the left. Thus, right-sided neglect is less common than left-sided neglect.

Heilman and co-workers, in contrast to Kinsbourne, propose that the right hemisphere is dominant for arousal and spatial attention (Heilman, 1979; Heilman & Van Den Abell, 1980). Patients with right brain damage have greater electroencephalographic slowing than those with left brain damage. They also demonstrate diminished galvanic skin responses compared with normal control subjects or patients with left hemisphere damage (Heilman, Schwartz, & Watson, 1978). This diminished arousal interacts with hemispheric biases in directing attention. The right hemisphere is thought to be capable of directing attention into both hemispaces, while the left hemisphere directs attention only into contralateral space. Thus, after right brain damage, the left hemisphere is ill equipped to direct attention into left hemispace. However, after left brain damage, the right is capable of directing attention into both hemispaces and neglect does not occur with the same severity as after right brain damage. Mesulam (1981, 1990), emphasizing the distributed nature of neural networks dedicated to spatial attention, also proposed a similar hemispheric organization for spatial attention.

Posner and colleagues proposed an influential model of spatial attention composed of elementary operations, such as engaging, disengaging, and shifting (Posner, Walker, Friedrich, & Rafal, 1984; Posner & Dehaene, 1994). They reported that patients with right superior parietal damage are selectively impaired in disengaging attention from right-sided stimuli before they shift and engage left-sided stimuli. This disengage deficit is likely to account for some symptoms of visual extinction. In more recent versions of this theory, Posner and colleagues proposed a posterior and an anterior attentional network, which bears considerable resemblance to Heilman's and Mesulam's ideas of distributed networks. Some parts of this network are preferentially dedicated to selecting stimuli in space for perception and others to selecting stimuli in space on which to act.

Representational Theories

Representational theories propose that the inability to form adequate contralateral mental representations of space underlies the clinical phenomenology in neglect (Bisiach, 1993). In a classic observation, Bisiach and Luzzatti (1978) asked two patients to imagine the Piazza del Duomo in Milan, Italy, from two perspectives: looking into the square toward the cathedral and looking from the cathedral into the square (figure 1.5). In each condition, the patients only reported landmarks to the right of their imagined position in the piazza. Neglect for images evoked from memory may be dissociated from neglect of stimuli in extrapersonal space (Anderson, 1993; Coslett, 1997). In addition to difficulty in evoking contralateral representations from memory, patients with neglect may also be impaired in forming new contralateral representations (Bisiach, Luzzatti, & Perani, 1979). Rapid eye movements in sleeping neglect patients are restricted ipsilaterally (Doricchi, Guariglia, Paolucci, & Pizzamiglio, 1993), raising the intriguing possibility that these patients' dreams are spatially restricted.

Attentional versus Representational Theories

Although representational theories are often contrasted with attentional theories, it is not clear that attentional and representational theories of neglect are really in conflict (see the contributions in Halligan & Marshall, 1994, for related discussions). Sensory-attentional and representational theories seem to be describing different aspects of the same phenomena. Awareness of external stimuli occurs by mentally reconstructing objects in the world. It is therefore not clear that describing attention directed in external space avoids the need to consider mental representations. Similarly, mental representations, even when internally evoked, are selectively generated and maintained. It is not clear how describing spatially selective representation avoids the need to consider spatial attention. Attentional theories refer to the process and dynamics that support mental representations. Representational theories refer to the structural features of the disordered system. Each theoretical approach seems inextricably linked to the other.

Biological Correlates of Neglect

Neglect is seen with a variety of lesions involving different cortical and subcortical structures. It is also associated with dysregulation of specific neurotransmitter systems.

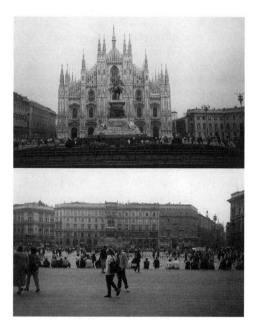

Figure 1.5
Two views of the Piazza del Duomo in Milan, Italy.

Cortical Lesions

Neglect is more common and more severe in cases of right than left hemisphere damage (Gainotti, Messerli, & Tissot, 1972). The characteristic lesion involves the right inferior parietal lobe, Brodmann areas 39 and 40 (Heilman, Watson, & Valenstein, 1994). Recently, Karnath and colleagues (Karnath, Ferber & Himmelbach, 2001) have suggested that lesions to the right superior temporal gyrus are associated most commonly with extrapersonal neglect in the absence of visual field defects. Neglect may also be observed after dorsolateral prefrontal (Heilman & Valenstein, 1972; Husain & Kennard, 1996; Maeshima, Funahashi, Ogura, Itakura, & Komai, 1994) and cingulate gyrus lesions (Watson, Heilman, Cauthen, & King, 1973). Severe neglect is more likely if the posterior-superior longitudinal fasciculus and the inferior-frontal fasciculus are damaged in addition to these cortical areas (Leibovitch et al., 1998).

The cortical areas associated with neglect are supramodal or polymodal areas into which unimodal association cortices project (Mesulam, 1981). This observation underscores the idea that neglect is a spatial disorder, not one of primary sensory processing (such as a visual field defect). The polymodal nature of the deficit means that neglect may be evident in different sensory and motor systems, without necessarily being restricted to one modality.

Subcortical Lesions

Subcortical lesions in the thalamus, basal ganglia, and midbrain may also produce neglect. Neglect in humans is associated with decreased arousal (Heilman et al., 1978). Interruptions of ascending monoaminergic or cholinergic projections may in part mediate this clinical manifestation (Watson, Heilman, Miller, & King, 1974).

The extension of the reticular system into the thalamus is a thin shell of neurons encasing much of the thalamus and is called the "nucleus reticularis." The nucleus reticularis neurons inhibit relays of sensory information from the thalamus to the cortex. In turn, descending projections from the polymodal association cortices inhibit the nucleus reticularis. Therefore damage to these systems may result in a release of the inhibitory action of the nucleus reticularis on thalamic relay nuclei, producing impairment of contralesional sensory processing (Watson, Valenstein, & Heilman, 1981). Damage to the pulvinar, a large nucleus located posteriorily in the thalamus, which has reciprocal connections with the posterior parietal lobule, may result in neglect. Lesions of the basal ganglia, which are tightly linked to prefrontal and cingulate cortices, may also produce neglect (Hier, Davis, Richardson, & Mohr, 1977).

Distributed Neural Networks

The clinical observation that lesions to disparate cortical and subcortical structures produce neglect led Heilman and co-workers to propose that a distributed network mediates spatially directed attention (Heilman, 1979; Watson et al., 1981). The limbic connections to the anterior cingulate may provide an anatomical basis for poor alertness for stimuli in contralesional locations (Watson et al., 1973) or poor motivation (Mesulam, 1990) in neglect patients.

Mesulam (1981, 1990), emphasizing the monosynaptic interconnectivity of the different brain regions associated with neglect, also proposed a similar model suggesting that different regions within a large-scale network control different aspects of an individual's interaction with the spatial environment. He suggested that dorsolateral prefrontal damage produces abnormalities of contralesional exploratory behavior and that posterior parietal damage produces the perceptual disorder seen in neglect.

The appealingly straightforward idea that lesions in different locations within this distributed network are associated with different behavioral manifestations of neglect is not entirely supported by the evidence (Chatterjee, 1998). The most commonly cited association is that parietal lesions produce the perceptual aspects of neglect and frontal lesions produce the response or motor aspects of neglect. Some studies report this association and others do not (Binder, Marshall, Lazar, Benjamin, & Mohr, 1992; Coslett, Bowers, Fitzpatrick, Haws, & Heilman, 1990; McGlinchey-Berroth et al., 1996). One study of a large number of patients even reports parietal lesions associated with a bias to respond ipsilesionally (Bisiach, Ricci, Lualdi, & Colombo, 1998a).

Neurochemistry of Neglect

Distributed neural networks are usually thought of in terms of anatomical connections. However, neurotransmitter systems also form distributed networks with more diffuse effects. Rather than influencing specific cognitive domains, these diffuse systems seem to influence the state of brain functions across many domains. Dopaminergic systems are of critical importance in neglect. In rats, lesions to ascending dopaminergic pathways produce behavioral abnormalities that resemble neglect (Marshall & Gotthelf, 1979), and the dopaminergic agonist, apomorphine, ameliorates these deficits. This improvement can be blocked by pretreatment with spiroperidol, a dopamine receptor blocking agent (Corwin et al., 1986).

These observations led to a small open trial of the dopamine agonist, bromocriptine, in two patients with neglect (Fleet, Valenstein, Watson, & Heilman, 1987). Both patients' performances improved during bedside assessments of neglect. One patient's husband reported improvement in her activities of daily living. Recent reports suggest that bromocriptine may produce greater improvement than methylphenidate (Hurford, Stringer, & Jann, 1998) and may be more effective in treating the motor aspects of neglect behaviors than strictly perceptual ones (Geminiani, Bottini, & Sterzi, 1998). The efficacy of pharmacological treatment in the neglect syndrome has not been investigated systematically in large-scale studies.

Experimental Research on Neglect

Neglect has become an important probe in investigating several issues in cognitive neuroscience. The topics described next have in common the use of neglect and related disorders as a point of departure, although the issues addressed may be quite divergent.

Intention in Spatial Representations

Intentional systems select from among many locations those in which to act. This system is yoked to attentional systems, which select stimuli to be processed. There is a growing awareness that much of perception serves to guide actions in the world (Milner & Goodale, 1995). Some time ago, Watson and colleagues advanced the idea that neglect patients may have a premotor intentional deficit, a disinclination to initiate movements or move toward or into contralateral hemispace (Watson, Valenstein, & Heilman, 1978). Similarly, Rizzolatti and coworkers argued that attention facilitates perception by activating the circuits responsible for motor preparation (Rizzolatti, Matelli, & Pavesi, 1983).

In most situations, attention and intention are inextricably linked, since attention is usually directed to objects on which one acts. Several clever experiments have tried to dissociate attention from intention using cameras, pulleys, and mirrors (Bisiach, Geminiani, Berti, & Rusconi, 1990; Bisiach et al., 1995; Coslett et al., 1990; Milner, Harvey, Roberts, & Forster, 1993; Na et al., 1998; Tegner & Levander, 1991). The general strategy in these studies is to dissociate where patients are looking from where their limb is acting. When patients perform tasks in which these two are in conflict, in some patients neglect is determined by where they are looking and in others by where they are acting. Some patients behave as though they have a combination of the two forms of neglect.

Neglect as ipsilesional biases in limb movements is sometimes associated with frontal lesions (Binder et al., 1992; Coslett et al., 1990; Tegner &

Levander, 1991). However, patients with lesions restricted to the posterior parietal cortex can have intentional neglect (Mattingley, Husain, Rorden, Kennard, & Driver, 1998; Triggs, Gold, Gerstle, Adair, & Heilman, 1994). Mattingley and colleagues (Mattingley, Bradshaw, & Phillips, 1992) reported that slowness in the initiation of leftward movements is associated with right posterior lesions, whereas slowness in the execution of leftward movements is associated with right anterior and subcortical lesions. Most patients with neglect probably have mixtures of attentional and intentional neglect (Adair, Na, Schwartz, & Heilman, 1998b), which may be related in quite complex ways.

One problem in the interpretation of these studies is that attention versus intention may not be the relevant distinction. Rather, the "attention" experimental conditions may reflect the link of attention to eye movement and the "intention" conditions may reflect the link of attention to limb movements (Bisiach et al., 1995; Chatterjee, 1998). The relevant distinction may actually be between two perceptual-motor systems, one led by direction of gaze and the other by direction of limb movements. Such an interpretation would be consonant with single-cell neurophysiological data from monkeys, which show that attentional neurons in the posterior parietal cortex are selectively linked to eye or to limb movements (Colby, 1998).

Spatial Attention in Three Dimensions

Neglect is usually described along the horizontal (left-right) axis. However, our spatial environment also includes radial (near-far) and vertical (up-down) axes. Neglect may also be evident in these coordinate systems. Patients with left neglect frequently have a more subtle neglect for near space. On cancellation tasks they are most likely to omit targets in the left lower quadrant in which left and near neglect combine (Chatterjee et al., 1999; Mark & Heilman, 1997). Patients with bilateral lesions may have dramatic vertical and radial neglect (Butter, Evans, Kirsch, & Kewman, 1989;

Mennemeier, Wertman, & Heilman, 1992; Rapcsak, Fleet, Verfaellie, & Heilman, 1988). Bilateral lesions to temporal-parietal areas may produce neglect for lower and near peripersonal space, whereas bilateral lesions to the ventral temporal structures are associated with neglect for upper and far extrapersonal space. Neglect in the vertical axis probably represents complex interplays between the visual and vestibular influences on spatial attention (Mennemeier, Chatterjee, & Heilman, 1994).

Left neglect may also vary, depending on whether the stimuli are located in close peripersonal space or in far extrapersonal space, suggesting that the organization of space in peripersonal space is distinct from the organization in further extrapersonal space (Previc, 1998). This notion of concentric shells of space around the body's trunk was suggested initially by Brain (1941), who proposed that peripersonal space is a distinct spatial construct defined by the reach of one's limbs.

Spatial Reference Frames

Objects in extrapersonal space are anchored to different reference frames. These frames are generally divided into viewer-, object-, and environment-centered reference frames. For example, we can locate a chair in a room in each of these frames. A viewer-centered frame would locate the chair to the left or right of the viewer. This frame itself is divided into retinal, head-centered, or body-centered frames. An object-centered frame refers to the intrinsic spatial coordinates of the object itself, its top or bottom or right and left. These coordinates are not altered by changes in the position of the viewer. The top of the chair remains its top regardless of where the viewer is located.

An environment-centered reference frame refers to the location of the object in relation to its environment. The chair would be coded with respect to other objects in the room and how it is related to gravitational coordinates. The vestibular system through the otolith organs probably plays an important role in establishing the orientation of an object in relationship to the environmental vertical axis

(Mennemeier et al., 1994; Pizzamiglio, Vallar, & Doricchi, 1997). Several reports demonstrate that neglect may occur in any of these reference frames (Behrmann, Moscovitch, Black, & Mozer, 1994; Chatterjee, 1994; Driver & Halligan, 1991; Farah, Brun, Wong, Wallace, & Carpenter, 1990; Hillis & Caramazza, 1995; Ladavas, 1987), suggesting that spatial attention operates across these different reference frames.

Cross-Modal and Sensorimotor Integration of Space

Humans have a coherent sense of space in which they perceive objects and act (Driver & Spence, 1998). Neglect studies suggest that multiple spatial representations are embedded within this sense of space. Presumably, multiple sensory modalities interact in complex ways to give rise to multiple representations of space.

Rubens and colleagues (Rubens, 1985) demonstrated that left-sided vestibular stimulation improves extrapersonal neglect. Presumably, vestibular inputs influence visual and spatial attention in complex ways. Vestibular stimulation can also improve contralesional somatosensory awareness (Vallar, Bottini, Rusconi, & Sterzi, 1993) and may transiently improve anosognosia as well (Cappa, Sterzi, Guiseppe, & Bisiach, 1987). Spatial attention may also be influenced by changes in posture, which are presumably mediated by otolith vestibular inputs (Mennemeier et al., 1994). Similarly, proprioceptive inputs from neck muscles can influence spatial attention (Karnath, Sievering, & Fetter, 1994; Karnath, Schenkel, & Fischer, 1991) and serve to anchor viewer-centered reference frames to an individual's trunk.

Recent studies of patients with tactile extinction have also focused on cross-modal factors in awareness. Visual input when close to the location of tactile stimulation may improve contralesional tactile awareness (di Pellegrino, Basso, & Frassinetti, 1998; Ladavas, Di Pellegrino, Farne, & Zeloni, 1998; Vaishnavi et al., 1999). Similarly, the intention to move may also improve contralesional

tactile awareness (Vaishnavi et al., 1999). Since patients with neglect may have personal neglect (Bisiach et al., 1986) or a deficit of their own body schema (Coslett, 1998), the question of how body space is integrated with extrapersonal space also arises. Tactile sensations are experienced as being produced by an object touching the body, an aspect of peripersonal space. Visual sensations are experienced as being produced by objects at a distance from the body, in extrapersonal space. The integration of tactile and visual stimulation may contribute to the coordination of extrapersonal and peripersonal space (Vaishnavi, Calhoun, & Chatterjee, 2001).

Guiding movements by vision also involves integrating visual signals for movement. This visual-motor mapping can be altered if a subject wears prisms that displace stimuli to the left or right of their field of view. Recent work suggests that patients with neglect who are wearing prisms that displace visual stimuli to their right remap ballistic movements leftward, and that this remapping can be useful in rehabilitation (Rossetti et al., 1998).

Psychophysics, Attention, and Perception in Neglect

What is the relationship between the magnitude of stimuli and the magnitude of patients' representations of these stimuli? This question features prominently in psychophysical studies dating back to the seminal work of Gustav Fechner in the nineteenth century (Fechner, 1899). How do we understand the kinds of spatial distortions (Anderson, 1996; Karnath & Ferber, 1999; Milner & Harvey, 1995) and "anisometries" (Bisiach, Ricci, & Modona, 1998b) shown in the perception of neglect patients? It turns out that patients are not always aware of the same proportion of space. Nor are they always aware of the same quantity of stimuli. Rather, their awareness is systematically related to the quantity of stimuli presented (Chatterjee et al., 1992b).

The evidence that neglect patients are systematically influenced by the magnitude of the stimuli with which they are confronted has been studied the most in the context of line bisection (Bisiach, Bulgarelli, Sterzi, & Vallar, 1983). Patients make larger errors on larger lines. Marshall and Halligan demonstrated that psychophysical laws could describe the systematic nature of these performances (Marshall & Halligan, 1990). Following this line of reasoning, Chatterjee showed that patients' performances on line bisection, cancellation, single-word reading tasks, and weight judgments can be described mathematically by power functions (Chatterjee, 1995, 1998; Chatterjee et al., 1994a, 1992b; Chatterjee, Mennemeier, & Heilman, 1994b). In these functions, $\psi = K\phi^\beta$, ϕ represents the objective magnitude of the stimuli, and ψ represents the subjective awareness of the patient. The constant K and exponent β are derived empirically.

Power function relationships are observed widely in normal psychophysical judgments of magnitude estimates across different sensory stimuli (Stevens, 1970). An exponent of one suggests that mental representations within a stimulus range are proportionate to the physical range. Exponents less than one, which occur in the normal judgments of luminance magnitudes, suggest that mental representations are compressed in relation to the range of the physical stimulus. Exponents greater than one, as in judgments of pain intensity, suggest that mental representations are expanded in relation to the range of the physical stimulus.

Chatterjee and colleagues showed that patients with neglect, across a variety of tasks, have power functions with exponents that are lower than those of normal patients. These observations suggest that while patients remain sensitive to changes in sensory magnitudes, their awareness of the size of these changes is blunted. For example, the exponent for normal judgments of linear extension is very close to one. By contrast, neglect patients have diminished exponents, suggesting that they, unlike normal subjects, do not experience horizontal lines of increasing lengths as increasing proportionately. It should be noted that these observations also mean that nonlinear transformations of the magnitude of sensations into mental representations occur within the central nervous system and not simply at the level of sensory receptors, as implied by Stevens (1972).

Crossover in Neglect

Halligan and Marshall (Halligan & Marshall, 1988; Marshall & Halligan, 1989) discovered that patients with neglect tended to bisect short lines to the left of the objective midpoint and seemed to demonstrate ipsilesional neglect with these stimuli. This crossover behavior is found in most patients (Chatterjee et al., 1994a) with neglect, and is not explained easily by most neglect theories. In fact, Bisiach referred to it as "a repressed pain in the neck for neglect theorists." Using performance on single-word reading tasks, Chatterjee (1995) showed that neglect patients sometimes confabulate letters to the left side of short words, and thus read them as longer than their objective length. He argued that this crossover behavior represents a contralesional release of mental representations. This idea has been shown to be plausible in a formal computational model (Monaghan & Shillcock, 1998).

The crossover in line bisection is also influenced by the context in which these lines are seen. Thus, patients are more likely to cross over and bisect to the left of the true midpoint if these bisections are preceded by a longer line (Marshall, Lazar, Krakauer, & Sharma, 1998). Recently, Chatterjee and colleagues (Chatterjee, Ricci, & Calhoun, 2000; Chatterjee & Thompson, 1998) showed that a crossoverlike phenomenon also occurs with weight judgments. Patients in general are likely to judge right-sided weights as heavier than left-sided weights. However, with lighter weight pairs, this bias may reverse to where they judge the left side to be heavier than the right. These results indicate that crossover is a general perceptual phenomenon that is not restricted to the visual system.

Implicit Processing in Neglect

The general view of the hierarchical nature of visual and spatial processing is that visual information is processed preattentively before attentional systems are engaged. If neglect is an attentional disorder, then some information might still be processed preattentively. Neglect patients do seem able to process some contralesional stimuli preattentively, as evidenced by their abilities to make figure-ground distinctions and their susceptibility to visual illusions (Driver et al., 1992; Mattingley et al., 1997; Ricci et al., 2000).

How much can stimuli be processed and yet not penetrate consciousness? Volpe and colleagues (Volpe, Ledoux, & Gazzaniga, 1979) initially reported that patients with visual extinction to pictures shown simultaneously were still able to make same-different judgments more accurately than would be expected if they were simply guessing. Since then, others have reported that pictures neglected on the left can facilitate processing of words centrally located (and not neglected) if the pictures and words belong to the same semantic category, such as animals (McGlinchey-Berroth, Milberg, Verfaellie, Alexander, & Kilduff, 1993). Similarly, lexical decisions about ipsilesional words are aided by neglected contralesional words (Ladavas, Paladini, & Cubelli, 1993). Whether neglected stimuli may be processed to higher levels of semantic knowledge and still be obscured from the patient's awareness remains unclear (Bisiach & Rusconi, 1990; Marshall & Halligan, 1988).

Functional Neuroimaging Studies of Spatial Attention and Representation

Positron emission tomography (PET) and functional magnetic resonance imaging (fMRI) studies offer insights into neurophysiological changes occurring during specific cognitive tasks. Functional imaging has the advantage of using normal subjects. These methods address several issues relevant to neglect.

Hemispheric Asymmetries

Heilman and colleagues (Heilman & Van Den Abell, 1980) as well as Mesulam (1981) postulated that the right hemisphere deploys attention diffusely to the right and left sides of space, whereas the left hemisphere directs attention contralesionally. From such a hemispheric organization of spatial attention, one would predict relatively greater right than left hemisphere activation when attention shifts in either direction. By contrast, the left hemisphere should be activated preferentially when attention is directed to the right.

Normal subjects do show greater right hemispheric activation with attentional shifts to both the right and left hemispaces, and greater left hemisphere activations with rightward shifts (Corbetta, Miezen, Shulman, & Peterson, 1993; Gitelman et al., 1999; Kim et al., 1999). Because intentional neglect follows right brain damage, one might expect similar results for motor movements. Right hemisphere activation is seen with exploratory movements, even when directed into right hemispace (Gitelman et al., 1996). Despite these asymmetries, homologous areas in both hemispheres are often activated, raising questions about the functional significance of left hemisphere activation in these tasks.

Frontal-Parietal Networks

Most functional imaging studies of visual and spatial attention find activation of the intraparietal sulcus (banks of BA 7 and BA 19) and adjacent regions, especially the superior parietal lobule (BA 7). Corbetta and colleagues (Corbetta et al., 1993) used PET and found the greatest increases in blood flow in the right superior parietal lobule (BA 7) and dorsolateral prefrontal cortex (BA 6) when subjects were cued endogenously to different locations. They found bilateral activation, but the activation was greater in the hemisphere contralateral to the attended targets. The right inferior parietal cortex (BA 40), the superior temporal sulcus (BA 22), and the anterior cingulate were also active (BA 24), but not consistently.

Nobre and colleagues (Nobre, Sebestyen, Gitelman, & Mesulam, 1997), also using PET, found that an exogenous shift in attention was associated with activation around the intraparietal sulcus. Taking advantage of fMRI's better spatial resolution, Corbetta and colleagues (Corbetta, 1998) confirmed activation of the intraparietal sulcus as well as the postcentral and precentral sulcus with shifts of attention. This activation was found even when explicit motor responses were not required, suggesting that these areas can be attentionally engaged without motor preparation. They also found similar blood flow increases in the right intraparietal sulcus and precentral cortex when attention was directed at a peripheral location in a sustained manner, rather than just shifting to a peripheral location.

The dorsolateral prefrontal cortex is also activated in most studies in which visual attention is shifted to different locations. These activations seem to center around the frontal eye fields (BA 6/8) and the adjacent areas. Working memory or inhibition of eye movement might be associated with dorsolateral prefrontal cortex activity. Gitelman and co-workers (Gitelman et al., 1999) showed that activation of these areas on attentional tasks is probably not due to these processes. However, the studies did not completely control for eye movements, which could be contributing to these activations. Nonetheless, given that dorsolateral prefrontal cortex lesions also produce disorders of attention, it is likely that these areas are linked to the posterior parietal regions involved in directing spatial attention.

Supramodal, Space-Based, and Object-Based Attention

A long-standing question about the organization of attention is whether there is a supramodal all-purpose attention module, or whether attention is better viewed as a collection of different modules

tied to distinct sensory and motor systems. To address this question, Wojciulik and Kanwisher (1999) used fMRI in three different tasks of visual attention. These tasks involved shifting attention, matching objects in different locations, and conjoining visual features of an object at a specific location. They found that the intraparietal sulcus was activated in all three tasks. While one cannot prove the null hypothesis that the intraparietal sulcus is involved in all attentional tasks, they suggest that this area might mediate a general attention and selection module. Similarly, Coull and Frith (1998) in a PET study found that while the superior parietal lobule was more responsive to spatial than nonspatial attention, the intraparietal sulcus was responsive to both.

The most striking aspect of neglect syndromes is that patients are unaware of contralesional space and of objects that inhabit that space. A central tenet of visual neuroscience is the relative segregation of visual information into a dorsal "where" stream and a ventral "what" stream (Ungerleider & Mishkin, 1982). The dorsal stream processes the spatial locations of objects of interest, whereas the ventral stream processes features necessary to identify the object. Somehow humans integrate these streams of information to be aware of both the "where" and "what" of objects.

Attention modulates the activity of neural structures in the ventral stream dedicated to identifying objects. Patients with prefrontal damage are impaired in discriminating contralesional visual targets. This impairment is associated with diminished event-related potentials at 125 ms and lasting for another 500 ms (Barcelo, Suwazono, & Knight, 2000). These event-related potentials are linked to extrastriate processing, which is associated with tonic activation as well as the selection of features and the postselection analyses of objects.

The earliest point in visual processing at which attentional modulation can occur is not clear. Several studies suggest that the primary visual cortex might be modulated by attention (Brefczynski & DeYoe, 1999; Gandhi, Heeger, &

Boynton, 1999; Sommers, Dale, Seiffert, & Tootell, 1999). However, Martinez and colleagues (Martninez et al., 1999) using data from event-related potentials point out that attentional modulation in the visual system is evident only after 70–75 ms. Since the initial sensory input to the primary visual cortex occurs at about 50–55 ms, they suggest that primary visual activation may be due to feedback activity rather than attentional modulation. The behavioral significance of such feedback, if that is what is being observed, remains to be explored.

Activity in neural structures downstream in ventral visual processing is clearly modulated by attention. Cognitively demanding tasks can inhibit activity in visual motion areas, even when the moving stimuli are irrelevant to the task at hand (Rees, Frith, & Lavie, 1997). Baseline activity in these early visual processing areas can also be modulated by attentional sets. Normally, stimuli suppress the processing of other stimuli located in close proximity. Similarly, subjects instructed to attend to color have increased activity in color areas (V4) and when asked to attend to motion have increased activity in motion areas (V5), even when the stimuli themselves are not colored or moving (Chawla, Rees, & Friston, 1999). Kastner and colleagues (Kastner, De Weerd, Desimone, & Ungerleider, 1998) showed that fMRI activation of areas within occipitotemporal regions is associated with this normal suppression. This suppression, however, diminishes when spatial attention is directed to locations encompassing both stimuli, suggesting an overall enhancement of processing of stimuli in those areas.

The appropriate experimental paradigms and methods of analysis in functional imaging studies of spatial attention are still being worked out. In this early stage of the field's development, some findings are difficult to reconcile with the rest of the literature. One might reasonably surmise that the parietal cortex mediates attention directed in space and the occipital and temporal cortices mediate attention directed to features and objects. However, in a PET study, Fink and colleagues (Fink, Dolan, Halligan, Marshall, & Frith, 1997) did not find this

functional anatomical relationship. They found that attention directed in space activated the right prefrontal (BA 9) and inferior temporal-occipital (BA 20) cortex, whereas attention directed at objects activated the left striate and peristriate cortex (BA 17/18). Both types of attention activated the left and right medial superior parietal cortex (BA 7/19), the left lateral inferior parietal cortex (BA 40/7), the left prefrontal cortex (BA 9), and the cerebellar vermis.

Animal Studies of Spatial Attention and Representation

Animal studies offer insight into mechanisms of spatial attention that are not obtained easily by studying humans. Lesions in animals can be made with considerable precision, in contrast to lesions in humans, which are often determined by vascular anatomy (in the case of stroke) rather than by cortical or functional anatomy. Neurophysiological studies in animals can address the activity and responsiveness of single neurons, in contrast to functional neuroimaging in humans, which offers insight into the neurophysiology at the level of neural networks.

Lesion Studies

Animal lesion studies confirm the idea that distributed neural networks involving the parietal and frontal cortices mediate spatial attention and awareness. In rodents, lesions of the posterior parietal or frontal cortex (medial agranular cortex) or the dorsolateral striatum produce a syndrome similar to neglect (Burcham, Corwin, Stoll, & Reep, 1997; Corwin & Reep, 1998). These rodents are more likely to orient ipsilesionally than contralesionally to visual, tactile, or auditory stimuli. This orientation bias recovers to a considerable degree over days to weeks. Dopamine antagonists impede spontaneous recovery and dopamine agonists enhance recovery (Corwin et al., 1986), probably by influencing striatal function (Vargo, Richard-Smith, & Corwin, 1989).

In macaque monkeys, lesions to the frontal peri-arcuate areas and around the inferior parietal lobule result in neglect, at least transiently (Duel, 1987; Milner, 1987). These monkeys are more likely to orient toward and act on stimuli in ipsilesional space. Single-cell recordings of neurons around the intraparietal sulcus and prefrontal cortices (reviewed later) suggest that these regions are critical in the maintenance of spatial representations and preparation for actions directed at specific locations. From this, one would expect that lesions in these areas would produce profound neglect in animals. Yet such cortical lesions produce only mild and transient neglect (Milner, 1987). If anything, biased behavior seems more obvious with frontal lesions, which seems at odds with human lesion studies in which posterior lesions are associated more often with neglect.

In monkeys, cortical lesions with remote metabolic abnormalities are more likely to be associated with neglect (Duel, 1987). Frontal lesions producing neglect are associated with decreased glucose utilization in the caudate nucleus and the ventral anterior and dorsomedial thalamic nuclei. Parietal lesions producing neglect are associated with decreased glucose metabolism in the pulvinar and the lateral posterior thalamic nuclei and in the deeper layers of the superior colliculus. It is interesting that recovery in these animals is also associated with recovery of these remote metabolic abnormalities. This idea that distributed abnormalities are needed to produce neglect is reiterated in a more recent study by Gaffan and Hornak (1997). They found in monkeys that transecting white matter tracts underlying the posterior parietal cortex was important in producing more persistent neglect.

Watson and colleagues (Watson, Valenstein, Day, & Heilman, 1994) reported that damage to monkeys' superior temporal sulcus produced more profound neglect than damage to the inferior parietal lobule. They suggest that the superior temporal sulcus in the monkey may serve as an important convergence zone for processing both the dorsal and the ventral visual streams integrating the "where" and "what" of objects. Damage to this area might

then be associated with greater contralesional neglect since the "what" and "where" of contralesional objects are no longer conjoined. This study highlights the difficulties in establishing the appropriate homology between the monkey and the human posterior temporoparietal cortex. While neglect in humans is associated most commonly with lesions to the inferior posterior parietal cortex, Brodmann's areas 39 and 40, it is not clear which, if any regions, are the appropriate monkey analog to these areas.

Finally, Gaffan and Hornak (1997) emphasize the importance of memory in monkeys' behavioral manifestations of overt neglect. They find that neglect is associated with complete commissurotomy and optic tract lesions, but not with isolated optic tract, parietal, or frontal cortex lesions. They interpret this finding in the following way: Sectioning the optic tract makes one hemisphere blind to visual information. This hemisphere acquires visual information from the other hemisphere through interhemispheric commissures. If each hemisphere maintains a representation of contralateral space, then a monkey without access to information about contralesional space will act as if this space did not exist. With an isolated optic tract lesion, information about contralesional space is acquired through the nonlesioned hemisphere because with multiple ocular fixations, objects in contralesional space sometimes fall on the ipsilesional side of fixation. The idea that short-term memories of contralesional stimuli influence spatial behavior had not been considered previously in animal models.

Single-Cell Neurophysiological Studies

Single-cell neurophysiological studies record the activity of neurons in animals, often monkeys that are engaged in various perceptual, motor, or cognitive tasks. These studies support the idea that neurons in parietal and frontal association cortices mediate spatial attention and representations. These neurons form a distributed network dedicated to a variety of spatial behaviors, including attention and intention regarding spatial locations, memory of spatial locations, and facilitation of perception of objects in different locations.

Parietal Neurons

In the 1970s, Mountcastle and co-workers found neurons in the parietal cortex of monkeys that were responsive when the animals attended to lights in their peripheral vision despite gazing toward a central location (Mountcastle, Lynch, Georgopolous, Sakata, & Acuna, 1975). They found that neurons in the posterior parietal cortex responded to a variety of spatial behaviors, including fixation, smooth pursuit, saccades, and reaching (Mountcastle, 1976). Neurons in different regions (ventral, medial, lateral) of the posterior intra-parietal sulcus and nearby regions, such as areas 5, 7a, and 7b, seem to be critical to the mediation of spatial attention. These neurons form a mosaic linked to different sensory and motor systems. For example, lateral intraparietal (LIP) neurons are less responsive to tactile stimuli or the directional aspects of moving visual stimuli than ventral in-traparietal (VIP) neurons (Duhamel, Colby, & Goldberg, 1998).

Many posterior parietal and frontal neurons are responsive to combinations of visual and tactile stimuli (Colby & Duhamel, 1991). VIP neurons are responsive to aligned visual and tactile receptive fields when they move in specific directions. Medial intraparietal (MIP) neurons are especially respon-sive to joint rotations and movements of limbs. Other neurons in area 7a integrate visual and vestibular input, and neurons in the lateral intra-parietal area integrate visual and proprioceptive input from neck muscles (Andersen, 1995b; Snyder, Grieve, Brotchie, & Andersen, 1998).

Generally, neurons within the posterior parietal cortex link specific sensations to different motor systems, although there is disagreement on whether neurons within the LIP sulcus are purely attentional or whether these neurons are necessarily linked to eye movements (Andersen, Bracewell, Barash, Gnadt, & Fogassi, 1990; Colby & Goldberg, 1999).

Reference Frames

The integration of different sensory modalities in the posterior parietal cortex is presumably involved in constructing different kinds of reference frames (Brotchie, Anderson, Snyder, & Goodman, 1995). From studies of people with neglect, we know that viewer-centered reference frames can be anchored to retinotopic, head-, or body-centered coordinates. From animal studies it appears unlikely that a different pool of neurons code retinal and head-centered coordinates. Andersen and colleagues suggest that head-centered coordinates are derived from the interaction of retinal and eye position signals. The amplitude of a neuron's response to stimulation of a retinal location is modulated by eye position. Within area 7a, neurons compute the location of a stimulus in head-centered coordinates from these interactions (Andersen, Essick, & Siegel, 1985). Anderson et al. suggest that other areas, including the lateral intraparietal sulcus, area V3, the pulvinar, nucleus and parts of the premotor and prefrontal cortex may code different kinds of spatial reference frames in a similar fashion (Andersen, 1995a). Pouget and Sejnowski (1997) use basis functions to offer a slightly different computational solution to the mediation of different reference frames encoded within the same array of neurons.

In addition to reference frames divided along viewer-centered coordinates, space can be parti-tioned as concentric shells around the body, with close peripersonal space being coded distinctly from distant extrapersonal space (Previc, 1998). In monkeys, this segregation of space may be medi-ated by the link between attentional neurons and multiple motor systems (Snyder, Batista, & Andersen, 1997). Rizzolatti adopts the strong posi-tion that all attentional circuits organize movements to specific sectors of space. He claims that the facil-itation of perception by attention is a consequence of circuits activated in preparation for moving (Rizzolatti & Berti, 1993; Rizzolatti et al., 1988).

Neurons within the monkey intraparietal sulcus are tuned to actions involving different motor systems, such as the mouth, eyes, or hands. In combination with their connections to frontal regions, these neurons integrate the visual fields with the tactile fields of specific body parts and with the actions of these body parts (Gross & Graziano, 1995). The parietal and frontal interconnections are anatomically segregated along a ventral-to-dorsal axis (Petrides & Pandya, 1984). Neurons within the VIP sulcus are responsive to visual stimuli within 5 cm of the monkey's face (Colby, Duhamel, & Goldberg, 1993). These neurons project to area F4 of area 6 in the premotor cortex, an area that contributes to head and mouth movements (Fogassi et al., 1996; Graziano, Yap, & Gross, 1994) and may mediate the construction of very close peripersonal space. Neurons in the MIP sulcus are responsive to visual stimuli within reaching distance (Graziano & Gross, 1995). These neurons project to ventral premotor cortices that mediate visually guided arm movements (Caminiti, Ferraina, & Johnson, 1996; Gentilucci et al., 1988) and are sensitive to stimuli in arm-centered rather than retinotopic coordinates (Graziano et al., 1994). This area has direct connections to the putamen, which also has such arm-centered neurons (Graziano et al., 1994). These putamenal neurons may be involved in the decision processes by which different kinds of movements are selected (Merchant, Zainos, Hernandez, Salinas, & Romo, 1997).

Neurons within the monkey LIP sulcus (Duhamel, Colby, & Goldberg, 1992) may be connected to saccadic mechanisms of the frontal eye fields and the superior colliculus. Neurons in the superior colliculus are responsive to behaviorally relevant stimuli when linked to saccadic eye movements (Wurtz & Goldberg, 1972; Wurtz & Munoz, 1995). These networks probably link sensations to eye movements and construct distant extrapersonal space.

Space-Based and Object-Based Attention

Neuroimaging studies in humans have shown that visual or spatial attention can influence the processing of objects in the ventral stream. This influence is presumably involved in binding the "what" and "where" of things. Single-cell monkey physiological studies also support such modulation. Neurons in area V4 are sensitive to specific stimuli located within their receptive fields (Moran & Desimone, 1985). Their firing increases when the animal attends to that location. This stronger response to the stimulus for which the neuron is already tuned, when the animal attends to it, suggests a physiological correlate of the enhanced perception of objects when attention is directed to the location of those objects.

Conclusions and Future Directions

Convergence

There is a remarkable convergence of some ideas across different disciplines with highly varied traditions and methods. Four related ideas about spatial attention and representation recur and are summarized here.

Distributed Networks

Neural networks involving different and noncontiguous parts of the brain mediate spatial attention. Rather than being localized to a single brain location, spatial attention is mediated by the parietal and frontal and probably cingulate cortices, as well as the basal ganglia, thalamus, and superior colliculus.

Multiple Representations of Space

The brain constructs multiple representations of space, despite our intuitions of space as a homogeneous medium that surrounds us. These representations involve the body and different kinds of extrapersonal space. Extrapersonal space can be viewed as concentric shells around the body, closer to the trunk, within reach of our limbs, or further away in more distant space. Extrapersonal space can also be partitioned into retinotopic, head-centered, and trunk-centered coordinates that all have the viewer as the primary referent. Viewer-independent reference frames are anchored to the spatial axes of the object itself or to axes intrinsic to the environment.

Attention and Intention

Attention and intention are tightly linked. The extent to which perception and actions are coordinated in the formation and sustenance of spatial representations is remarkable. The actions themselves, whether they are eye movements, head movements, or limb movements in space, are also related to notions of different kinds of reference frames.

Attention and Perception

Attention and perception may not be as distinct as is often thought. Processing of relatively early stages of perception seems to be modulated by attention, although the precise boundaries between the two remain to be worked out.

Unresolved Issues

Despite this convergence of ideas, I would like to mention some issues that in my view warrant further consideration. Some questions involve research in neglect directly and others involve the relationship of findings in neglect and other approaches.

Contralesional Hyperorientation in Neglect

Why do patients with right brain damage sometimes "hyperorient" into contralesional space, rather than neglect contralesional space? We are used to thinking of neglect as the tendency to orient toward or act in ipsilesional space. However, in some cases patients seem to be drawn contralesionally. The most robust of these contralesional productive behaviors is the crossover phenomenon, in which patients bisect short lines (usually less than 4 cm) to the left of the midline. However, there are other dramatic instances of contralesional hyperorientation (Chatterjee, 1998). Some patients bisect long lines in contralesional space (Adair, Chatterjee, Schwartz, & Heilman, 1998a; Kwon & Heilman, 1991). Some patients will point into contralesional

space when asked to indicate the environmental midline (Chokron & Bartolomeo, 1998). What has happened to left-sided representations or to motor systems directed contralesionally to produce this paradoxical behavior?

Memory, Attention, and Representation

How does memory interact with attention to affect online processing of stimuli in neglect? Functional imaging studies and neurophysiological studies suggest that there is considerable overlap between circuits dedicated to spatial attention and spatial working memory. Monkey lesion studies indicate an important role for spatial memories in online processing (Gaffan & Hornak, 1997). We recently reported that memory traces of contralesional stimuli might have a disproportionate influence on online representations in patients with neglect (Chatterjee et al., 2000). A conceptual framework that relates spatial memory and attention in influencing online perception remains to be articulated.

Frontal and Parietal Differences

How different are the roles of the frontal and parietal cortices in spatial attention? The notion that parietal neglect is attentional and frontal neglect is intentional has great appeal. Unfortunately, the empirical evidence for such a clear dichotomy is mixed at best. It is not even clear that these distinctions make conceptual sense, since what has been called "attentional neglect" involves eye movements and what has been called "intentional neglect" involves limb movements. Single-cell neurophysiological studies suggest that neurons within both parietal and frontal cortices mediate spatial actions. It may be the case that the actions are more clearly segregated in the frontal cortex than in the parietal cortex. However, it is not clear that one should expect clean behavioral dissociations from lesions to the frontal and parietal cortices. Perhaps eye and limb movements may be coded within the same array of neurons, as suggested by Andersen and colleagues (Andersen, 1995a) and Pouget and

Sejnowski (1997) for the coding of visual reference frames. If that were the case, it is not clear how lesions would bias behavior toward different forms of neglect. Furthermore, the ways in which frontal and parietal areas interact based on their interconnections is not well understood. In humans, damage to the posterior superior longitudinal fasciculus and the inferior frontal fasciculus is associated with more severe and long-lasting neglect. Similarly in monkeys, transection of the white matter underlying the parietal cortex is also associated with greater neglect.

Distinctions within the Parietal Cortex

What are the roles of different regions within the posterior parietotemporal lobes? Lesion studies in humans suggest that damage to the inferior parietal lobule or the superior temporal gyrus produces the most consistent and profound disorder of spatial attention and representation. Lesion studies in humans suggest that damage to the inferior parietal lobule or superior temporal gyrus produces the most consistent and profound disorder of spatial attention and representation. By contrast, functional imaging studies activate more *dersal* regions within the intraparietal sulcus and the superior parietal sulcus most consistently. Why this discrepancy? Perhaps the greater dorsal involvement in functional imaging studies is related to the design of the studies, which emphasize shifts of visual attention. Perhaps experimental probes emphasizing the integration of both "what" and "where" information would be more likely to involve the inferior parietal cortex. Recent functional imaging data suggest that the temporal-parietal junction may be preferentially activated when subjects detect targets, rather than simply attend to locations (Corbetta et al., 2000). Monkey lesion studies may not be able to resolve the discrepancy for two reasons. As mentioned below, the appropriate anatomical monkey–human homologs are not clear, and neglectlike symptoms occur only transiently following parietal lesions in monkeys.

Monkey and Human Homologs

What are the appropriate anatomical homologs between humans and monkeys? Human lesion studies focus on the inferior parietal lobule. It is not clear that an analogous structure exists in monkeys (Watson et al., 1994). Both human functional imaging studies and monkey neurophysiology emphasize the role of the intraparietal sulcus. However, it is not clear that these two structures are homologous across species.

In summary, we know a great deal about spatial attention and representation. Across the varied disciplines there is a remarkable convergence of the kinds of questions being asked and solutions being proposed. However, many questions remain. A comprehensive and coherent understanding of spatial attention and representation is more likely with the recognition of insights gleaned from different methods.

Acknowledgments

This work was supported by National Institutes & Health grout RO1 NS37539. I would like to thank Lisa Santer for her critical reading of early drafts of this chapter.

References

Adair, J., Chatterjee, A., Schwartz, R., & Heilman, K. (1998a). Ipsilateral neglect: Reversal of bias or exaggerated cross-over phenomenon? *Cortex, 34,* 147–153.

Adair, J. C., Na, D. L., Schwartz, R. L., & Heilman, K. M. (1998b). Analysis of primary and secondary influences on spatial neglect. *Brain and Cognition, 37,* 351–367.

Albert, M. L. (1973). A simple test of visual neglect. *Neurology, 23,* 658–664.

Andersen, R. A. (1995a). Coordinate transformation and motor planning in parietal cortex. In M. S. Gazzaniga (Ed.), *The cognitive neurosciences* (pp. 519–532). Cambridge, MA: MIT Press.

Andersen, R. A. (1995b). Encoding of intention and spatial location in the posterior parietal cortex. *Cerebral Cortex, 5,* 457–469.

Andersen, R. A., Bracewell, R. M., Barash, S., Gnadt, J. W., & Fogassi, L. (1990). Eye position effects on visual, memory, and saccade-related activity in areas LIP and 7a of macaque. *Journal of Neuroscience, 10*, 1176–1196.

Andersen, R. A., Essick, G. K., & Siegel, R. M. (1985). Encoding of spatial locations by posterior parietal neurons. *Science, 230*, 456–458.

Anderson, B. (1993). Spared awareness for the left side of internal visual images in patients with left-sided extrapersonal neglect. *Neurology, 43*, 213–216.

Anderson, B. (1996). A mathematical model of line bisection behaviour in neglect. *Brain, 119*, 841–850.

Barcelo, F., Suwazono, S., & Knight, R. (2000). Prefrontal modulation of visual processing in humans. *Nature Neuroscience, 3*, 399–403.

Behrmann, M., Moscovitch, M., Black, S. E., & Mozer, M. (1994). Object-centered neglect in patients with unilateral neglect: Effects of left-right coordinates of objects. *Journal of Cognitive Neuroscience, 6*, 1–16.

Bender, M. B., & Furlow, C. T. (1945). Phenomenon of visual extinction and homonomous fields and psychological principles involved. *Archives of Neurology and Psychiatry, 53*, 29–33.

Beschin, N., & Robertson, I. H. (1997). Personal versus extrapersonal neglect: A group study of their dissociation using a reliable clinical test. *Cortex, 33*, 379–384.

Binder, J., Marshall, R., Lazar, R., Benjamin, J., & Mohr, J. (1992). Distinct syndromes of hemineglect. *Archives of Neurology, 49*, 1187–1194.

Bisiach, E. (1993). Mental representation in unilateral neglect and related disorders: The twentieth Bartlett Memorial lecture. *Quarterly Journal of Experimental Psychology, 46A*, 435–461.

Bisiach, E., Bulgarelli, C., Sterzi, R., & Vallar, G. (1983). Line bisection and cognitive plasticity of unilateral neglect of space. *Brain and Cognition, 2*, 32–38.

Bisiach, E., Geminiani, G., Berti, A., & Rusconi, M. L. (1990). Perceptual and premotor factors of unilateral neglect. *Neurology, 40*, 1278–1281.

Bisiach, E., & Luzzatti, C. (1978). Unilateral neglect of representational space. *Cortex, 14*, 129–133.

Bisiach, E., Luzzatti, C., & Perani, D. (1979). Unilateral neglect, representational schema and consciousness. *Brain, 102*, 609–618.

Bisiach, E., Perani, D., Vallar, G., & Berti, A. (1986). Unilateral neglect: Personal and extrapersonal. *Neuropsychologia, 24*, 759–767.

Bisiach, E., Ricci, R., Lualdi, M., & Colombo, M. R. (1998a). Perceptual and response bias in unilateral neglect: Two modified versions of the Milner landmark task. *Brain and Cognition, 37*, 369–386.

Bisiach, E., Ricci, R., & Modona, M. N. (1998b). Visual awareness and anisometry of space representation in unilateral neglect: A panoramic investigation by means of a line extension task. *Consciousness and Cognition, 7*, 327–355.

Bisiach, E., & Rusconi, M. L. (1990). Breakdown of perceptual awareness in unilateral neglect. *Cortex, 26*, 643–649.

Bisiach, E., Tegnér, R., Làdavas, E., Rusconi, M. L., Mijovic, D., & Hjaltason, H. (1995). Dissociation of ophthalmokinetic and melokinetic attention in unilateral neglect. *Cerebral Cortex, 5*, 439–447.

Brain, W. R. (1941). Visual disorientation with special reference to lesions of the right hemisphere. *Brain, 64*, 224–272.

Brefczynski, J. A., & DeYoe, E. A. (1999). A physiological correlate of the "spotlight" of visual attention. *Nature Neuroscience, 2*, 370–374.

Brotchie, P. R., Anderson, R. A., Snyder, L. H., & Goodman, S. J. (1995). Head position signals used by parietal neurons to encode locations of visual stimuli. *Nature, 375*, 232–235.

Burcham, K. J., Corwin, J. V., Stoll, M. L., & Reep, R. L. (1997). Disconnection of medial agranular and posterior patietal cortex produces multimodal neglect in rats. *Behavioral Brain Research, 90*, 187–197.

Butter, C. M., Evans, J., Kirsch, N., & Kewman, D. (1989). Altitudinal neglect following traumatic brain injury. *Cortex, 25*, 135–146.

Caminiti, R., Ferraina, S., & Johnson, P. (1996). The source of visual information to the primate frontal lobe: A novel role for the superior parietal lobule. *Cerebral Cortex, 6*, 319–328.

Cappa, S., Sterzi, R., Guiseppe, V., & Bisiach, E. (1987). Remission of hemineglect and anosagnosia during vestibular stimulation. *Neuropsychologia, 25*, 775–782.

Chatterjee, A. (1994). Picturing unilateral spatial neglect: Viewer versus object centred reference frames. *Journal of Neurology, Neurosurgery and Psychiatry, 57*, 1236–1240.

Chatterjee, A. (1995). Cross over, completion and confabulation in unilateral spatial neglect. *Brain, 118*, 455–465.

Chatterjee, A. (1998). Motor minds and mental models in neglect. *Brain and Cognition, 37*, 339–349.

Chatterjee, A., Dajani, B. M., & Gage, R. J. (1994a). Psychophysical constraints on behavior in unilateral spatial neglect. *Neuropsychiatry, Neuropsychology and Behavioral Neurology, 7,* 267–274.

Chatterjee, A., & Mennemeier, M. (1996). Anosognosia for hemiplegia: Patient retrospections. *Cognitive Neuropsychiatry, 1,* 221–237.

Chatterjee, A., Mennemeier, M., & Heilman, K. M. (1992a). Search patterns and neglect: A case study. *Neuropsychologia, 30,* 657–672.

Chatterjee, A., Mennemeier, M., & Heilman, K. M. (1992b). A stimulus-response relationship in unilateral neglect: The power function. *Neuropsychologia, 30,* 1101–1108.

Chatterjee, A., Mennemeier, M., & Heilman, K. M. (1994b). The psychophysical power law and unilateral spatial neglect. *Brain and Cognition, 25,* 92–107.

Chatterjee, A., Ricci, R., & Calhoun, J. (2000). Weighing the evidence for cross over in neglect. *Neuropsychologia, 38,* 1390–1397.

Chatterjee, A., & Thompson, K. A. (1998). Weigh(t)ing for awareness. *Brain and Cognition, 37,* 477–490.

Chatterjee, A., Thompson, K. A., & Ricci, R. (1999). Quantitative analysis of cancellation tasks in neglect. *Cortex, 35,* 253–262.

Chawla, D., Rees, G., & Friston, K. (1999). The physiological basis of attentional modulation in extrastriate visual areas. *Nature Neuroscience, 2,* 671–676.

Chokron, S., & Bartolomeo, P. (1998). Position of the egocentric reference and directional movements in right brain-damaged patients. *Brain and Cognition, 46,* 34–38.

Colby, C. L. (1998). Action-oriented spatial reference frames in cortex. *Neuron, 20,* 15–24.

Colby, C., & Duhamel, J.-R. (1991). Heterogeneity of extrastriate visual areas and multiple parietal areas in the macaque monkey. *Neuropsychologia, 29,* 497–515.

Colby, C. L., Duhamel, J.-R., & Goldberg, M. E. (1993). Ventral intraparietal area of the macaque: Anatomic location and visual response properties. *Journal of Neurophysiology, 69,* 902–914.

Colby, C. L., & Goldberg, G. E. (1999). Space and attention in parietal cortex. *Annual Review of Neuroscience, 23,* 319–349.

Corbetta, M. (1998). Frontoparietal cortical networks for directing atention and the eye to visual locations: Identical, independent, or overlapping neural systems. *Proceedings of the National Academy of Sciences U.S.A., 95,* 831–838.

Corbetta, M., Kincade, J. M., Ollinger, J. M., McAvoy, M. P., & Shulman, G. M. (2000). Voluntary orienting is dissociated from target detection in human posterior parietal cortex. *Nature Neuroscience, 3,* 292–296.

Corbetta, M., Miezen, F. M., Shulman, G. L., & Peterson, S. E. (1993). A PET study of visuospatial attention. *Journal of Neuroscience 11,* 1202–1226.

Corwin, J. V., Kanter, S., Watson, R. T., Heilman, K. M., Valenstein, E., & Hashimoto, A. (1986). Apomorphine has a therapeutic effect on neglect produced by unilateral dorsomedial prefrontal cortex lesions in rats. *Experimental Neurology, 36,* 683–698.

Corwin, J. V., & Reep, R. L. (1998). Rodent posterior parietal cortex as a component of a cortical mediating directed spatial attention. *Psychobiology, 26,* 87–102.

Coslett, H. B. (1997). Neglect in vision and visual imagery: A double dissociation. *Brain, 120,* 1163–1171.

Coslett, H. B. (1998). Evidence for a disturbance of the body schema in neglect. *Brain and Cognition, 37,* 529–544.

Coslett, H. B., Bowers, D., Fitzpatrick, E., Haws, B., & Heilman, K. M. (1990). Directional hypokinesia and hemispatial inattention in neglect. *Brain, 113,* 475–486.

Coull, J. T., & Frith, C. D. (1998). Differential activation of right superior parietal cortex and intraparietal sulcus by spatial and nonspatial attention. *Neuroimage, 8,* 176–187.

Critchley, M. (1974). Misoplegia or hatred of hemiplegia. *Mt. Sinai Journal of Medicine, 41,* 82–87.

di Pellegrino, G., Basso, G., & Frassinetti, F. (1998). Visual extinction as a spatio-temporal disorder of selective attention. *Neuroreport, 9,* 835–839.

Doricchi, F., Guariglia, C., Paolucci, S., & Pizzamiglio, L. (1993). Disturbance of the rapid eye movements (REM) of REM sleep in patients with unilateral attentional neglect: Clue for the understanding of the functional meaning of REMs. *Electroencephalography and Clinical Neurophysiolog, 87,* 105–116.

Driver, J., Baylis, G., & Rafal, R. (1992). Preserved figure-ground segregation and symmetry perception in visual neglect. *Nature, 360,* 73–75.

Driver, J., & Halligan, P. W. (1991). Can visual neglect operate in object-centered coordinates? An affirmative single-case study. *Cognitive Neuropsychology, 8,* 475–496.

Driver, J., & Spence, C. (1998). Cross-modal links in spatial attention. *Philosophical Transactions of the Royal Society of London, Sen. B, 353*, 1319–1331.

Duel, R. (1987). Neural dysfunction during hemineglect after cortical damage in two monkey models. In M. Jeannerod (Ed.), *Neurophysiological and neuropsychological aspects of spatial neglect* (pp. 315–334). Amsterdam: Elsevier.

Duhamel, J., Colby, C. L., & Goldberg, M. E. (1992). The updating of representation of visual space in parietal cortex by intended eye movements. *Science, 255*, 90–92.

Duhamel, J.-R., Colby, C. L., & Goldberg, M. E. (1998). Ventral intraparietal area of the macaque: Confluent visual and somatic response properties. *Journal of Neurophysiology, 79*, 126–136.

Farah, M. J., Brun, J. L., Wong, A. B., Wallace, M. A., & Carpenter, P. A. (1990). Frames of reference for allocating attention to space: Evidence from the neglect syndrome. *Neuropsychologia, 28*, 335–347.

Fechner, G. T. (1899). *Elemente der Psychophysik*, Vol. II. (H. E. Leipzig: Breitkopfund Härtel.

Feinberg, T., Haber, L., & Stacy, C. (1990). Ipsilateral extinction in the hemineglect syndrome. *Archives of Neurology, 47*, 802–804.

Fink, G. R., Dolan, R. J., Halligan, P. W., Marshall, J. C., & Frith, C. D. (1997). Space-based and object-based visual attention: Shared and specific neural domains. *Brain, 120*, 2013–2028.

Fleet, W. S., Valenstein, E., Watson, R. T., & Heilman, K. M. (1987). Dopamine agonist therapy for neglect in humans. *Neurology, 37*, 1765–1770.

Fogassi, L., Gallese, L., Fadiga, L., Luppino, G., Matelli, M., & Rizzolatti, G. (1996). Coding of peripersonal space in inferior premotor cortex (area F4). *Journal of Neurophysiology, 76*, 141–157.

Gaffan, D., & Hornak, J. (1997). Visual neglect in the monkey: Representation and disconnection. *Brain, 120*, 1647–1657.

Gainotti, G., Messerli, P., & Tissot, R. (1972). Qualitative analysis of unilateral and spatial neglect in relation to laterality of cerebral lesions. *Journal of Neurology, Neurosurgery and Psychiatry, 35*, 545–550.

Gandhi, S. P., Heeger, D. J., & Boynton, G. M. (1999). Spatial attention affects brain activity in human primary visual cortex. *Proceedings of the National Academy of Sciences U.S.A., 96*, 3314–3319.

Geminiani, G., Bottini, G., & Sterzi, R. (1998). Dopaminergic stimulation in unilateral neglect. *Journal of Neurology, Neurosurgery and Psychiatry, 65*, 344–347.

Gentilucci, M., Fogassi, L., Luppino, G., Matelli, M., Camarda, R., & Rizzolatti, G. (1988). Functional organization of inferior area 6 in the macaque monkey: I. Somatotopy and the control of proximal movements. *Experimental Brain Research, 71*, 475–490.

Gitelman, D. R., Alpert, N. M., Kosslyn, S., Daffner, K., Scinto, L., Thompson, W., & Mesulam, M.-M. (1996). Functional imaging of human right hemispheric activation for exploratory movements. *Annals of Neurology, 39*, 174–179.

Gitelman, D., Nobre, A., Parish, T., LaBar, K., Kim, Y.-H., Meyer, J., & Mesulam, M.-M. (1999). Large-scale distributed network for covert spatial attention: Further anatomical delineation based on stringent behavioral and cognitive controls. *Brain, 122*, 1093–1106.

Graziano, M. S. A., & Gross, C. G. (1995). The representation of extrapersonal space: A possible role for bimodal, visual-tactile neurons. In M. S. Gazzaniga (Ed.), *The cognitive neurosciences* (pp. 1021–1034). Cambridge, MA: MIT Press.

Graziano, M. S. A., Yap, G. S., & Gross, C. G. (1994). Coding of visual space by premotor neurons. *Science, 266*, 1054–1056.

Gross, C. G., & Graziano, M. S. A. (1995). Multiple representations of space in the brain. *Neuroscientist, 1*, 43–50.

Halligan, P. W., & Marshall, J. C. (1988). How long is a piece of string? A study of line bisection in a case of visual neglect. *Cortex, 24*, 321–328.

Halligan, P. W., & Marshall, J. C. (1992). Left visuo-spatial neglect: A meaningless entity? *Cortex, 28*, 525–535.

Halligan, P. W., & Marshall, J. C. (1994). Spatial neglect: Position papers on theory and practice. Hillsdale, NJ: Lawrence Erlbaum Associates.

Halligan, P. W., & Marshall, J. C. (1998). Visuo-spatial neglect: The ultimate deconstruction. *Brain and Cognition, 37*, 419–438.

Halligan, P. W., Marshall, J. C., & Wade, D. T. (1992). Left on the right: Allochiria in a case of left visuo-spatial neglect. *Journal of Neurology, Neurosurgery and Psychiatry, 55*, 717–719.

Heilman, K. M. (1979). Neglect and related disorders. In K. M. H. a. E. Valenstein (Ed.), *Clinical neuropsychology* (pp. 268–307). New York: Oxford University Press.

Heilman, K. M., Pandya, D. N., & Geschwind, N. (1970). Trimodal inattention following parietal lobe ablations. *Transactimes of the American Neurological Association, 95*, 259–261.

Heilman, K. M., Schwartz, H. D., & Watson, R. T. (1978). Hypoarousal in patients with the neglect syndrome and emotional indifference. *Neurology, 28*, 229–232.

Heilman, K. M., & Valenstein, E. (1972). Frontal lobe neglect in man. *Neurology, 22*, 660–664.

Heilman, K. M., & Valenstein, E. (1979). Mechanisms underlying hemispatial neglect. *Annals of Neurology, 5*, 166–170.

Heilman, K. M., & Van Den Abell, T. (1980). Right hemisphere dominance for attention: The mechanisms underlying hemispheric assymmetries of inattention (neglect). *Neurology, 30*, 327–330.

Heilman, K. M., Watson, R. T., & Valenstein, E. (1994). Localization of lesions in neglect and related disorders. In A. Kertesz (Ed.), *Localization and neuroimaging in neuropsychology* (pp. 495–524). New York: Academic Press.

Hier, D. B., Davis, K. R., Richardson, E. P., & Mohr, J. P. (1977). Hypertensive putaminal hemorrhage. *Annals of Neurology, 1*, 152–159.

Hillis, A. E., & Caramazza, A. (1995). A framework for interpreting distinctive patterns of hemispatial neglect. *Neurocase, 1*, 189–207.

Hurford, P., Stringer, A., & Jann, B. (1998). Neuropharmacologic treatment of hemineglect: A case report comparing bromocriptine and methylphenidate. *Archives of Physical Medicine and Rehabilitation, 79*, 346–349.

Husain, M., & Kennard, C. (1996). Visual neglect associated with frontal lobe infarction. *Journal of Neurology, 243*, 652–657.

Karnath, H.-O., & Ferber, S. (1999). Is space representation distorted in neglect? *Neuropsychologia, 37*, 7–15.

Karnath, H.-O., Ferber, S., & Himmelbach, M. (2001). Spatial awareness is a function of the temporal not the posterior parietal lobe. *Nature, 411*, 950–953.

Karnath, H.-O., Sievering, D., & Fetter, M. (1994). The interactive contribution of neck muscle proprioception and vestibular stimulation to subjective "straight ahead" orientation in man. *Experimental Brain Research, 101*, 140–146.

Karnath, H. O., Schenkel, P., & Fischer, B. (1991). Trunk orientation as the determining factor of the "contralateral" deficit in the neglect syndrome and as the physical anchor of the internal representation of body orientation in space. *Brain, 114*, 1997–2014.

Kastner, S., De Weerd, P., Desimone, R., & Ungerleider, L. G. (1998). Mechanisms of directed attention in the human extrastriate cortex as revealed by functional MRI. *Science, 282*, 108–111.

Kim, Y.-H., Gitelman, D. R., Nobre, A. C., Parrish, T. B., LaBar, K. S., & Mesulam, M.-M. (1999). The large-scale neural network for spatial attention displays multifunctional overlap but differential asymmetry. *Neuroimage, 9*, 269–277.

Kinsbourne, M. (1970). A model for the mechanisms of unilateral neglect of space. *Transactions of the American Neurological Association, 95*, 143–147.

Kinsbourne, M. (1987). Mechanisms of unilateral neglect. In M. Jeannerod (Ed.), *Neurophysiological and neuropsychological aspects of spatial neglect* (pp. 69–86). New York: North-Holland.

Kinsbourne, M., & Warrington, E. K. (1962). Variety of reading disability associated with right hemisphere lesions. *Journal of Neurology, Neurosurgery and Psychiatry, 25*, 339–344.

Kwon, S. E., & Heilman, K. M. (1991). Ipsilateral neglect in a patient following a unilateral frontal lesion. *Neurology, 41*, 2001–2004.

Ladavas, E. (1987). Is the hemispatial damage produced by right parietal lobe damage associated with retinal or gravitational coordinates. *Brain, 110*, 167–180.

Ladavas, E., Di Pellegrino, G., Farne, A., & Zeloni, G. (1998). Neuropsychological evidence of an integrated visuotactile representation of peripersonal space in humans. *Journal of Cognitive Neuroscience, 10*, 581–589.

Ladavas, E., Paladini, R., & Cubelli, R. (1993). Implicit associative priming in a patient with left visual neglect. *Neuropsychologia, 31*, 1307–1320.

Leibovitch, F. S., Black, S. E., Caldwell, C. B., Ebert, P. L., Ehrlich, L. E., & Szalai, J. P. (1998). Brain-behavior correlations in hemispatial neglect using CT and SPECT. *Neurology, 50*, 901–908.

Maeshima, S., Funahashi, K., Ogura, M., Itakura, T., & Komai, N. (1994). Unilateral spatial neglect due to right frontal lobe haematoma. *Journal of Neurology, Neurosurgery and Psychiatry, 57*, 89–93.

Mark, V. W., & Heilman, K. M. (1997). Diagonal neglect on cancellation. *Neuropsychologia, 35*, 1425–1436.

Marshall, J. C., & Halligan, P. W. (1988). Blindsight and insight in visuospatial neglect. *Nature, 336*, 766–767.

Marshall, J. C., & Halligan, P. W. (1989). When right goes left: An investigation of line bisection in a case of visual neglect. *Cortex*, *25*, 503–515.

Marshall, J. C., & Halligan, P. W. (1990). Line bisection in a case of visual neglect: Psychophysical studies with implications for theory. *Cognitive Neuropsychology*, *7*, 107–130.

Marshall, J. C., & Halligan, P. W. (1993). Visuo-spatial neglect: A new copying test to assess perceptual parsing. *Journal of Neurology*, *240*, 37–40.

Marshall, J. F., & Gotthelf, T. (1979). Sensory inattention in rats with 6-hydroxydopamine-induced degeneration of ascending dopaminergic neurons: Apomorphine-induced reversal of deficits. *Experimental Neurology*, *1986*, 683–689.

Marshall, R. S., Lazar, R. M., Krakauer, J. W., & Sharma, R. (1998). Stimulus context in hemineglect. *Brain*, *121*, 2003–2010.

Martninez, A., Anllo-Vento, L., Sereno, M. I., Frank, L. R., Buxton, R. B., Dubowitz, D. J., Wong, E. C., Hinrichs, H. J., & Hillyard, S. A. (1999). Involvement of striate and extrastriate visual cortical areas in spatial attention. *Nature Neuroscience*, *2*, 364–369.

Mattingley, J. B., Bradshaw, J. L., & Phillips, J. G. (1992). Impairments of movement initiation and execution in unilateral neglect. *Brain*, *115*, 1849–1874.

Mattingley, J. B., Davis, G., & Driver, J. (1997). Preattentive filling-in of visual surfaces in parietal extinction. *Science*, *275*, 671–674.

Mattingley, J., Husain, M., Rorden, C., Kennard, C., & Driver, J. (1998). Motor role of the human inferior parietal lobe in unilateral neglect patients. *Nature*, *392*, 179–182.

McGlinchey-Berroth, R., Bullis, D. P., Milberg, W. P., Verfaellie, M., Alexander, M., & D'Esposito, M. (1996). Assessment of neglect reveals dissociable behavioral but not neuroanatomic subtypes. *Journal of the International Neuropsychological Society*, *2*, 441–451.

McGlinchey-Berroth, R., Milberg, W. P., Verfaellie, M., Alexander, M., & Kilduff, P. T. (1993). Semantic processing in the neglected visual field: Evidence from a lexical decision task. *Cognitive Neuropsychology*, *10*, 79–108.

Mennemeier, M., Chatterjee, A., & Heilman, K. M. (1994). A comparison of the influences of body and environment-centred references on neglect. *Brain*, *117*, 1013–1021.

Mennemeier, M., Wertman, E., & Heilman, K. M. (1992). Neglect of near peripersonal space: Evidence for multi-directional attentional systems in humans. *Brain*, *115*, 37–50.

Merchant, H., Zainos, A., Hernandez, A., Salinas, E., & Romo, R. (1997). Functional properties of primate putamen neurons during the categorization of tactile stimuli. *Journal of Neurophysiology*, *77*, 1132–1154.

Mesulam, M.-M. (1981). A cortical network for directed attention and unilateral neglect. *Annals of Neurology*, *10*, 309–325.

Mesulam, M.-M. (1990). Large-scale neurocognitive networks and distributed processing for attention, language and memory. *Annals of Neurology*, *28*, 597–613.

Milner, A. D., & Goodale, M. (1995). *The visual brain in action*. New York: Oxford University Press.

Milner, A. D., & Harvey, M. (1995). Distortion of size perception in visuospatial neglect. *Current Biology*, *5*, 85–89.

Milner, A. D., Harvey, M., Roberts, R. C., & Forster, S. V. (1993). Line bisection error in visual neglect: Misguided action or size distortion? *Neuropsychologia*, *31*, 39–49.

Milner, A. D. (1987). Animal models of neglect. In M. Jeannerod (Ed.), *Neurophysiological and neuropsychological aspects of spatial neglect* (pp. 259–288). Amsterdam: Elsevier.

Monaghan, P., & Shillcock, R. (1998). The cross-over effect in unilateral neglect. Modelling detailed data in the line-bisection task. *Brain*, *121*, 907–921.

Moran, J., & Desimone, R. (1985). Selective attention gates visual processing in extrastriate cortex. *Science*, *229*, 782–784.

Mountcastle, V. B. (1976). The world around us: Neural command functions for selective attention. *Neurosciences Research Program Bulletin*, *14*, 1–47.

Mountcastle, V. B., Lynch, J. C., Georgopolous, A., Sakata, H., & Acuna, C. (1975). The influence of attentive fixation upon the excitability of the light-sensitive neurons of the posterior parietal cortex. *Journal of Neuroscience*, *1*, 1218–1245.

Na, D. L., Adair, J. D., Williamson, D. J. G., Schwartz, R. L., Haws, B., & Heilman, K. M. (1998). Dissociation of sensory-attentional from motor-intentional neglect. *Journal of Neurology, Neurosurgery, and Psychiatry*, *64*, 331–338.

Nobre, A. C., Sebestyen, G. N., Gitelman, D. R., & Mesulam, M.-M. (1997). Functional localization of the system for visuospatial attention using positron emission tomography. *Brain, 120*, 5151–5533.

Petrides, M., & Pandya, D. N. (1984). Projections to the frontal cortex from the posterior parietal region in the rhesus monkey. *Journal of Comparative Neurology, 288*, 105–116.

Pizzamiglio, L., Vallar, G., & Doricchi, F. (1997). Gravitational inputs modulate visuospatial neglect. *Experimental Brain Research, 117*, 341–345.

Posner, M. I., & Dehaene, S. (1994). Attentional networks. *Trends in Neuroscience, 17*, 75–79.

Posner, M., Walker, J., Friedrich, F., & Rafal, R. (1984). Effects of parietal injury on covert orienting of attention. *Journal of Neuroscience, 4*, 1863–1874.

Pouget, A., & Sejnowski, T. J. (1997). Lesion in a basis function model of parietal cortex: Comparison with hemineglect. In P. Thier & H.-O. Karnath (Eds.), *Parietal lobe contributions to Orientation in 3 D Space* (pp. 521–538). Heidelberg: Springer-Verlag.

Previc, F. H. (1998). The neuropsychology of 3-D space. *Psychological Bulletin, 124*, 123–163.

Rapcsak, S. Z., Fleet, W. S., Verfaellie, M., & Heilman, K. M. (1988). Altitudinal neglect. *Neurology, 38*, 277–281.

Rapcsak, S., Verfaellie, M., Fleet, W., & Heilman, K. (1989). Selective attention in hemispatial neglect. *Archives of Neurology, 46*, 172–178.

Rapcsak, S. Z., Watson, R. T., & Heilman, K. M. (1987). Hemispace-visual field interactions in visual extinction. *Journal of Neurology, Neurosurgery and Psychiatry, 50*, 1117–1124.

Rees, G., Frith, C., & Lavie, N. (1997). Modulating irrelevant motion perception by varying attentional load in an unrelated task. *Science, 278*, 1616–1619.

Ricci, R., Calhoun, J., & Chatterjee, A. (2000). Orientation bias in unilateral neglect: Representational contributions. *Cortex, 36*, 671–677.

Ricci, R., Vaishnavi, S., & Chatterjee, A. (1999). A deficit of preattentive vision: Experimental observations and theoretical implications. *Neurocase, 5*, 1–12.

Rizzolatti, G., & Berti, A. (1993). Neural mechanisms in spatial neglect. In I. H. Robertson & J. C. Marshall (Eds.), *Unilateral neglect: Clinical and experimental studies* (pp. 87–105). Hillsdale, NJ: Lawrence Erlbaum Associates.

Rizzolatti, G., Camarda, R., Fogassi, L., Gentilucci, M., Luppino, G., & Matelli, M. (1988). Functional organization of inferior area 6 in the macaque monkey: II. Area F5

and the control of distal movements. *Experimental Brain Research, 71*, 491–507.

Rizzolatti, G., Matelli, M., & Pavesi, G. (1983). Deficits in attention and movement following the removal of postarcuate (area 6) and prearcuate (area 8) cortex in macaque monkeys. *Brain, 106*, 655–673.

Rossetti, Y., G, R., Pisella, L., Farne, A., Li, L., Boisson, D., & Perenin, M. (1998). Prism adaptation to a rightward optical deviation rehabilitates left spatial neglect. *Nature, 395*, 166–169.

Rubens, A. (1985). Caloric stimulation and unilateral neglect. *Neurology, 35*, 1019–1024.

Schenkenberg, T., Bradford, D. C., & Ajax, E. T. (1980). Line bisection and unilateral visual neglect in patients with neurologic impairment. *Neurology, 30*, 509–517.

Seki, K., & Ishiai, S. (1996). Diverse patterns of performance in copying and severity of unilateral spatial neglect. *Journal of Neurology, 243*, 1–8.

Snyder, L. H., Batista, A. P., & Andersen, R. A. (1997). Coding of intention in the posterior parietal cortex. *Nature, 386*, 167–170.

Snyder, L. H., Grieve, K. L., Brotchie, P., & Andersen, R. A. (1998). Separate body and world-referenced representations of visual space in parietal cortex. *Nature, 394*, 887–891.

Sommers, D. C., Dale, A. M., Seiffert, A. E., & Tootell, R. B. H. (1999). Functional MRI reveals spatially specific attentional modulation in human primary visual cortex. *Proceedings of the National Academy of Sciences U.S.A., 96*, 1663–1668.

Stevens, S. S. (1970). Neural events and the psychophysical power law. *Science, 170*, 1043–1050.

Stevens, S. S. (1972). A neural quantum in sensory discrimination. *Science, 177*, 749–762.

Tegner, R., & Levander, M. (1991). Through the looking glass. A new technique to demonstrate directional hypokinesia in unilateral neglect. *Brain, 114*, 1943–1951.

Triggs, W. J., Gold, M., Gerstle, G., Adair, J., & Heilman, K. M. (1994). Motor neglect associated with a discrete parietal lesion. *Neurology, 44*, 1164–1166.

Ungerleider, L. G., & Mishkin, M. (1982). Two cortical visual systems. In D. J. Ingle, M. A. Goodale, & R. J. W. Mansfield (Eds.), *Analysis of visual behavior* (pp. 549–586). Cambridge, MA: MIT Press.

Vaishnavi, S., Calhoun, J., & Chatterjee, A. (1999). Cross-modal and sensorimotor integration in tactile awareness. *Neurology, 53*, 1596–1598.

Vaishnavi, S., Calhoun, J., & Chatterjee, A. (2001). Binding personal and peripersonal space: Evidence from tactile extinction. *Journal of Cognitive Neuroscience*. *13*, 181–189.

Vallar, G., Bottini, G., Rusconi, M. L., & Sterzi, R. (1993). Exploring somatosensory hemineglect by vestibular stimulation. *Brain*, *116*, 71–86.

Vallar, G., Daini, R., & Antonucci, G. (2000). Processing of illusion of length in spatial hemineglect: A study of line bisection. *Neuropsychologia*, *38*, 1087–1097.

Vargo, J. M., Richard-Smith, M., & Corwin, J. V. (1989). Spiroperidol reinstates asymmetries in neglect in rats recovered from left or right dorsomedial prefrontal cortex lesions. *Behavioral Neuroscience*, *103*, 1017–1027.

Vecera, S., & Behrmann, M. (1997). Spatial attention does not require preattentive grouping. *Neuropsychology*, *11*, 30–43.

Volpe, B. T., Ledoux, J. E., & Gazzaniga, M. S. (1979). Information processing of visual stimuli in an "extinguished" field. *Nature*, *282*, 722–724.

Watson, R. T., Heilman, K. M., Cauthen, J. C., & King, F. A. (1973). Neglect after cingulectomy. *Neurology*, *23*, 1003–1007.

Watson, R. T., Heilman, K. M., Miller, B. D., & King, F. A. (1974). Neglect after mesencephalic reticular formation lesions. *Neurology*, *24*, 294–298.

Watson, R. T., Valenstein, E., Day, A., & Heilman, K. M. (1994). Posterior neocortical systems subserving awareness and neglect: Neglect associated with superior temporal sulcus but not area 7 lesions. *Archives of Neurology*, *51*, 1014–1021.

Watson, R. T., Valenstein, E., & Heilman, K. M. (1978). Nonsensory neglect. *Annals of Neurology*, *3*, 505–508.

Watson, R. T., Valenstein, E., & Heilman, K. M. (1981). Thalamic neglect. *Archives of Neurology*, *38*, 501–506.

Wojciulik, E., & Kanwisher, N. (1999). The generality of parietal involvement in visual attention. *Neuron*, *23*, 747–764.

Wurtz, R. H., & Goldberg, M. E. (1972). Activity of superior colliculus in behaving monkey: III. Cells discharging before eye movements. *Journal of Neurophysiology*, *35*, 575–586.

Wurtz, R. H., & Munoz, D. P. (1995). Role of monkey superior colliculus in control of saccades and fixation. In M. S. Gazzaniga (Ed.), *The cognitive neurosciences* (pp. 533–548). Cambridge, MA: MIT Press.

Bálint's Syndrome: A Disorder of Visual Cognition

Robert Rafal

Case Report

R.M. had suffered from two strokes, both due to cardiac emboli from hypertensive heart disease. The first occurred in June 1991 at the age of 54 and produced infarction in the right parietal lobe and a small lesion in the right cerebellum. He recovered from a transient left hemiparesis and left hemispatial neglect. The second stroke, in March 1992, involved the left parietal lobe and left him functionally blind. Five months after the second stroke, he was referred to a neurologist for headaches. At that time, neurological examination revealed a classical Bálint's syndrome without any other deficits of cognitive, motor, or sensory function.

The patient had normal visual acuity; he could recognize colors, shapes, objects, and faces and could read single words. He suffered severe spatial disorientation, however, and got lost easily anywhere except in his own home. Although he was independent in all activities of daily living, he could not maintain his own household and had to be cared for by his family. He had to be escorted about the hospital. When shown two objects, he often saw only one. When he did report both, he did so slowly and seemed to see them sequentially. Depth perception was severely impaired and he could not judge the distance of objects from him or tell which of two objects was closer to him. Optic ataxia was pronounced. He could not reach accurately toward objects, and was unable to use a pencil to place a mark within a circle. He could not make accurate saccades to objects and he could not make pursuit eye movements to follow the most slowly moving object. Visual acuity was 20/15 in both eyes. Perimetry at the time of the initial neurological exam revealed an altitudinal loss of the lower visual fields. Two years later, however, visual fields were full. Contrast sensitivity and color vision were normal. Three-dimensional experience of shapes in random dot stereograms was preserved and he experienced depth from shading.

His headaches were controlled with amitriptyline, and anticoagulation treatment with warfarin was instituted to prevent further strokes. By June 1995, the patient was able to live independently in a duplex next door to his brother's daughter, and needed only intermittent help in his daily activities. He was able to take unescorted walks in his neighborhood, to get about in his own house without help,

watch television, eat and dress himself, and carry on many activities of daily living. He was slower than normal in these activities, but was able to lead a semi-independent life.

A magnetic resonance imaging (MRI) scan in 1994 with three-dimensional reconstruction revealed nearly symmetrical lesions in each parieto-occipital region (Friedman-Hill, Robertson, & Treisman, 1995). The lesions were concentrated primarily in Brodmann areas 7 and 39, and possibly included some of areas 5 and 19. In addition, there was a small (volume $<0.3\,cm^3$) lesion in Brodmann area 6 of the right hemisphere and asymmetrical cerebellar lesions (volume = $0.3\,cm^3$ left hemisphere, $6.0\,cm^3$ right hemisphere). The damage preserved the primary visual cortex and all the temporal lobe. The supramarginal gyri were intact on both sides, as were somatosensory and motor cortices.

The syndrome represented by this patient was first described by the Hungarian neurologist Rezsö Bálint (Bálint, 1909; Harvey, 1995; Harvey & Milner, 1995; Husain & Stein, 1988). While visual acuity is preserved and patients are able to recognize objects placed directly in front of them, they are unable to interact with, or make sense of, their visual environment. They are lost in space. Fleeting objects that they can recognize, but that they cannot locate or grasp, appear and disappear, and their features are jumbled together. These patients are helpless in a visually chaotic world.

Holmes and Horax (1919) provided a detailed analysis of the syndrome that remains definitive. They emphasized two major components of the syndrome: (1) simultanagnosia—a constriction, not of the visual field, but of visual attention, which restricts the patient's awareness to only one object at a time and (2) spatial disorientation—a loss of all spatial reference and memory that leaves the patients lost in the world and unable to look at objects (which Bálint called "psychic paralysis of gaze") or to reach for them (which Bálint called "optic ataxia").

This chapter reviews the clinical and neuropsychological aspects of this intriguing syndrome.

It reviews its anatomical basis and some of the diseases that cause it. It then details the independent component symptoms of Bálint's syndrome. It concludes with a synthesis that attempts to summarize what Bálint's syndrome tells us about the role of attention and spatial representation in perception and action.

Anatomy and Etiology of Bálint's Syndrome

Bálint's syndrome is produced by bilateral lesions of the parieto-occipital junction. The lesions characteristically involve the dorsorostral occipital lobe (Brodmann area 19), and often, but not invariably (Karnath, Ferber, Rorden, & Driver, 2000), the angular gyrus, but may spare the supramarginal gyrus and the superior temporal gyrus. Figure 2.1 shows a drawing of the lesions in the patient reported by Bálint in 1909 (Husain & Stein, 1988). The supramarginal gyrus and the posterior part of the superior temporal gyrus are affected in the right hemisphere, but spared on the left. The superior parietal lobule is only minimally involved in either hemisphere. Figure 2.2 (Friedman-Hill, Robertson, & Treisman, 1995) shows the reconstructed MRI scan of the patient (R. M.) with Bálint's syndrome described in the case report. The lesion involves the parieto-occipital junction and part of the angular gyrus of both hemispheres, but spares the temporal lobe and supramarginal gyrus. A review of other recent cases of Bálint's syndrome emphasizes the consistent involvement of the posterior parietal lobe and parieto-occipital junction as critical in producing the syndrome (Coslett & Saffran, 1991; Pierrot-Deseillgny, Gray, & Brunet, 1986; Verfaellie, Rapcsak, & Heilman, 1990).

Thus Bálint's syndrome is associated with diseases in which symmetric lesions of the parieto-occipital junction are typical. For example, Luria (1959) and Holmes and Horax (1919) have reported this syndrome after patients received penetrating wounds from projectiles entering laterally and traversing the coronal plane through the parieto-occipital regions. Strokes successively injuring both hemispheres in the distribution of posterior parietal branches of the middle cerebral artery are another common cause (Coslett & Saffran, 1991; Friedman-Hill et al., 1995; Pierrot-Deseillgny et al., 1986). Because the parieto-occipital junction lies in the watershed territory between the middle and the posterior cerebral arteries, Bálint's syndrome is a common sequela of infarction due to global cerebral hypoperfusion. Another symmetrical pathology is the "butterfly" glioma—a malignant tumor origi-

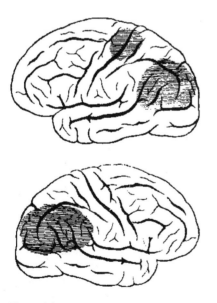

Figure 2.1
Bálint's drawing of the brain of the patient he described. (Husain and Stein, 1988).

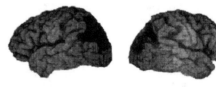

Figure 2.2
MRI of patient R.M.

nating in one parietal lobe and spreading across the corpus callosum to the other side.

Radiation necrosis may develop after radiation of a parietal lobe tumor in the opposite hemisphere in the tract of the radiation port. Cerebral degenerative disease, prototypically Alzheimer's disease, may begin in the parieto-occipital regions, and there is now a growing literature reporting cases of classic Bálint's syndrome that are due to degenerative diseases (Benson, Davis, & Snyder, 1988; Hof, Bouras, Constintinidis, & Morrison, 1989, 1990; Mendez, Turner, Gilmore, Remler, & Tomsak, 1990).

The Symptom Complex of Bálint's Syndrome

Bálint's initial description of this syndrome emphasized in his patient the constriction of visual attention, resulting in an inability to perceive more than one object at a time, and optic ataxia, the inability to reach accurately toward objects. Bálint used the term *optic ataxia* to distinguish it from the tabetic ataxia of neurosyphilis; tabetic ataxia is an inability to coordinate movements based on proprioceptive input, while optic ataxia describes an inability to coordinate movements based on visual input. Many similar patients have since been reported (Coslett & Saffran, 1991; Girotti et al., 1982; Godwin-Austen, 1965; Kase, Troncoso, Court, Tapia, & Mohr, 1977; Luria, 1959; Luria, Pravdina-Vinarskaya, & Yarbuss, 1963; Pierrot-Deseillgny et al., 1986; Tyler, 1968; Williams, 1970).

In addition to noting the simultanagnosia and optic ataxia reported by Bálint, Holmes and Horax emphasized spatial disorientation as the cardinal feature of the syndrome. Holmes and Horax offered their case "for the record . . . as an excellent example of a type of special disturbance of vision . . . which sheds considerable light on . . . those processes which are concerned in the integration and association of sensation" (Holmes & Horax, 1919, p. 285).

Constriction of Visual Attention: Simultanagnosia

In their 1919 report of a 30-year-old World War I veteran who had a gunshot wound through the parieto-occipital regions, Holmes & Horax observed that "the essential feature was his inability to direct attention to, and to take cognizance of, two or more objects" (Holmes & Horax, 1919, p. 402). They argued that this difficulty "must be attributed to a special disturbance or limitation of attention" (p. 402). Because of this constriction of visual attention (what Bálint referred to as the psychic field of gaze), the patient could attend to only one object at a time regardless of the size of the object. "In one test, for instance, a large square was drawn on a sheet of paper and he recognized it immediately, but when it was again shown to him after a cross had been drawn in its center he saw the cross, but identified the surrounding figure only after considerable hesitation; his attention seemed to be absorbed by the first object on which his eyes fell" (Holmes & Horax, 1919, p. 390).

Another useful clinical test uses overlapping figures (figure 2.3). The degree to which local detail can capture the patient's attention and exclude all other objects from his or her attention can be quite

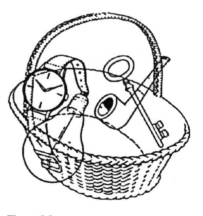

Figure 2.3
Overlapping figures used to test for simultaneous agnosia.

astonishing. I was testing a patient one day, drawing geometric shapes on a piece of paper and asking her to tell me what she saw. She was doing well at reporting simple shapes until at one point she shook her head, perplexed, and told me, "I can't see any of those shapes now, doctor, the watermark on the paper is so distracting."

The visual experience of the patient with Bálint's syndrome is a chaotic one of isolated snapshots with no coherence in space or time. Coslett and Saffran report a patient whom television programs bewildered "because she could only 'see' one person or object at a time and, therefore, could not determine who was speaking or being spoken to. She reported watching a movie in which, after a heated argument, she noted to her surprise and consternation that the character she had been watching was suddenly sent reeling across the room, apparently as a consequence of a punch thrown by a character she had never seen" (Coslett & Saffran, 1991, p. 1525).

Coslett and Saffran's patient also illustrated how patients with Bálint's syndrome are confounded in their efforts to read: "Although she read single words effortlessly, she stopped reading because the 'competing words' confused her" (Coslett & Saffran, 1991, p. 1525). Luria's patient reported that he "discerned objects around him with difficulty, that they flashed before his eyes and sometimes disappeared from his field of vision. This [was] particularly pronounced in reading: the words and lines flashed before his eyes and now one, now another, extraneous word suddenly intruded itself into the text." The same occurred in writing: "[T]he patient was unable to bring the letters into correlation with his lines or to follow visually what he was writing down: letters disappeared from the field of vision, overlapped with one another and did not coincide with the limits of the lines" (Luria, 1959, p. 440). Coslett and Saffran's patient "was unable to write as she claimed to be able to see only a single letter; thus when creating a letter she saw only the tip of the pencil and the letter under construction and "lost" the previously constructed letter" (Coslett & Saffran, 1991, p. 1525).

Figure 2.4 shows the attempts of one of Luria's patients to draw familiar objects. When the patient's attention was focused on the attempt to draw a part of the object, the orientation of that part with regard to the rest of the object was lost, and the rendering was reduced to piecemeal fragments.

Patients are unable to perform the simplest everyday tasks involving the comparison of two objects. They cannot tell which of two lines is longer, nor which of two coins is bigger. Holmes and Horax's patient could not tell, visually, which of two pencils was bigger, although he had no difficulty doing so if he touched them. Holmes and Horax made the important observation that although their patient could not explicitly compare the lengths of two lines or the angles of a quadrilateral shape, he had no difficulty distinguishing shapes whose identity is implicitly dependent upon such comparisons: "Though he failed to distinguish any difference in the length of lines, even if it was as great as 50 percent, he could always recognize whether a quadrilateral rectangular figure was a square or not. . . . [H]e did not compare the lengths of its sides but 'on the first glance I see the whole figure and know whether it is a square or not'. . . . He could also appreciate . . . the size of angles; a rhomboid even when its sides stood at almost right angles was 'a square shoved out of shape' " (Holmes & Horax, 1919, p. 394).

Holmes and Horax appreciated the importance of their observations for the understanding of normal vision: "It is therefore obvious that though he could not compare or estimate linear extensions he preserved the faculty of appreciating the shape of bidimensional figures. It was on this that his ability to identify familiar objects depended" (Holmes & Horax, 1919, p. 394). "[T]his is due to the rule that the mind when possible takes cognizance of unities" (Holmes & Horax, 1919, p. 400).

Spatial Disorientation

Holmes and Horax considered spatial disorientation to be a symptom independent from simultanagnosia, and to be the cardinal feature of the syn-

Drawing

Elephant

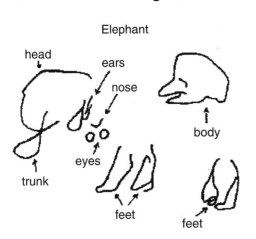

"I can visualize it well ... but
my hands don't move properly"

Copying

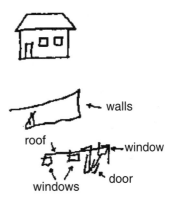

Figure 2.4
Drawing by the patient described by Luria (1959).

drome: "The most prominent symptom . . . was his inability to orient and localize correctly objects which he saw" (Holmes & Horax, 1919, pp. 390–391). Patients with Bálint's syndrome cannot indicate the location of objects, verbally or by pointing (optic ataxia, to be discussed later). Holmes and Horax emphasized that the defect in visual localization was not restricted to visual objects in the outside world, but also extended to a defect in spatial memory: "[H]e described as a visualist does his house, his family, a hospital ward in which he had previously been, etc. But, on the other hand, he had complete loss of memory of topography; he was unable to describe the route between the house in a provincial town in which he had lived all his life and the railways station a short distance away, explaining 'I used to be able to see the way but I can't see it now. . . .' He was similarly unable to say how he could find his room in a barracks in which he had been stationed for some months, or describe

the geography of trenches in which he had served" (Holmes & Horax, 1919, p. 389).

This gentleman was clearly lost in space: "On one occasion, for instance, he was led a few yards from his bed and then told to return to it; after searching with his eyes for a few moments he identified the bed, but immediately started off in a wrong direction" (Holmes & Horax, 1919, p. 395). This patient showed, then, no recollection of spatial relationships of places he knew well before his injury, and no ability to learn new routes: "He was never able to give even an approximately correct description of the way he had taken, or should take, and though he passed along it several times a day he never 'learned his way' as a blind man would" (Holmes & Horax, 1919, p. 395).

Holmes and Horax concluded that "The fact that he did not retain any memory of routes and topographical relations that were familiar to him before he received his injury and could no longer recall them, suggests that the cerebral mechanisms concerned with spatial memory, as well as those that subserve the perception of spatial relations, must have been involved" (Holmes & Horax, 1919, p. 404).

Impaired Oculomotor Behavior

Oculomotor behavior is also chaotic in Bálint's syndrome, with striking disturbances of fixation, saccade initiation and accuracy, and smooth-pursuit eye movements. The patient may be unable to maintain fixation, may generate apparently random saccadic eye movements (Luria et al., 1963), and may seem unable to execute smooth-pursuit eye movements. The disorder of eye movements in Bálint's syndrome is restricted to visually guided eye movements. The patient can program accurate eye movements when they are guided by sound or touch: "When, however, requested to look at his own finger or to any point of his body which was touched he did so promptly and accurately" (Holmes & Horax, 1919, p. 387).

Holmes and Horax suggested that the oculomotor disturbances seen in Bálint's syndrome were secondary to spatial disorientation: "Some influence might be attributed to the abnormalities of the movements of his eyes, but . . . these were an effect and not the cause" (Holmes & Horax, 1919, p. 401). "All these symptoms were secondary to and dependent upon the loss of spatial orientation by vision" (Holmes & Horax, 1919, p. 405). They described, similarly, the behavior of a patient with Bálint's syndrome when he was tested for smooth-pursuit eye movements: "When an object at which he was staring was moved at a slow and uniform rate he could keep his eyes on it, but if it was jerked or moved abruptly it quickly disappeared" (Holmes & Horax, 1919, p. 387).

Optic Ataxia

Figure 2.5 shows misreaching in Bálint's syndrome. Even after the patient sees the comb, he doesn't look directly at it, and his reaching is inaccurate in depth

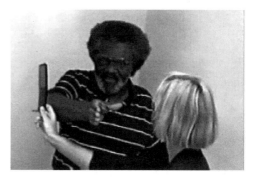

Figure 2.5
Optic ataxia in Bálint's syndrome.

as well as being off to the side. He groped for the comb until his hand bumped into it. Given a pencil and asked to mark the center of a circle, the patient with Bálint's syndrome typically won't even get the mark within the circle—and may not be able to even hit the paper. In part this may be because the patient cannot take cognizance, simultaneously, of both the circle and the pencil point; but it is also clear that the patient doesn't know where the circle is.

Holmes and Horax considered optic ataxia, like the oculomotor impairment, to be secondary to the patient's "inability to orient and localize correctly in space objects which he saw. When . . . asked to take hold of or point to any object, he projected his hand out vaguely, generally in a wrong direction, and had obviously no accurate idea of its distance from him" (Holmes & Horax, 1919, p. 391).

Holmes and Horax again observed that the lack of access to a representation of space was specific to vision. Their patient was able to localize sounds and he did have a representation of peripersonal space based on kinesthetic input: "The contrast between the defective spatial guidance he received from vision and the accurate knowledge of space that contact gave him, was excellently illustrated when he attempted to take soup from a small bowl with a spoon; if he held the bowl in his own hand he always succeeded in placing the spoon accurately in it, . . . but when it was held by a observer or placed on a table in front of him he could rarely bring his spoon to it at once, but had to grope for it till he had located it by touch" (Holmes & Horax, 1919, pp. 391 and 393).

Impaired Depth Perception

Holmes and Horax (1919) also attributed impaired depth perception to spatial disorientation. They viewed the loss of depth perception in Bálint's syndrome as a consequence of the loss of topographic perception, and as a failure to have any appreciation of distance. In their patient they attributed the loss of blinking in response to a visual threat to the patient's inability to recognize the nearness of the threatening object. Difficulty in judging distances also causes another serious problem for patients— they collide with objects when they walk about.

The impairment of depth perception in Bálint's syndrome seems to be due to a failure to appreciate the relative location of two objects, or of the patient and the object he or she is looking at. Size cues seem not to help the patient judge the distance to an object. However, Holmes and Horax commented that their patient's lack of a sense of distance did not indicate a lack of appreciation of metrics in general since he could: "indicate by his two hands the extension of ordinary standards of linear measurement, as an inch, a foot, or a yard . . . and he could indicate the lengths of familiar objects, as his rifle, bayonet, etc. (Holmes & Horax, 1919, p. 393).

Nosological Consideration: Bálint's Syndrome, Its Neighbors and Relatives

The clinical picture described here is that of Bálint's syndrome when it is quite dense and in its pure form. It reflects the typical presentation of a patient with bilateral lesions restricted to the parieto-occipital junction. While strokes and head trauma may occasionally cause discretely restricted and symmetrical lesions, it is more commonly the case that lesions will not respect these territories and will cause more extensive damage to the occipital, parietal, and temporal lobes.

Coexisting visual field deficits, hemispatial neglect, apperceptive or associative agnosia, prosopagnosia, alexia, and other cognitive deficits are often present in association with Bálint's syndrome or some of its constituent elements.

The patient reported by Bálint (1909), for example, also had left hemispatial neglect, possibly owing to extension of the lesion into the right temporoparietal junction (figure 2.1): "[T]he attention of the patient is always directed [by approximately 35 or 40 degrees] to the right-hand side of space when he is asked to direct his attention to another object after having fixed his gaze on a first one, he tends to the right-hand rather than the left-hand side" (cited by Husain and Stein, 1988, p. 90). In other cases in which a constriction of visual attention is also associated with object agnosia, the tendency of the patient to become locked on parts of objects may contribute to observed agnosic errors and may result in diagnostic confusion with integrative agnosia (Riddoch & Humphreys, 1987).

It is also the case that a given patient may have optic ataxia, spatial disorientation, or simultanagnosia without other elements of Bálint's syndrome. Thus, spatial disorientation may occur without simultanagnosia (Stark, Coslett, & Saffran, 1996); optic ataxia may occur without simultanagnosia or spatial disorientation (Perenin & Vighetto, 1988); and simultanagnosia may occur without spatial disorientation (Kinsbourne & Warrington, 1962, 1963; Rizzo & Robin, 1990). It should be borne in mind that in such cases, the observed symptoms may result from very different mechanisms than those that produce them in Bálint's syndrome. Thus, while optic ataxia and oculomotor impairment may be attributable to a loss of spatial representation in patients with Bálint's syndrome caused by bilateral parieto-occipital lesions, optic ataxia from superior parietal lesions may reflect disruption of the neural substrates mediating visuomotor transformations (Milner & Goodale, 1995).

Similarly, simultanagnosia may be caused by very different kinds of lesions for different reasons. The term *simultanagnosia* was originated specifically to describe a defect in integrating complex visual scenes (Wolpert, 1924). As defined by Wolpert, the term includes, but is more general than, the constriction of attention seen in Bálint's syndrome. It is seen in conditions other than Bálint's syndrome and may result from unilateral lesions.

Hécaen and de Ajuriaguerra describe the difficulties of one of their patients (case 1) on being offered a light for a cigarette: "[W]hen the flame was offered to him an inch or two away from the cigarette held between his lips, he was unable to se the flame because his eyes were fixed on the cigarette" (Hécaen & de Ajuriaguerra, 1956, p. 374). However, the mechanism underlying simultanagnosia in such cases may be different than that which causes simultanagnosia in Bálint's syndrome.

Unlike in Bálint's syndrome, simultanagnosia caused by unilateral left temporoparietal lesions appears to be due to a perceptual bottleneck caused by slowing of visual processing as measured by rapid, serial, visual presentation (RSVP) tasks (Kinsbourne & Warrington, 1962, 1963). In contrast, patients with Bálint's syndrome may be able to recognize a series of individual pictures flashed briefly in an RSVP test (Coslett & Saffran, 1991).

Implications of Bálint's Syndrome for Understanding Visual Cognition

Bálint's syndrome holds valuable lessons for understanding the neural processes involved in controlling attention, representing space, and providing coherence and continuity to conscious visual experience: (1) attention makes a selection from object-based representations of space; (2) independent neural mechanisms that operate in parallel orient attention within objects and between objects; (3) the candidate objects on which attention operates are generated preattentively by early vision in the absence of explicit awareness; and (4) attention is involved in affording explicit (conscious) access to the spatial representations needed for goal-directed action and for binding features of objects.

Object- and Space-Based Attention

An appreciation of simultanagnosia in Bálint's syndrome has proven influential in helping to resolve one of the major theoretical controversies in visual attention research. The issue at stake was whether visual attention acts by selecting locations or objects. Work by Michael Posner and others (Posner, 1980; Posner, Snyder, & Davidson, 1980) showed that allocating attention to a location in the visual field enhanced the processing of the visual signals that appeared at the attended location.

Object-based models of attention, in contrast, postulate that preattentive processes parse the visual scene to generate candidate objects (more on this later) and that attention then acts by selecting one such object for further processing that can guide goal-directed action. These models are supported by experiments in normal individuals that show better discrimination of two features belonging to the same object than of features belonging to two different objects (Duncan, 1984) and that these object-based effects are independent of the spatial location of their features (Baylis & Driver, 1995; Vecera & Farah, 1994).

Physiological recordings have shown that an object-based attentional set can modulate processing in the extrastriate visual cortex (Chelazzi, Duncan, Miller, & Desimone, 1998). Recent neuroimaging studies have confirmed that attentional selection of one of two objects results in activation of brain regions representing other unattended features of that object (O'Craven, Downing, & Kanwisher, 2000).

Object-based models predict that brain lesions could produce an object-based simultanagnosia that is independent of location. This is precisely the kind of simultanagnosia that was observed in patients with Bálint's syndrome decades before this debate was joined by psychologists and physiologists. Moreover, recent experimental work by Humphreys and colleagues has shown that simultanagnosia can be manifest in nonspatial domains. In two patients with parietal lobe lesions and poor spatial localization, these authors observed that pictures extinguished words and closed shapes extinguished open shapes (Humphreys, Romani, Olson, Riddoch, & Duncan, 1994). Thus the object-based attention deficit in this syndrome cannot be attributed simply to the effects of parietal lobe lesions in disrupting access to spatial representations.

Neural Representations of Objects in Space

The spatial representations upon which attention operates are determined by objects, or "candidate" objects, derived from a grouped array of features by early vision (Vecera & Farah, 1994), and are not simple Cartesian coordinates of empty space centered on the observer (Humphreys, 1998). Humphreys has recently posited that attention operates on spatial representations determined by objects, and that there are separate mechanisms, operating in parallel, for shifting attention within objects and between objects (Humphreys, 1998). Shifting attention within an object implies shifting attention between locations within the object.

Figure 2.6 shows stimuli that Cooper and Humphreys (2000) used to study shifts of attention within and between objects in patient G.K. with Bálint's syndrome. In conditions 1 and 2, G.K.'s task was to report whether the upright segments were the same or different lengths. For the stimuli in condition 1, in which the comparison was

between two parts of the same object, G.K. was correct on 84% of the trials, whereas in condition 2 in which the judgment required comparison of two separate objects, performance was at chance level (54%).

Visual Processing Outside of Conscious Awareness

The interaction of spatial and object representations in determining the allocation of attention requires that candidate objects be provided by preattentive processes that proceed in the absence of awareness. Cumulative observations in patients with hemispatial neglect (see chapter 1) have indeed provided growing evidence that early vision does separate figure from ground, group features, and assign primary axes; it even extracts semantic information that can assign attentional priorities for subsequent processing. Here some examples are considered in which implicit measures of processing in Bálint's syndrome have provided strong evidence for extensive processing of visual information outside of awareness.

Preattentive Representation of Space

Spatial disorientation is a cardinal feature of Bálint's syndrome, and one view of the constriction

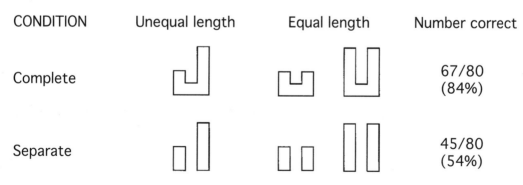

Figure 2.6
Figures used by Cooper and Humphreys (2000) to demonstrate grouping in Bálint's syndrome.

of visual attention posits that it, too, is due to a loss of a neural representation of space on which attention may act (Friedman-Hill et al., 1995). However, as we have seen from the work of Humphreys et al. (1994), simultanagnosia may also occur for nonspatial information, such as shifting between words and pictures. Moreover, recent observations in patients with both hemispatial neglect (Danziger, Kingstone, & Rafal, 1998) and Bálint's syndrome (Robertson, Treisman, Friedman-Hill, & Grabowecky, 1997) have shown that parietal damage does not eliminate representations of spatial information, but rather prevents explicit access to this information.

Robertson et al. (1997) showed that although patient R.M. could not explicitly report the relative location of two objects, he nevertheless exhibited a spatial Stroop interference effect. That is, although he could not report whether the word "up" was in the upper or lower visual field, he was, nevertheless, slower to read "up" if it appeared in the lower visual field than in the upper visual field.

Preattentive Grouping of Features and Alignment of Principal Axis

As described earlier, observations by Luria (Luria, 1959) and by Humphreys & Riddoch (1993) have revealed that there is less simultanagnosia when shapes in the visual field are connected. Other recent observations by Humphreys and his colleagues in patient G.K. have confirmed that grouping based on brightness, collinearity, surroundedness, and familiarity also are generated preattentively, as is grouping based on alignment of a principal axis. Figure 2.7 shows G.K.'s performance in reporting two items; it shows that performance is better when the items are grouped on the basis of brightness, collinearity, connectedness, surroundness, and familiarity (Humphreys, 1998).

Preattentive Processing of Meaning of Words

As is the case in hemispatial neglect, neglected objects do appear to be processed to a high level of semantic classification in patients with Bálint's

syndrome. Furthermore, although this information is not consciously accessible to the patient, it does influence the perception of objects that are seen. For example, Coslett & Saffran (1991) simultaneously presented pairs of words or pictures briefly to their patient, and asked her to read or name them. When the two stimuli were not related semantically, the patient usually saw only one of them, but when they were related, she was more likely to see them both. Hence, both stimuli must have been processed to a semantic level of representation, and the meaning of the words or objects determined whether one or both would be perceived.

Words are an example of hierarchical stimuli in which letters are present at the local level and the word at the global level. We (Baylis, Driver, Baylis, & Rafal, 1994) showed patient R.M. letter strings and asked him to report all the letters he could see. Since he could only see one letter at a time, he found this task difficult and, with the brief exposure durations used in the experiment, he usually only saw a few of the letters. However, when the letter string constituted a word, he was able to report more letters than when it did not. That is, even when the patient was naming letters and ignoring the word, the word was processed and helped to bring the constituent letters to his awareness.

Attention, Spatial Representation, and Feature Integration: Gluing the World Together

I discussed earlier how a single object seen by a patient is experientially mutable in time. It has no past or future. Any object that moves disappears. In addition, objects seen in the present can be perplexing to the patient, because other objects that the patient does not see, and their features, are processed and impinge upon the experience of the attended object. Normally, the features of an object, such as its color and its shape, are correctly conjoined, because visual attention selects the location of the object and glues together all the features sharing that same location (Treisman & Gelade, 1980). For the patient with Bálint's syndrome, however, all locations are the same, and all the

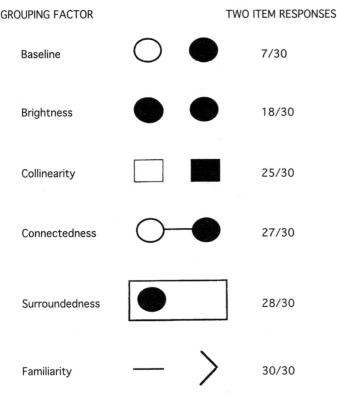

GROUPING FACTOR   TWO ITEM RESPONSES

Baseline   7/30

Brightness   18/30

Collinearity   25/30

Connectedness   27/30

Surroundedness   28/30

Familiarity   30/30

Figure 2.7
Figures used by Humphreys (1998) to demonstrate grouping in Bálint's syndrome.

features that impinge on the patient's awareness are perceptually conjoined into that object.

Friedman-Hill et al. (1995) showed R.M. pairs of colored letters and asked him to report the letter he saw and its color. R.M. saw an exceptional number of illusory conjunctions (Treisman & Schmidt, 1982), reporting the color of the letter that he did not see as being the color of the letter that he did report. Lacking access to a spatial representation in which colocated features could be coregistered by his constricted visual attention, visual features throughout the field were free floating and conjoined arbitrarily. Since a spatial Stroop effect was observed in patient R.M. (see earlier discussion), Robertson and her colleagues (1997) argued that spatial information did exist and that feature binding relies on a relatively late stage where implicit spatial information is made explicitly accessible. Subsequent observations in patient R.M. showed, however, that feature binding also occurred implicitly. Wojciulik & Kanwisher (1998) used a modification of a Stroop paradigm in which R.M. was shown two words, one of which was colored, and asked to report the color and ignore the words. Although he was not able to report explicitly which word was colored, there was nevertheless a larger Stroop interference effect (i.e., he was slower to name the color) when a word had an incongruent color. Thus, there was implicit evidence that the word and its color had been bound, even though R.M. had no explicit access to the conjunction of features.

Conclusions and Future Directions

Lost in space, and stuck in a perceptual present containing only one object that he or she cannot find or grasp, the patient with Bálint's syndrome is helpless in a visually chaotic world. Objects appear and disappear and their features become jumbled together. Contemporary theories of attention and perception help us to understand the experience of these patients. At the same time, their experience provides critical insights into the neural basis of visual attention and perception, and how they operate together normally to provide coherent perceptual experience and efficient goal-directed behavior.

Some of the critical issues remain unresolved and await future research. It remains unclear whether simultanagnosia and spatial disorientation are independent symptoms in Bálint's syndrome, or whether the apparent constriction of visual attention is a secondary consequence of the lack of access to an explicit representation of space. The identification of individual cases in which these two symptoms are dissociated would resolve this question. It is also important to learn more about the impairment in feature binding that causes the generation of illusory conjunctions, and whether this deficit is an integral component of the syndrome or, rather, is present only in some patients with a lesion in a specific part of the parietal-occipital association cortex. Furthermore, if the component symptoms of the syndrome are found to be dissociable, we will need to know more about the neural substrates of each.

References

Bálint, R. (1909). Seelenlahhmung edes "schauens," optische ataxie, raumliche storung der aufmerksamkeit. *Montschrife Pscyhiatrie und Neurologie, 25*, 51–81.

Baylis, G. C., & Driver, J. (1995). One-sided edge-assignment in vision: 1. Figure-ground segmentation and attention to objects. *Current Directions in Psychological Science, 4*, 201–206.

Baylis, G. C., Driver, J., Baylis, L. L., & Rafal, R. D. (1994). Perception of letters and words in Bálint's syndrome: Evidence for the unity of words. *Neuropsychologia, 32*, 1273–1286.

Benson, D. F., Davis, R. J., & Snyder, B. D. (1988). Posterior cortical atrophy. *Archives of Neurology, 45*, 789–793.

Chelazzi, L., Duncan, J., Miller, E. K., & Desimone, R. (1998). Responses of neurons in inferior temporal cortex during memory-guided visual search. *Journal of Neurophysiology, 80*, 2918–2940.

Cooper, C. G., & Humphreys, G. W. (2000). Coding space within but not between objects: Evidence from Bálint's syndrome. *Neuropsychologia 38*, 723–733.

Coslett, H. B., & Saffran, E. (1991). Simultanagnosia. To see but not two see. *Brain, 113*, 1523–1545.

Danziger, S., Kingstone, A., & Rafal, R. (1998). Reflexive orienting to signals in the neglected visual field. *Psychological Science, 9*, 119–123.

Duncan, J. (1984). Selective attention and the organization of visual information. *Journal of Experimental Psychology: General, 113*, 501–517.

Friedman-Hill, S. R., Robertson, L. C., & Treisman, A. (1995). Parietal contributions to visual feature binding: Evidence from a patient with bilateral lesions. *Science, 269*, 853–855.

Girotti, F., Milanese, C., Casazza, M., Allegranza, A., Corridori, F., & Avanzini, G. (1982). Oculomotor disturbances in Bálint's syndrome: Anatomoclinical findings and electrooculographic analysis in a case. *Cortex, 16*, 603–614.

Godwin-Austen, R. B. (1965). A case of visual disorientation. *Journal of Neurology, Neurosurgery and Psychiatry, 28*, 453–458.

Harvey, M. (1995). Psychic paralysis of gaze, optic ataxia, spatial disorder of attention. Translated from Bálint (1909). *Cognitive Neuropsychology, 12*, 266–282.

Harvey, M., & Milner, A. D. (1995). Bálint's patient. *Cognitive Neuropsychology, 12*, 261–264.

Hécaen, H., & de Ajuriaguerra, J. (1956). Agnosie visuelle pour les objects inanimes par lesion unilaterle gauche. *Review Neurologique, 94*, 222–233.

Hof, P. R., Bouras, C., Constintinidis, J., & Morrison, J. H. (1989). Bálint's syndrome in Alzheimer's disease: Specific disruption of the occipito-parietal visual pathway. *Brain Research*, *493*, 368–375.

Hof, P. R., Bouras, C., Constantinidis, J., & Morrison, J. H. (1990). Selective disconnection of specific visual association pathways in cases of Alzheimer's disease presenting with Bálint's syndrome. *Journal of Neuropathology and Experimental Neurology*, *49*, 168–184.

Holmes, G., & Horax, G. (1919). Disturbances of spatial orientation and visual attention, with loss of stereoscopic vision. *Archives of Neurology and Psychiatry*, *1*, 385–407.

Humphreys, G. W. (1998). Neural representation of objects in space: A dual coding account. *Philosophical Transactions of the Royal Society of London, Ser. B*, *353*, 1341–1351.

Humphreys, G. W., & Riddoch, M. J. (1993). Interactive attentional systems in unilateral visual neglect. In I. H. Robertson & J. C. Marshall (Eds.), *Unilateral neglect: Clinical and experimental studies* (pp. 139–168). Hillsdale, NJ: Lawrence Erlbaum Associates.

Humphreys, G. W., Romani, C., Olson, A., Riddoch, M. J., & Duncan, J. (1994). Non-spatial extinction following lesions of the parietal lobe in humans. *Nature*, *372*(6504), 357–359.

Husain, M., & Stein, J. (1988). Rezso Bálint and his most celebrated case. *Archives of Neurology 45*, 89–93.

Karnath, H.-O., Ferber, S., Rorden, C., & Driver, J. (2000). The fate of global information in dorsal simultanagnosia. *NeuroCase 6*, 295–306.

Kase, C. S., Troncoso, J. F., Court, J. E., Tapia, F. J., & Mohr, J. P. (1977). Global spatial disorientation. *Journal of the Neurological Sciences*, *34*, 267–278.

Kinsbourne, M., & Warrington, E. K. (1962). A disorder of simultaneous form perception. *Brain*, *85*, 461–486.

Kinsbourne, M., & Warrington, E. K. (1963). The localizing significance of limited simultaneous visual form perception. *Brain*, *86*, 461–486.

Luria, A. R. (1959). Disorders of "simultaneous perception" in a case of bilateral occipito-parietal brain injury. *Brain*, *83*, 437–449.

Luria, A. R., Pravdina-Vinarskaya, E. N., & Yarbuss, A. L. (1963). Disorders of ocular movement in a case of simultanagnosia. *Brain*, *86*, 219–228.

Mendez, M. F., Turner, J., Gilmore, G. C., Remler, B., & Tomsak, R. L. (1990). Bálint's syndrome in Alzheimer's disease: Visuospatial functions. *International Journal of Neuroscience*, *54*, 339–346.

Milner, A. D., & Goodale, M. A. (1995). *The visual brain in action*. Oxford: Oxford University Press.

O'Craven, K., Downing, P., & Kanwisher, N. (2000). fMRI evidence for objects as the units of attentional selection. *Nature 401*, 584–587.

Perenin, M.-T., & Vighetto, A. (1988). Optic ataxia: A specific disruption in visuomotor mechanisms. I. Different aspects of the deficit in reaching for objects. *Brain*, *111*, 643–674.

Pierrot-Deseillgny, C., Gray, F., & Brunet, P. (1986). Infarcts of both inferior parietal lobules with impairment of visually guided eye movements, peripheral visual inattention and optic ataxia. *Brain*, *109*, 81–97.

Posner, M. I. (1980). Orienting of attention. *Quarterly Journal of Experimental Psychology*, *32*, 3–25.

Posner, M. I., Snyder, C. R. R., & Davidson, B. (1980). Attention and the detection of signals. *Journal of Experimental Psychology: General*, *109*, 160–174.

Riddoch, M. J., & Humphreys, G. W. (1987). A case of integrative visual agnosia. *Brain*, *110*, 1431–1462.

Rizzo, M., & Robin, D. A. (1990). Simultanagnosia: A defect of sustained attention yields insights on visual information processing. *Neurology*, *40*, 447–455.

Robertson, L. C., Treisman, A., Friedman-Hill, S. R., & Grabowecky, M. (1997). The interaction of spatial and object pathways: Evidence from Bálint's syndrome. *Journal of Cognitive Neuroscience*, *9*, 295–317.

Stark, M., Coslett, H. B., & Saffran, E. (1996). Impairment of an egocentric map of locations: Implications for perception and action. *Cognitive Neuropsychology*, *13*, 481–523.

Treisman, A., & Gelade, G. (1980). A feature integration theory of attention. *Cognitive Psychology*, *12*, 97–136.

Treisman, A., & Schmidt, N. (1982). Illusory conjunctions in the perception of objects. *Cognitive Psychology*, *14*, 107–141.

Tyler, H. R. (1968). Abnormalities of perception with defective eye movements (Bálint's syndrome). *Cortex*, *3*, 154–171.

Vecera, S. P., & Farah, M. J. (1994). Does visual attention select objects or locations? *Journal of Experimental Psychology: General, 123*, 146–160.

Verfaellie, M., Rapcsak, S. Z., & Heilman, K. M. (1990). Impaired shifting of attention in Bálint's syndrome. *Brain and Cognition, 12*, 195–204.

Williams, M. (1970). *Brain damage and the mind.* Baltimore: Penguin Books.

Wojciulik, W., & Kanwisher, N. (1998). Implicit but not explicit feature binding in a Bálint's patient. *Visual Cognition, 5*, 157–182.

Wolpert, I. (1924). Die simultanagnosie: Storung der geamtauffassung. *Zeitschrift für die gesante Neurologie und Psychiatrie, 93*, 397–415.

3   Amnesia: A Disorder of Episodic Memory

Michael S. Mega

Memory is traditionally divided into implicit and explicit processes (figure 3.1). Implicit functions are not under conscious control, while explicit functions are available to our subjective awareness. Implicit processes include classic conditioning or associative learning (such as the conditioned eye-blink response), procedural memory or skill learning (such as riding a bike or learning the rotary pursuit task), and the effects of priming that facilitate the acquisition of information in the modality specific to the presentation of the information. Explicit memory includes both our recall of everything that has happened to us—called "episodic memory," and all the information about the meanings of things—called "semantic memory." The emphasis here is on patients' complaints of explicit memory impairments.

Explicit memory is heuristically divided into the subprocesses of acquisition, storage, and retrieval of information. Disorders of learning are assumed to arise from deficits in either acquisition or storage; thus poor spontaneous recall could arise from two distinct problems—either a failure in learning new information or a deficit in retrieval.

Classically, the amnesic syndrome has been defined as the presence of a significant isolated memory disorder in the absence of disturbed attention, language, visuospatial, or executive function (executive function is the ability to manipulate previously acquired knowledge). Although the exact dysfunctional subprocess producing amnesia is controversial (Bauer, Tobias, & Valenstein, 1993), it is clinically useful to describe amnesia as a failure to learn new information, which is distinct from a retrieval deficit identified by normal recognition.

Recognition, in turn, may depend on two subprocesses: a feeling of familiarity and an explicit recollection of some context associated with the recognized item (Gardiner & Parkin, 1990; Horton, Pavlick, & Moulin-Julian, 1993; Mandler, 1980). The recognition tasks that patients with hippocampal and perirhinal lesions preferentially fail on are those that make greater demands on the later recollection-based subprocess (Aggleton & Shaw, 1996; Squire & Shimamura, 1986). Successful recognition performance, after spontaneous recall has failed, also draws on intact prefrontal resources. A profound encoding or recognition impairment appears to require both medial temporal and prefrontal disconnection or destruction (Aggleton & Mishkin, 1983; Gaffan & Parker, 2000).

Case Report

On the first evaluation a 75-year-old right-handed female was accompanied by her husband to our clinic complaining of a 3–5-year history of declines in memory. The history was mainly provided by the patient's husband, who claimed that 5 years prior to presentation he first noticed abnormalities in his wife's ability to operate a new video-cassette recorder and new 35-mm camera. There was also a decline in her ability to cook large meals for dinner parties that began 3 years prior to presentation. Approximately 2 years prior to presentation, he began noticing difficulty with his wife's memory so that she was unable to shop for food without a detailed list. She would frequently forget conversations that transpired between them or episodes that might have occurred days prior. Approximately 6 months prior to presentation, the patient's husband noted that she forgot what cards were played in their bridge club when previously she had been an excellent player. The patient agreed with the history of memory problems, but felt that her cooking was unaffected. Both the patient and her husband denied any problems with language function, visuospatial function, or any change in personality or mood. The patient continued to be quite active socially, as well as taking part in community activities. Despite her memory problem, she was still capable of functioning almost independently with copious list keeping.

On initial examination the patient had a normal general medical exam. The patient was well nourished, cooperative, well groomed, and in no apparent distress. The patient's attention was intact with six digits forward, five digits in reverse. The Mini Mental State Exam (MMSE) (Folstein, Folstein, & McHugh, 1975) score was 28/30; the

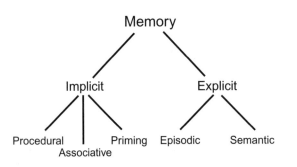

Figure 3.1
Conceptual organization and terminology of general memory function.

patient missed two of the recall questions. Language was normal for fluency, comprehension, and repetition; and naming was intact, with fifteen out of fifteen items on a modified Boston Naming Test correctly identified. Verbal fluency showed nineteen animals produced in 1 minute, and reading and writing ability were entirely normal. Memory testing using a ten-word list (Fillenbaum et al., 1997) showed a learning curve of four, six, and eight after three trials; and after a 10-minute interval with interference, the patient spontaneously recalled one out of ten items. Recognition performance, using ten target items and ten foils, produced five additional items, with three false positives.

Visuospatial function showed no problems in copying two-dimensional figures and some mild strategy difficulty but good copying of a three-dimensional cube. Executive function showed no problems with calculation ability for two-digit addition and multiplication; however, word problems showed some hesitancy and difficulty in response, although the answers were eventually correct. Frontal system evaluation showed no perseveration or loss of set; reciprocal programs, go-no-go, and alternating programs were all intact. The rest of the neurological examination, including cranial nerves, motor and sensory function, coordination, reflexes, and gait was normal.

On the initial evaluation the patient underwent formal neuropsychological testing, functional imaging with [^{18}F]fluorodeoxyglucose positron emission tomography (FDG-PET) and structural imaging with 3-D coronal volumetric and double echo magnetic resonance imaging (MRI).

Neuropsychological evaluation revealed a normal Wechsler Adult Intelligence Scale-Revised (WAIS-R)

(Wechsler, 1955), a full-scale IQ with normal scores on all subscales except for arithmetic, which was 1 standard deviation (S.D.) below age and education norms. Language evaluation was intact on the Boston Naming Test (Kaplan, Goodglass, & Weintraub, 1984), with a score of 59/60. Controlled oral word fluency (FAS) (Benton & Hamsher, 1976 revised 1978) and animal naming were intact, but in the low average range.

Memory testing showed impairments on the California Verbal Learning Test (CVLT), which demonstrated encoding and storage abnormalities greater than 1.5 S.D. below age- and education-matched norms. Weschler memory (Wechsler Memory Scale, WMS) (Wechsler, 1945), logical memory, and paragraph recall showed significant abnormalities in the first and second paragraph delayed-recall scores. Nonverbal memory was also impaired as noted by the 30-minute delay on the Rey-Osterrieth Complex Figure Recall (Osterrieth, 1944; Rey, 1941) as well as the Benton Visual Retention Test (Benton, 1974). Executive function showed spotty performance, with normal trails A and B but Stroop B declines at approximately 1 S.D. below age- and education-matched norms. The Ruff figural fluency task showed low normal performance (Jones-Gotman & Milner, 1977). Interpretation of neuropsychological testing concluded that the patient did not meet the criteria for dementia according to DSM-IV (APA, 1994); however, the patient did meet the criteria for amnesic disorder.

FDG-PET showed essentially normal metabolism in the frontal, parietal, and occipital cortices as well as subcortical structures, but indicated decreased metabolism in medial temporal lobe regions, the loss in the left being greater than in the right (figure 3.2). MRI analysis showed no significant cerebrovascular disease either cortically or

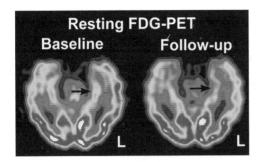

Figure 3.2
Oblique axial slices through the long axis of the hippocampus of a FDG-PET scan (registered to the University of California at Los Angeles (UCLA) Alzheimer's Disease Atlas) of a patient at baseline evaluation for an isolated memory complaint (*left*) and at follow-up 18 months later (*right*), showing progressive left medial (arrow) and lateral temporal dysfunction.

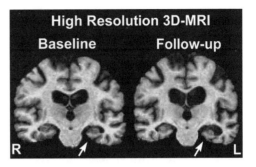

Figure 3.3
Coronal 3-D MRI at baseline evaluation and at follow-up 18 months later (registered to the UCLA Alzheimer's Disease Atlas) showing progressive atrophy in the left hippocampus (arrow) for the patient described in the case report.

subcortically and no masses or cortical atrophy; however, there was mild to moderate volume loss in medial temporal structures as determined by qualitative assessment of the MRI resliced parallel to the long axis of the hippocampus (de Leon et al., 1997; de Leon et al., 1993) (figure 3.3) Laboratory evaluation showed a normal chemistry panel-20, complete blood cell count, thyroid-stimulating hormone, B_{12} and folate levels, a negative fluorescent triponamae antibody absorbed test, and a normal erthrocyte sedimentation rate.

The history, examination, and diagnostic studies at initial evaluation described here are consistent with an amnesic disorder. The patient met criteria at that time for mild cognitive impairment (MCI) (Petersen et al., 1999) based on logical memory performance (a paragraph recall score of less than 8) and other memory scores (<1.5 S.D. below age- and education-matched norms). There were no other significant abnormalities, save for some mild to moderate executive dysfunction as reflected in both history and neuropsychological testing. The possibility of incipient Alzheimer's disease could not be ruled out at the time of initial evaluation.

A follow-up visit occurred approximately a year and a half after the time of initial presentation. The

interim history was significant for progressive declines in memory function with continued preservation of language and visuospatial function. Questionable executive dysfunction evolved, with difficulty in preparing meals, balancing her checkbook, and paying household bills. No significant change in personality or mood occurred over this interim period. Repeat neuropsychological testing was significant for progressive decline in both verbal and visual memory, with more than 2 standard deviations below age and education mean scores on memory tests, but still relative preservation in executive function and some improvement in visuospatial function, with continued unimpaired language function.

In comparison with the initial evaluation, PET showed progressive bilateral metabolic declines in medial temporal structures, with continued preservation of metabolism in the dorsolateral frontal, high parietal, and occipital cortices (figure 3.2). Structural imaging showed no evidence of new cerebral vascular disease, but showed progressive atrophy in medial temporal structures (figure 3.3).

Two years later, the patient collapsed at the breakfast table. Her husband called paramedics, but they were unable to revive her and she was pronounced dead on arrival at the local hospital, with pathological evaluation showing a myocardial infarction. Evaluation of the brain showed no evidence of significant Alzheimer's changes, but moderate cell loss in the CA1 fields of the hippocampus, with gliotic change on the left and less so on the right. A diagnosis was made of hippocampal sclerosis.

A Historical Perspective on Amnesia

The case described here illustrates a typical assessment strategy for a patient presenting with a progressive memory complaint. When a memory problem is reported with no clear etiology on bedside, laboratory, or imaging evaluation, it is often necessary to follow the patient and repeat the imaging and neuropsychological evaluation in 9 months to a year if the complaints persist. In the above case, worsening was observed at the follow-up exam compared with the baseline assessment and thus a degenerative disorder was most likely. The patient's initial performance on bedside memory testing using a ten-word list showed a adequate learning curve during three presentations of the same words revealing normal performance during the acquisition phase of learning new information. After a 10-minute interval with interference, the patient exhibited poor spontaneous recall, showing a defect in either storage or retrieval. It is important not to stop the evaluation at this point because in order to determine which of the above two defects are present, we must prompt the patient with cues; either category or recognition cues. When a patient with poor spontaneous recall significantly improves their performance with cues, then we have ruled out a disorder of learning and have identified a retrieval deficit as being responsible for their memory complaints. Care must be taken not to ignore the number of false positives a patient may produce with cueing. The patient described here correctly recognized half of the items with cueing, but had also said yes to several items that were foils (i.e., false-positive responses); this

reveals moderate guessing. When cueing does not improve recall, or when false positives nearly equal or surpass true positives on the recognition portion of the exam, patients should be considered amnesic. When recognition performance surpasses spontaneous recall, then patients are said to have a retrieval deficit.

The anatomical defects underlying a failure to learn information (i.e., amnesia) are different from those underlying a retrieval deficit. Amnesia results from damage to the medial temporal encoding system and its connections to the prefrontal cortex, whereas a retrieval deficit does not result from medial temporal damage (Teng & Squire, 1999), but from dorsolateral frontal cortical abnormalities.

The Medial Temporal Encoding System

An understanding of hippocampal anatomy is necessary before we attempt to interpret lesion and imaging findings (figure 3.4). In a normal adult brain, the distance from the tip of the temporal pole to the most caudal aspect of the hippocampal formation is about 7.5 cm, while the intraventricular portion of the hippocampus extends about 4 cm. The cytoarchitecture of the temporal pole (Brodmann's area 38) resembles that of the perirhinal cortex (areas 35 and 36) (Amaral & Insausti, 1990). The temporal polar portion of the perirhinal cortex is continuous with the ventral perirhinal cortex, which lines the banks of the collateral sulcus. The perirhinal cortex extends posteriorly to the anterior boundary of the lateral geniculate nucleus, where it is replaced caudally by the parahippocampal cortex (areas TF and TH). Medially, the amygdaloid complex lies posterior to the temporal pole, and the hippocampal formation is inferior to the amygdala in its most anterior extent and then caudal to the amygdala. The hippocampal formation is made up of four components: the dentate gyrus, hippocampus, subicular complex, and entorhinal cortex.

In 1900, Bechterew found that bilateral lesions of the hippocampus and diencephalic structures (the mamillary bodies and anterior thalamus) resulted in derangements of memory function. Both short- and

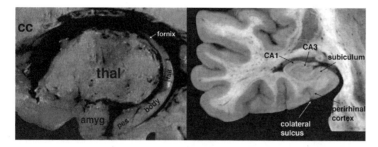

Figure 3.4
Anatomy of the hippocampus in relation to other brain regions (*left*) showing the anterior pes, body, and tail with extension into the fornix near the splenium of the corpus callosum (cc). The coronal section (*right*) shows the hippocampal fields transitioning from CA3 into CA2 and then CA1, which in turn extends into the subiculum and eventually into the entorhinal and perirhinal cortex within the banks of the collateral sulcus.

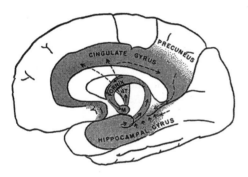

Figure 3.5
The medial circuit of Papez, as depicted by MacLean (1949), was proposed to support emotional processing (Papez, 1937).

long-term memory remained relatively intact; however, the process of registration of information was disturbed (Bechterew, 1900). In 1937, Papez proposed a mechanism of emotion based on a medial circuit (figure 3.5). He described three divisions in the brain through which "man's volitional energies" flow. First a "stream of movement" is conducted through the dorsal thalamus and the internal capsule to the corpus striatum and then out the central nervous system to the somatic motor neuron. Second, the "stream of thought" arises from

the thalamus and ascends the internal capsule to find expression in the lateral cerebral cortex involved in executive function (the ability to organize a solution to a complex problem). Third, there are impulses flowing through medial structures in a "stream of feeling" (Papez, 1987).

Papez conceived of a two-way circuit for the flow of emotion leading to internal or external expression. Information from external sensory receptors arrives at the primary sensory cortex and then is relayed to the hippocampal area and onward to the mamillary bodies via the fornix. From the mamillary bodies, information spreads throughout the hypothalamus, initiating emotional expression or affect. Impulses are also directed to the anterior nucleus of the thalamus, via the mamillothalamic tract, and then diffusely projected through the anterior limb of the internal capsule toward the cingulate gyrus. There, Papez thought, emotion as an internal state or mood is consciously perceived. Processing within the cingulate gyrus provides feedback to the hippocampus via the retrosplenial cortex, completing the circuit.

Papez observed that mood may be dissociated from affect since in decorticate subjects emotional states were displayed but not perceived by the subject. For Papez, the integration of emotional responsiveness with the dorsolateral frontal executive functions occurred in the medial cortex of the cingulate gyrus. There was no anatomical support for the closing connection of the cingulate gyrus to the hippocampus in Papez's circuit until 1975, when Shipley and Sørensen (1975) documented that the presubiculum, which receives a dense cingulate cortex outflow, projects heavily to layer III of the entorhinal cortex—the origin of the perforant pathway into hippocampal pyramidal cells (Witter & Amaral, 1991). The entorhinal cortex also is the conduit for highly processed sensory afferents. The perirhinal and parahippocampal cortices receive the result of a chain of feed-forward projections from the unimodal and polymodal sensory cortices (Freeman, Murray, O'Neill, & Mishkin, 1986; Mesulam & Mulson, 1982; Pandya & Yeterian, 1985; Suzuki & Amaral, 1994; Tranel, Brady, Van Hoesen, & Damasio, 1988; Van Hoesen, 1982; Webster, Ungerleider, & Bachevalier, 1991), providing 60% of the cortical input to the entorhinal cortex (Insausti, Amaral, & Cowan, 1987).

Papez incorrectly conceived his hippocampal circuit as exclusively subserving emotional processes. Bechterew's insight was more accurate. He observed that defects in episodic memory encoding occurred when elements of the hippocampal circuit were damaged (Bechterew, 1900). This explicit or conscious encoding of events by the hippocampal circuit stands in contrast to the subconscious processing that may occur in the amygdala when objects are imbued with emotional valence (Bechara et al., 1995; Blair, Morris, Frith, Perrett, & Dolan, 1999; Ikeda et al., 1998; Mori et al., 1999; Price, 1999).

The Dorsolateral Frontal Executive System

The superior dorsolateral prefrontal cortex (Brodmann areas 9 and 10) is the center of an executive cognitive network that links the posterior parietal lobe and anterior cingulate gyrus. Functionally, the dorsolateral prefrontal cortex subserves executive function (Cummings, 1993) and short-term or working memory (Baddeley, 1992, 1996, 1998)

(See Chapter 11, this volume). These functions include the ability to organize a behavioral response to solve a complex problem (including the strategies used in learning new information and systematically searching memory), activation of remote memories, self-direction and independence from environmental contingencies, shifting and maintaining behavioral sets appropriately, generating motor programs, and using verbal skills to guide behavior.

Damage to the dorsolateral frontal cortex produces deficits in executive function and working memory.

With regard to long-term memory performance, it is the organization and successful execution of the retrieval process during free recall that is most impaired by dorsolateral frontal lesions because of the disruption of the anatomically distributed dorsolateral network.

Regions reciprocally connected to the superior dorsolateral prefrontal areas 9 and 10 are the inferior prefrontal area 46 (Selemon & Goldman-Rakic, 1985), the superior prefrontal area 8, and area 7a of the caudal superior parietal lobe (Yeterian & Pandya, 1993). Parietal area 7a subserves visual spatial attention, visually guided reaching, and planning of visuospatial strategies. Major reciprocal connections with the anterior cingulate cortex (supracallosal areas 24, 24a' and b', and 32') (Mega & Cummings, 1997) also occur with prefrontal areas 8, 9, 10, and 46 (Morecraft & Van Hoesen, 1991; Vogt & Pandya, 1987). The anterior cingulate cortex is the center for directing attentional systems and coordinating the dorsolateral frontal and parietal heteromodal association network (Morecraft, Geula, & Mesulam, 1993). Areas reciprocally connected to the anterior cingulate cortex include the rostral insula and anterior parahippocampal areas. The rostral insular cortex is a transitional paralimbic region that integrates visceral alimentary input with olfactory and gustatory afferents (Mesulam & Mufson, 1985). Connections with anterior parahippocampal areas 35 and 36 allow the attentional network to influence multimodal sensory afferents entering the hippocampus.

An understanding of the distributed anatomy of the medial encoding circuit and the dorsolateral executive system will aid our interpretation of the results of human and nonhuman primate lesion studies producing memory dysfunction as well as those of functional neuroimaging studies that attempt to map explicit encoding and retrieval mechanisms in normal subjects.

Experimental Research on Episodic Memory

Lesion Studies

Medial Temporal Lesions

Although Bechterew (1900) first noted that bilateral lesions of the medial temporal lobes produced encoding defects, it was the detailed report 57 years later by Scoville and Milner (1957) on H.M., who underwent bilateral temporal lobectomy to relieve intractable seizures, that initiated the modern anatomical search for the encoding, storage, and retrieval systems. Speculation (Horel, 1978) that lesions outside the hippocampus proper might explain H.M.'s memory impairment combined with results from animal studies (Mishkin & Murray, 1994) implicate other medial temporal structures subserving memory. The perirhinal cortex became a focus of the medial temporal memory system in monkeys (Meunier, Bachevalier, Mishkin, & Murray, 1993; Suzuki, Zola-Morgan, Squire, & Amaral, 1993; Zola-Morgan, Squire, Amaral, & Suzuki, 1989c; Zola-Morgan, Squire, Clower, & Rempel, 1993) because the delayed matching and nonmatching-to-sample tasks (which are primarily recognition tests) were unimpaired if a hippocampal lesion did not also extend into the monkey's rhinal cortex (Zola-Morgan, Squire, Rempel, Clower, & Amaral, 1992).

In H.M., the surgical lesion included the medial temporal pole, most of the amygdaloid complex, and bilaterally all of the entorhinal cortex (figure 3.6). In addition, the anterior 2 cm of the dentate gyrus, hippocampus, and subicular complex were

removed. Given that the collateral sulcus and the cortex lining its banks are visible, then at least some of the posterioventral perirhinal cortex was intact in H.M. The posterior parahippocampal gyrus (areas TF and TH) was only slightly damaged rostrally. The lingual and fusiform gyri, lateral to the collateral sulcus, were also intact.

Another surgical case (P.B.) had the entire left temporal lobe removed in a two-stage procedure (Penfield & Milner, 1958) and suffered a life-long dense amnesia (Corkin, 1965). At autopsy P.B. also had preservation of the posterior 22 mm of the hippocampus and parahippocampal cortex (Penfield & Mathieson, 1974). Patients with ischemic lesions bilaterally confined to the CA1 field of the hippocampus (Cummings, Tomiyasu, Read, & Benson, 1984; Zola-Morgan, Squire, & Amaral, 1986) have clinically significant anterograde amnesia that is milder than that of H.M., and have significant retrograde amnesia that may last more than 25 years (Rempel-Clower, Zola, Squire, & Amaral, 1996).

Isolated hippocampal lesions occurring in childhood appear to disrupt only the encoding of declarative memories about past events, but not the encoding of information about the world (semantic memory) (Vargha-Khadem et al., 1997) that may depend upon parahippocampal integrity. Thus, if a bilateral lesion includes adjacent structures such as the temporal pole and the anterior perirhinal and entorhinal cortices (as in the case of H.M.), the amnesic syndrome and the resultant recognition deficit (Buffalo, Reber, & Squire, 1998) in humans is much more severe than that resulting from an isolated hippocampal lesion.

Similar studies on monkeys, which evaluated small lesions restricted to the hippocampal (Alvarez, Zola-Morgan, & Squire, 1995), entorhinal (Leonard, Amaral, Squire, & Zola-Morgan, 1995), or perirhinal and parahippocampal cortices (Suzuki et al., 1993; Zola-Morgan et al., 1989c), have confirmed that all these medial temporal structures—except the amygdale (Murray, 1991; Zola-Morgan, Squire, & Amaral, 1989a)—participate in recognition memory (Meunier et al., 1993; Zola-Morgan, Squire, & Amaral, 1989b; Zola-Morgan et al.,

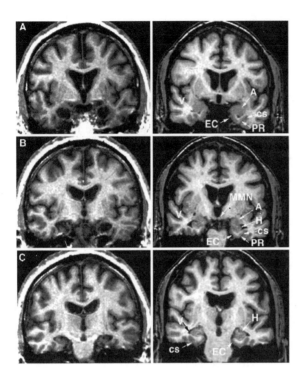

Figure 3.6
A coronal MRI of H.M. from rostral (*A*) to caudal (*C*) showing the extent of bilateral hippocampal ablation (*left*) compared with a normal 66-year-old subject (*right*); note the destruction of the amygdala (A), hippocampus (H), and entorhinal cortex (EC) anterior to the level of the mamillary bodies (MMN), with relative sparing of the posterior perirhinal cortex (PR) in the banks of the collateral sulcus(cs). V, temporal horn of lateral ventricle. (Adapted from Corkin et al., 1997.)

1989c; Zola-Morgan, Squire, & Ramus, 1994). The greatest recognition memory defect occurs when the perirhinal cortex is ablated along with the "H lesion" (hippocampus, dentate gyrus, and subicular complex) (Zola-Morgan et al., 1993), followed by the combined caudal entorhinal and perirhinal cortices and the H lesion (Mahut, Zola-Morgan, & Moss, 1982; Zola-Morgan et al., 1989c); this defect is greater than that resulting from the H lesion alone (Alvarez et al., 1995).

Restricted lesions of the perirhinal and parahippocampal (Suzuki et al., 1993; Zola-Morgan et al., 1989c) or entorhinal and perirhinal cortices (Meunier et al., 1993) produce chronic multimodal memory deficits similar to those of a bilateral medial temporal lobectomy (Suzuki et al., 1993). Thus each of these medial temporal regions makes a contribution to the mnemonic process, with the resultant recognition memory defect becoming more severe with the removal of each additional processing region (Zola-Morgan et al., 1994). What the unique functions are, if any, within each region is not known (Eichenbaum, Otto, & Cohen, 1994; Gaffan, 1994a).

Diencephalic Lesions

Hippocampal output from the subiculum, via the fornix, enters the mamillary body (primarily the medial mamillary nucleus) and projects to the anterior thalamic nuclei (Aggleton, Desimone, & Mishkin, 1986). The anterior thalamic region also receives direct hippocampal input via the fornix (Aggleton et al., 1986) and has reciprocal connections with the cingulate gyrus and anterior reticularus thalami (Gonzalo-Ruiz, Morte, & Lieberman, 1997). The dorsomedial thalamic nucleus receives more widespread afferents from the amygdala, basal forebrain, and brainstem, and has reciprocal connections with the prefrontal cortex and reticularus thalami (Aggleton & Mishkin, 1984; Ilinsky, Jouandet, & Goldman-Rakic, 1985; Kuroda, Yokofujita, & Murakami, 1998; Russchen, Amaral, & Price, 1987). Lesions of the diencephalon often affect both the anterior and the dorsomedial thalamus; thus the isolation of hippocampal outflow within the Papez circuit rarely occurs and the added disruption of the frontal subcortical circuits and amygdalo-olfactory system (Mega, Cummings, Salloway, & Malloy, 1997) through the dorsomedial thalamus is common.

Wernicke-Korsakoff's syndrome (Korsakoff, 1889), which is often the result of thiamine deficiency in alcoholics, drew attention to the diencephalon in memory function. These and other cases of amnesia associated with third ventricular tumors (Foerster & Gagel, 1933; Grünthal, 1939; Lhermitte, Doussinet, & de Ajuriaguerra, 1937; Sprofkin & Sciarra, 1952; Williams & Pennybacker, 1954) pointed to the mamillary bodies or thalamus as critical to memory function. Mamillary body damage was thought to be involved in the amnesia of alcoholic Korsakoff's psychosis since this region suffers the most concentrated pathology in the disease (Torvik, 1987). The mamillary bodies and thalamus were evaluated in forty-three cases (Victor, Adams, & Collins, 1971) of Wernicke's encephalopathy; five patients who recovered without evidence of memory loss were found to

have mamillary body damage but no thalamic damage; the remaining thirty-eight cases, with enduring memory disturbance, all had additional dorsomedial thalamic damage. These findings identified the thalamus as the pivotal diencephalic structure subserving memory function. Furthermore, mamillary body damage was not correlated with memory impairment in Korsakoff patients (Charness & DeLaPaz, 1987; Davila, Shear, Lane, Sullivan, & Pfefferbaum, 1994; Estruch et al., 1998; Shear, Sullivan, Lane, & Pfefferbaum, 1996), and isolated lesions in animals produced only spatial memory disturbances, without recognition difficulty (Aggleton, Neave, Nagle, & Hunt, 1995; Neave, Nagle, & Aggleton, 1997; Parker & Gaffan, 1997b; Sziklas & Petrides, 1997).

A thalamic infarction produces lethargy, confusion (Cole, Winkelman, Morris, Simon, & Boyd, 1992), apathy (Kritchevsky, Graff-Radford, & Damasio, 1987), and amnesia (Cole et al., 1992; Peru & Fabbro, 1997; Shuren, Jacobs, & Heilman, 1997), depending on the lesion size. Severe dorsomedial degeneration occurs in fatal familial insomnia (Lugaresi, Tobler, Gambetti, & Montagna, 1998) and results in failure to generate electro encephalographic (EEG) sleep patterns, underscoring its role in arousal. The dorsomedial thalamic damage in Korsakoff patients, as reflected by imaging (Charness, 1993; McDowell & LeBlanc, 1984; Shimamura, Jernigan, & Squire, 1988) and histology (Mair, Warrington, & Weiskrantz, 1979; Mayes, Meudell, & Pickering, 1988; Torvik, 1985; Victor et al., 1989), may require additional neuronal loss in the anterior thalamic nuclei (Harding, Halliday, Caine, & Kril, 2000) to produce permanent memory impairment.

Lesions of the entire magnocellular division of the dorsomedial thalamus in monkeys, which disrupt all prefrontal efferents (Russchen et al., 1987), compared with isolated medial magnocellular lesions (Parker, Eacott, & Gaffan, 1997) that destroy only the entorhinal and perirhinal inputs (Aggleton et al., 1996), produce significant impairment of object recognition (Gaffan & Parker, 2000).

Initial reports of the patient N.A., who developed amnesia from a penetrating injury with a fencing foil (Teuber, Milner, & Vaughan, 1968), suggested restricted dorsomedial thalamic damage (Squrie & Moore, 1979). However, with the use of high-resolution magnetic resonance imaging (MRI), N.A.'s lesion was found to affect only the ventral aspect of the dorsomedial nucleus, with more severe damage to the intralaminar nuclei, mamillothalamic tract, and internal medullary lamina (Squire, Amaral, Zola-Morgan, Kritchevsky, & Press, 1989). Lesions isolated to the internal medullary lamina and the mamillothalamic tract appear capable of producing thalamic amnesia (Cramon, Hebel, & Schuri, 1985; Gentilini, DeRenzi, & Crisi, 1987; Graff-Radford, Tranel, Van Hoesen, & Brandt, 1990; Malamut, Graff-Radfore, Chawluk, Grossman, & Gur, 1992; Winocur, Oxbury, Roberts, Agnetti, & Davis, 1984) more severe than lesions that affect only the dorsomedial thalamus and spare the former structures (Cramon et al., 1985; Graff-Radford et al., 1990; Kritchevsky et al., 1987).

Anterior thalamic lesions on the right, sparing the dorsomedial nucleus (Daum & Ackermann, 1994; Schnider, Gutbrod, Hess, & Schroth, 1996), can cause memory dysfunction similar to that of Korsakoff's amnesia. Thus limited damage to the anterior thalamus can produce permanent deficits in episodic memory, supporting previous studies emphasizing the importance of this region for the memory deficit in alcoholic Korsakoff's psychosis (Kopelman, 1995; Mair et al., 1979; Mayes et al., 1988). The lateral dorsal nucleus (a member of the anterior thalamic nuclei) projects to the retrosplenial cortex and is focally affected in Alzheimer's disease (Xuereb et al., 1991). These findings are also consistent with the severe memory deficits caused by lesions of the anterior thalamic nuclei in laboratory animals (Aggleton et al., 1995; Aggleton & Sahgal, 1993; Aggleton & Saunders, 1997; Parker & Gaffan, 1997a); the degree of memory dysfunction is related to the extent of the lesion (Aggleton & Shaw, 1996).

The basal forebrain is also considered part of the diencephalon and includes the nucleus accumbens, olfactory tubercle, nucleus of the stria terminalis, and the preoptic area. It also includes the cell groups that provide acetylcholine (ACh) to the telencephalon: the septum (Ch1), the vertical (Ch2) and horizontal (Ch3) diagonal bands of Broca, and the basal nucleus of Meynert (Ch4) (Mesulam, Mufson, Levey, & Wainer, 1983). These neurons play an important role in attention (anterior cingulate cortex—vertical diagonal band of Broca), memory (hippocampus—medial septum and diagonal band) (Lewis & Shute, 1967), aversive conditioning (amygdala—nucleus basalis of Meynert, nbM), and the ability to use learned responses (dorsolateral frontal cortex—nbM).

The basal forebrain was long noted to be damaged in repair or rupture of an aneurysm of an anterior communicating artery (Lindqvist & Norlen, 1966; Talland, Sweet, & Ballantine, 1967), but isolated lesions are rare. Results from three patients who had discrete lesions in the basal forebrain suggest that the critical anatomical lesion may be confined to the nuclei of the medial septum and diagonal band (Abe, Inokawa, Kashiwagi, & Yanagihara, 1998; Damasio, Graff-Radford, Eslinger, Damasio, & Kassell, 1985; Morris, Bowers, Chatterjee, & Heilman, 1992), producing a disconnection of cholinergic innervation to the hippocampus. Though spontaneous recall was impaired in these patients, recognition memory was relatively spared.

In summary, for diencephalic lesions to produce profound abnormalities in recall and recognition, a mamillothalamic—anterior thalamus (Papez's circuit) disconnection should be combined with a dorsomedial thalamic—prefrontal disconnection. Relatively few human cases have been presented as exceptions to this generalization (Daum & Ackermann, 1994; Mair et al., 1979; Mayes et al., 1988; Schnider et al., 1996). Future combined structural and functional imaging assessments may be needed to determine if prefrontal disconnection has occurred in such cases as well.

Retrosplenial and Fornix Lesions

Lesions of the posterior cingulate gyrus disrupt memory function in animals and humans. The closing link in Papez's circuit, from the anterior thalamic efferents traveling through the cingulum to Brodmann areas 23 and 29/30, is the posterior cingulate projection sent to the presubiculum. Anterior cingulotomy will not disrupt this memory circuit, but rarely pathological lesions will extend into, and beyond, the posterior cingulate gyrus. If the lesion extends inferior to the splenium of the corpus callosum, it may also disrupt the fornix, thus disconnecting the efferents from the hippocampus to the diencephalon. If the lesion extends posteriorly, it may damage the supracommissural portion of the hippocampus—the gyrus fasciolaris and the fasciola cinerea. A lesion restricted to the left posterior cingulate gyrus, the cingulum, and the splenium of the corpus callosum (possibly sparing the fornix) resulted in a severe amnesia after the bleeding of an arteriovenous malformation (Valenstein et al., 1987). A left-sided lesion that extended beyond the posterior cingulate gyrus into the fornix and supracommissural hippocampus after repair of an arteriovenous malformation resulted in a transient nonverbal but permanent verbal amnesia (Cramon & Schuri, 1992). Disruption of septohippocampal pathways in the cingulum and fornix were thought by the authors to play a significant role in the patient's clinical deficit, but the supracommissural hippocampus was also damaged. Another case involving the right retrosplenial region produced a predominantly visual amnesia (Yasuda, Watanabe, Tanaka, Tadashi, & Akiguchi, 1997), but verbal memory was affected.

Isolation of the cingulum within the posterior cingulate gyrus on the left by a cryptic angioma hemorrhage produced only a transient encoding deficit (Cramon, Hebel, & Ebeling, 1990), suggesting that the supracommissural hippocampus or fornix must also be damaged for persistent deficits to occur. Splenial tumors are also capable of producing memory impairment, perhaps via compression of the fornix (Rudge & Warrington, 1991).

The questionable effect that fornix lesions in humans have on memory (Cairns & Mosberg, 1951; Dott, 1938; Garcia-Bengochea, De La Torre, Esquivel, Vieta, & Fernandec, 1954; Garcia-

Bengochea & Friedman, 1987; Woolsey & Nelson, 1975) has been attributed to the lesions being partial, or to poor psychometric evaluations (Gaffan & Gaffan, 1991). Bilateral disruption of the fornix, with ensuing memory decline, has resulted from tumors (Calabrese, Markowitsch, Harders, Scholz, & Gehlen, 1995; Heilman & Sypert, 1977), trauma (D'Esposito, Verfaellie, Alexander, & Katz, 1995; Grafman, Sclazar, Weingartner, Vance, & Ludlow, 1985), vascular disease (Botez-Marquard & Botez, 1992), and surgical transection (Aggleton et al., 2000; Hassler & Riechert, 1957; Sweet, Talland, & Ervin, 1959).

Unilateral damage to the left fornix has also produced verbal memory impairment (Cameron & Archibald, 1981; Gaffan & Gaffan, 1991; Tucker, Roeltgen, Tully, Hartmann, & Boxell, 1988). When memory impairment does occur, recall is usually affected more than simple list recognition (Aggleton et al., 2000; McMackin, Cockburn, Anslow, & Gaffan, 1995). Recognition tasks that require the encoding of individual items within a complex scene ("object in place" tasks) are poorly performed in both monkeys (Gaffan, 1994b) and humans (Aggleton et al., 2000) with fornix transection.

An analysis of rare circumscribed lesions in humans could not determine if lesions in the posterior cingulate cortex, rather than the fornix, cingulum, or neighboring members of Papez's circuit, result in amnesia. Excitotoxic lesions in animals that destroy neurons but spare fibers of passage can clarify this issue. Based on posterior cingulate cortical lesions made using the selective cytotoxin, quisqualic acid (Sutherland & Hoesing, 1993), animal studies reveal that posterior cingulate cortical neurons are necessary for the acquisition and retention of spatial and nonspatial memory.

Lesion Summary

Lesion studies in both animals and humans have demonstrated that the individual components of Papez's circuit all contribute to general memory function. As a general rule, however, for significant encoding defects to occur (as reflected by poor performance on generic recognition tasks), either perirhinal lesions must be present in isolation or other members of Papez's circuit must be lesioned in combination with disruption of prefrontal-subcortical circuits. Thus, the combination of relatively preserved recognition memory with poor spontaneous recall seems to require an intact perirhinal cortex and at least a partially spared prefrontal system.

When recognition memory, using the immediate recognition memory test (RMT) (Warrington, 1984) for both words and pictures, is evaluated across a spectrum of human lesions that produce isolated spontaneous memory dysfunction, the most impaired patients are those that are postencephalitic or have Korsakoff syndrome (Aggleton & Shaw, 1996). These data support the combined Papez's circuit–prefrontal contribution to successful encoding since the first four lesion groups in that study often affect these two circuits; or these data suggest that the RMT task is a poor test of environmentally relevant recognition. Future studies should use recognition tasks that do not have a "ceiling effect" as prominent as that of the RMT to further probe the anatomical basis of recognition and encoding integrity.

Functional Neuroimaging Studies

The Encoding System

Functional imaging studies of normal subjects performing tasks of episodic encoding, retrieval, and recognition also support the importance of Papez's circuit and frontal lobe function in the memory process. Several reviews have recently summarized this field (Buckner & Koutstaal, 1998; Cabeza & Nyberg, 2000; Cohen et al., 1999; Gabrieli, 1998, 2001; Lepage, Habib, & Tulving, 1998; Schacter & Wagner, 1999).

Has functional imaging taught us anything we did not already know from lesion studies about the neuronal systems supporting encoding and retrieval? The explosive growth in functional imaging studies over the past 5 years has confirmed the involvement of medial temporal structures in the encoding process (figure 3.7). When studies vary the novelty of items presented by increasing the repetition of presentations, medial temporal activation is increased for scenes (Gabrieli, Brewer, Desmond, & Glover, 1997; Stern et al., 1996; Tulving, Markowitsch, Craik, Habib, & Houle, 1996), words

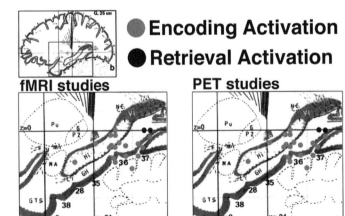

Figure 3.7
Regional mapping of the medial temporal activations found in encoding and retrieval tasks of episodic memory for both fMRI and PET studies of normal subjects. (Adapted from Schacter Wagner, 1999.)

(Kopelman, Stevens, Foli, & Grasby, 1998), object-noun pairs (Rombouts et al., 1997), and word pairs (Dolan & Fletcher, 1997). Bilateral activation usually occurs for scenes, whereas verbal activations are typically left-sided.

The magnitude of medial temporal activation is also correlated with the effectiveness of encoding, as reflected by a subject's recognition performance after the presentation and scanning phase; this correlative effect is bilateral for scenes (Brewer, Zhao, desmond, Glover, & Gabrieli, 1998) and left-sided for words (Wagner et al., 1998c); it has also been correlated with free recall for words even 24 hours after presentation (Alkire, Haier, Fallon, & Cahill, 1998). Distracter tasks (Fletcher et al., 1995) or varying the level of cognitive processing during the presentation of items to be learned can affect encoding success (Buckner & Koutstaal, 1998; Demb et al., 1995; Gabrieli et al., 1996).

Subsequent recall is significantly enhanced by judging the abstract quality or deeper associations of words, as opposed to their surface orthographic features. Such strategies of leveraging the associations of items to be remembered has been used since the ancient Greek orators. Increased medial temporal activation occurs with deeper semantic processing than with shallow letter or line inspection of words (Vandenberghe, Price, Wise, Josephs, & Frackowiak, 1996; Wagner et al., 1998c) or drawings (Henke, Buck, Weber, & Wieser, 1997; Vandenberghe et al., 1996), and with intentional memorization versus simple viewing of words (Kapur et al., 1996; Kelley et al., 1998), faces (Haxby et al., 1996; Kelley et al., 1998), or figures (Schacter et al., 1995).

Deep processing also recruits dorsolateral prefrontal regions during encoding (figure 3.8) (Buckner & Koutstaal, 1998). A differential activation of the prefrontal cortex occurs (Fiez, 1997; Poldrack et al., 1999) with a more posterior bilateral focus (in BA 6/44) for sensory-specific features of the encoding task (Klingberg & Roland, 1998; Zatorre, Meyer, Gjedde, & Evans, 1996), while a greater anterior left prefrontal focus (in BA 45/47) is found with increasing semantic

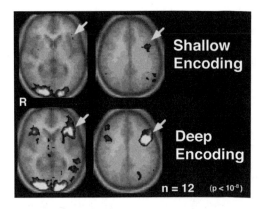

Figure 3.8
Functional MRI activation maps for "shallow" and "deep" encoding tasks, contrasted with fixation. Both tasks activate posterior visual areas, whereas only the deep encoding task shows increased activation of left inferior and dorsolateral frontal areas (arrows). These activations are at peak Talairach coordinates. (x, y, z) of -40, 9, 34 and -46, 6, 28 for the more dorsal activations and -40, 19, 3 and -43, 19, 12 for the more ventral prefrontal activations. (Adapted from Buckner and Koutstaal, 1998.)

demands (Demb et al., 1995; Fletcher, Shallice, & Dolan, 1998).

Although a lateralized pattern of activation is generally found for nonverbal (right frontal) (Kelley et al., 1998; McDermott, Buckner, Petersen, Petersen, Kelley, & Sanders, 1999; Wagner et al., 1998b) versus lexical (left frontal) (McDermott et al., 1999; Wagner et al., 1998b) stimuli, if visual stimuli can evoke semantic associations, then left anterior prefrontal activation tends to also occur (Haxby et al., 1996; Kelley et al., 1998), especially when longer retention times are provided for these semantic associations to form (Haxby, Ungerleider, Horwitz, Rapoport, & Grady, 1995). Right prefrontal activation is best correlated with successful encoding of scenes, as reflected by post-scanning recall performance (Brewer et al., 1998), while left prefrontal activations are best correlated with subsequent word recall (Wagner et al., 1998c).

Most functional imaging studies are focused on the assessment of activity occurring on the same day of testing. Long-term dynamic changes occur with the eventual consolidation of learned information. Functional imaging studies have just begun to probe this dynamic consolidation process. After medial temporal regions are engaged with initial encoding, the anterior cingulate cortex and temporal cortices appear to mediate the retrieval of learned information. The anterior cingulate cortex has been consistently activated in paradigms that require sustained attention to novel tasks. In a subtraction-based paradigm of memory encoding combined with a motor task demanding sustained divided attention (Fletcher et al., 1995), the anterior cingulate cortex was singularly activated by the sustained vigilance demanded to divide the effort between the two tasks. Position emission topography activation studies using varied designs (Corbetta, Miezin, Dobmeyer, Shulman, & Petersen, 1991; Frith, Friston, Liddle, & Frackowiak, 1991; Jones, Brown, Friston, Qi, & Frackowiak, 1991; Pardo, Pardo, Haner, & Raichle, 1990; Petersen, Fox, Posner, Mintun, & Raichle, 1988, 1989; Talbot et al., 1991) consistently activated the anterior cingulate cortex when subjects were motivated to succeed in whatever task was given them. When motivation to master a task was no longer required, and accurate performance of a task became routine, the anterior cingulate cortex returned to a baseline activity level (Raichle et al., 1994).

In a radial arm maze task using mice trained successfully after encoding-associated activation of Papez's circuit (hippocampal-posterior cingulate cortex), the anterior cingulate, dorsolateral prefrontal, and temporal cortices (but not the hippocampus) were engaged during retrieval 25 days after learning (Bontempi, Laurent-Demir, Destrade, & Jaffard, 1999). Thus the hippocampal formation encodes or maintains new information until the consolidation process has ended. When the context of the maze was changed, and new learning had to occur, the hippocampus-posterior cingulate cortex was once again activated. In addition to its role in the consolidation of declarative memory, the post-

erior cingulate cortex is also active during associative learning in classic conditioning paradigms (Molchan, Sunderland, McIntosh, Herscovitch, & Schreurs, 1994).

The Retrieval System

The greater neocortical recruitment during retrieval of remote compared with recent memories seen in the mouse experiment (Bontempi et al., 1999) suggests that there are dynamic hippocampal–cortical interactions during the consolidation process, with a gradual reorganization of neural substrates resulting in a shift toward the neocortex during long-term memory storage (Buzsaki, 1998; Damasio, 1989; Knowlton & Fanselow, 1998; Squire & Alvarez, 1995; Teyler & DiScenna, 1986). Most human functional imaging studies test retrieval within minutes or hours of presentation. In such studies, the medial temporal cortex is activated during retrieval compared to a resting condition (Ghaem et al., 1997; Grasby et al., 1993; Kapur et al., 1995a; Roland & Gulyas, 1995), passive viewing (Maguire, Frackowiak, & Frith, 1996; Schacter et al., 1995, 1997b), or nonepisodic retrieval (Blaxton et al., 1996; Schacter, Alpert, Savage, Rauch, & Albert, 1996a; Schacter, Buckner, Koutstaal, Dale, & Rosen, 1997a; Squire et al., 1992).

When decisions are required as to whether current items were previously studied, the medial temporal cortex shows the greatest activation for prior items even though correct judgments are made about novel items (Fujii et al., 1997; Gabrieli et al., 1997; Maguire et al., 1998; Nyberg et al., 1995; Schacter et al., 1995; Schacter et al., 1997b). This is not the case for frontal lobe activations, which are present during both successful retrieval (Buckner, Koutstaal, Schacter, Wagner, & Rosen, 1998; Rugg, Fletcher, Frith, Frackowiak, & Dolan, 1996; Tulving, Kapur, Craik, Moscovitch, & Houle, 1994a; Tulving et al., 1996) and attempted retrieval (Kapur et al., 1995b; Nyberg et al., 1995; Rugg, Fletcher, Frith, Frackowiak, & Dolan, 1997; Wagner, Desmond, Glover, & Gabrieli, 1998a).

The frontal lobe's contribution to memory retrieval, as evidenced from functional imaging

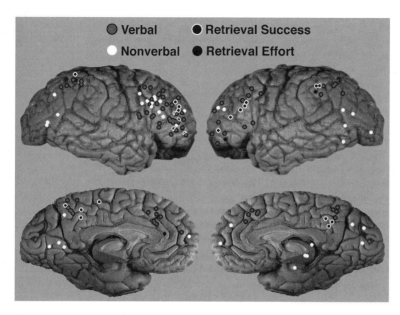

Figure 3.9
Summary of the peak regions of significance in functional imaging studies mapping the success and effort in the retrieval of verbal and nonverbal material. (Adapted from Carbeza and Nyberg, 2000.)

studies, may be related to the sequencing of search strategies (Alkire et al., 1998; Gabrieli, 1998; Schacter, Savage, Alpert, Rauch, & Albert, 1996c; Ungerleider, 1995), strategic use of knowledge (Wagner et al., 1998a), and working memory processes that facilitate successful retrieval (Desmond, Gabrieli, & Glover, 1998; Gabrieli et al., 1996; Thompson-Schill, D'Espsito, Aguirre, & Farah, 1997). This multiple processing interpretation of frontal lobe activations associated with memory retrieval evolved from a refinement of the hemispheric encoding–retrieval asymmetry (HERA) model, which proposed a dichotomy between left prefrontal activations associated with encoding and right prefrontal activations associated with retrieval (figure 3.9). Although the right prefrontal cortex is activated in most retrieval tasks whether the tasks are verbal (Blaxton et al., 1996; Buckner et al., 1996; Buckner et al., 1995; Cabeza, Kapur, Craik, & McIntosh, 1997; Flectcher et al.,

1998; Kapur et al., 1995b; Nyberg et al., 1995; Petrides, Alivasatos, & Evans, 1995; Rugg et al., 1996; Schacter, Curran, Galluccio, Milberg, & Bates, 1996b; Shallice et al., 1994; Squire et al., 1992; Tulving et al., 1994b; Wagner et al., 1998a), or nonverbal (Haxby et al., 1996; Moscovitch, Kapur, Kohler, & Houle, 1995; Owen, Milner, Petrides, & Evans, 1996), a posterior focus (BA 9/46) appears to be stimulus dependent, and an anterior focus (BA 10) may be related to retrieval attempts (McDermott et al., 1999).

Event-related functional MRI (fMRI) allows a better assessment of the activation correlated with individual trials, and when applied to episodic retrieval tasks, a differential time course of the vascular response is observed in the right frontal lobe. A typical transient 4-second peak is noted in the posterior right frontal cortex after item presentation and response, while a sustained 10-second vascular response is observed in the right anterior frontal cortex after stimulus presentation (Buckner et al., 1998; Schacter et al., 1997a). This sustained hemodynamic response may represent a different process assisting general retrieval, perhaps an anticipatory mechanism awaiting the next presentation (Buckner et al., 1998) or a success monitoring process resulting from the last presentation (Rugg et al., 1996).

The exact contribution of the prefrontal cortex to memory retrieval is not known, but given that strategic memory judgments (temporal order, source memory, etc.) yield more extensive bilateral frontal activations—coupled with results from the lesion literature that demonstrate impaired strategic memory in patients with focal frontal lesions—it appears that multiple processes are provided by discrete frontal regions that combine to assist retrieval of episodic memory (Cabeza et al., 1997; Henson, Rugg, Shallice, Josephs, & Dolan, 1999; Nolde, Johnson, & D'Esposito, 1998a; Nolde, Johnson, & Raye, 1998b). Once consolidation has occurred, the retrieval of remotely acquired information involves the anterior cingulate cortex and other neocortical regions in accessing stored representations (Markowitsch, 1995; Mega & Cummings, 1997). This activation of the anterior cingulate cortex may be related to increased attention and internal search strategies and be combined with other cortical regions, such as temporal cortices, which aid the retrieval of autobiographic memory (Fink, 1996).

In summary, functional imaging studies have furthered our understanding of the neural basis of the memory function. It is only through functional imaging that cognitive neuroscience has begun to explore the spatially diverse regions simultaneously engaged in the encoding and retrieval processes. Thus, functional imaging complements the lesion literature and in some cases advances our understanding of the brain regions involved in psychological processes. Caution must be used, however, in interpreting the results from both sources of inquiry, since the refinement of our understanding of cognition must account for lesion results in patients and activation results in normal subjects.

Utilizing both avenues to test emerging hypotheses will produce more robust models of cognitive processes.

Conclusions and Future Directions

The results from clinical, animal, and imaging studies all support the importance of the medial temporal region and other components of Papez's circuit in the spontaneous recall of new information. Variable recognition deficits will be observed, and thus presumed encoding defects, with concomitant dysfunction of prefrontal-subcortical integrity. The most profound amnesia will occur with perirhinal destruction, or combined Papez's-prefrontal circuit damage. When isolated prefrontal damage is present, with Papez's circuit spared, spontaneous retrieval may be impaired, but recognition will likely be intact.

Future studies of the neuronal basis of normal memory function will identify the networks responsible for the encoding, consolidation, and retrieval of a variety of stimuli with functional imaging paradigms that probe anatomically connected but spatially separate regions. Investigating functionally coupled distributed brain regions may require combining the excellent spatial resolution of fMRI with the superior temporal resolution of magnetoencephalography along with novel statistical techniques that control the search for linked systems. Once a distinct network is identified that is reproducible across individuals for a given memory task, population-based studies will be necessary to determine the magnitude and distribution of normal signal response across demographic variables. Armed with the normal population's variability in performance and signal change, abnormalities can be defined with cross-sectional studies of patients with memory disorders and longitudinal studies of normal subjects who develop memory dysfunction. Such a growing body of data will benefit not only our theories of normal memory function but also our diagnosis of subtle memory defects, and perhaps their treatment.

References

Abe, K., Inokawa, M., Kashiwagi, A., & Yanagihara, T. (1998). Amnesia after a discrete basal forebrain lesion. *Journal of Neurology, Neurosurgery and Psychiatry, 65,* 126–130.

Aggleton, J. P., Desimone, R., & Mishkin, M. (1986). The origin, course, and termination of the hippocampothalamic projections in the macaque. *Journal of Comparative Neurology, 243,* 409–421.

Aggleton, J. P., McMackin, D., Carpenter, K., Hornak, J., Kapur, N., Haipin, S., Wiles, C. M., Kame, H., Brennan, P., Carton, S., & Gaffan, D. (2000). Differential cognitive effects of colloid cysts in the third ventricle that spare or compromise the fornix. *Brain, 123,* 800–815.

Aggleton, J. P., & Mishkin, M. (1983). Memory impairments following restricted medial thalamic lesions in monkeys. *Experimental Brain Research, 52,* 199–209.

Aggleton, J. P., & Mishin, M. (1984). Projections of the amygdala to the thalamus in the cynomolgus monkey. *Journal of Comparative Neurology, 222,* 56–68.

Aggleton, J. P., Neave, N., Nagle, S., & Hunt, P. R. (1995). A comparison of the effects of anterior thalamic, mamillary body and fornix lesions on reinforced spatial alternation. *Behavioral Brain Research, 68,* 91–101.

Aggleton, J. P., & Sahgal, A. (1993). The contribution of the anterior thalamic nuclei to anterograde amnesia. *Neuropsychologia, 31,* 1001–1019.

Aggleton, J. P., & Saunders, R. C. (1997). The relationships between temporal lobe and diencephalic structures implicated in anterograde amnesia. *Memory, 5,* 49–71.

Aggleton, J. P., & Shaw, C. (1996). Amnesia and recognition memory: A re-analysis of psychometric data. *Neuropsychologia, 34,* 51–67.

Alkire, M. T., Haier, R. J., Fallon, J. H., & Cahill, L. (1998). Hippocampal, but not amygdala, activity at encoding correlates with long-term, free recall of nonemotional information. *Proceedings of the National Academy of Sciences U.S.A., 95,* 14506–14510.

Aivarez, P., Zola-Morgan, S., & Squire, L. R. (1995). Damage limited to the hippocampal region produces long-lasting memory impairment in monkeys. *Journal of Neuroscience, 15,* 3796–3807.

Amaral, D. G., & Insausti, R. (1990). Hippocampal formation. In G. Paxinos (Ed.), *The human nervous system* (pp. 711–755). New York: Academic Press.

American Psychiatric Association (1994). *Diagnostic and statistical manual of mental disorders* (Fourth Edition: DSM IV.). Washington, DC: American Psychiatric Press.

Baddeley, A. D. (1992). Working memory. *Science, 255,* 556–559.

Baddeley, A. D. (1996). The fractionation of working memory. *Proceedings of the National Academy of Sciences U.S.A., 93,* 13468–13472.

Baddeley, A. D. (1998). Recent developments in working memory. *Current Opinion in Neurobiology, 8,* 234–238.

Bauer, R. M., Tobias, B., & Valenstein, E. (1993). Amnesic disorders, In K. M. Heilman & E. Valenstain (Eds.), *Clinical neuropsychology* (pp. 523–602). New York; Oxford University Press.

Bechara, A., Tranel, D., Damasio, H,, Adolphs, R., Rockland, C., & Damasio, A. R. (1995). Double dissociation of conditioning and declarative knowledge relative to the amygdala and hippocampus in humans. *Science, 269,* 1115–1118.

Bechterew, W. (1900). Demonstration eines gehirns mit zestörung der vorderen und inneren theile der hirnrinde beider schläfenlappen. *Neurologisches Centralblatt, 20,* 990–991.

Benton, A. L. (1974). *Revised visual retention test* (4th ed.). New York: Psychological Corp.

Benton, A. L., & Hamsher, K. (1976 revised 1978). *Multilingual aphasia examination.* Iowa City: University of Iowa.

Blair, R. J. R., Morris, J. S., Frith, C. D., Perrett, D. I., & Dolan, R. J. (1999). Dissociable neural responses to facial expressions of sadness and anger. *Brain, 122,* 883–893.

Blaxton, T. A., Bookheimer, S. Y., Zeffiro, T. A., Figlozzi, C. M., William, D. G., & Theodore, W. H. (1996). Functional mapping of human memory using PET: Comparisons of conceptual and perceptual tasks. *Canadian Journal of Experimental Psychology, 50,* 42–56.

Bontempi, B., Laurent-Demir, C., Destrade, C., & Jaffard, R. (1999). Time-dependent reorganization of brain circuitry underlying long-term memory storage. *Nature, 400,* 671–675.

Botez-Marquard, T., & Botez, M. I. (1992). Visual memory deficits after damage to the anterior commissure and right fornix, *Archives of Neurology, 49,* 321–324.

Brewer, J. B., Zhao, Z., Desmond, J. E., Glover, G. H., & Gabrieli, J. D. E. (1998). Making memories: Brain activity that predicts how well visual experience will be remembered. *Science, 281,* 1185–1187.

Buckner, R. L., Bandettini, P. A., O'Craven, K. M., Savoy, R. L., Petersen, S. E., Raichle, M. E., & Rosen, B. R. (1996). Detection of cortical activation during averaged single trials of a cognitive task using functional magnetic resonance imaging. *Proceedings of the National Academy of Sciences U.S.A.*, *93*, 14878–14883.

Buckner, R., & Koutstaal, W. (1998). Functional neuroimaging studies of encoding, priming, and explicit memory retrieval. *Proceedings of the National Academy of Sciences U.S.A.*, *95*, 891–898.

Buckner, R. L., Koutstaal, W., Schacter, D. L., Wagner, A. D., & Rosen, B. R. (1998). Functional-anatomic study of episodic retrieval using fMRI: I. Retrieval effort versus retrieval success. *Neuroimage*, *7*, 151–162.

Buckner, R. L., Petersen, S. E., Ojemann, J. G., Miezin, F. M., Squire, L. R., & Raichle, M. E. (1995). Functional anatomical studies of explicit and implicit memory retrieval tasks. *Journal of Neuroscience*, *15*, 12–29.

Buffalo, E. A., Reber, P. J., & Squire, L. R. (1998). The human perirhinal cortex and recognition memory. *Hippocampus*, *8*, 330–339.

Buzsaki, G. (1998). Memory consolidation during sleep: A neuropsychological perspective. *Journal of Sleep Research*, *7*, 17–23.

Cabeza, R., Kapur, S., Craik, F. I. M., & McIntosh, A. R. (1997). Functional neuroanatomy of recall and recognition: A PET study of episodic memory. *Journal of Cognitive Neuroscience*, *9*, 254–256.

Cabeza, R., & Nyberg, L. (2000). Imaging cognition II: An empirical review of 275 PET and fMRI studies. *Journal of Cognitive Neuroscience*, *12*, 1–47.

Cairns, H., & Mosberg, W. H. (1951). Colloid cyst of the third ventricle. *Surg Gynecology and Obstetrics*, *92*, 545–570.

Calabrese, P., Markowitsch, H. J., Harders, A. G., Scholz, M., & Gehlen, W. (1995). Fornix damage and memory. A case report. *Cortex*, *31*, 555–564.

Cameron, A. S., & Archibald, Y. M. (1981). Verbal memory deficit after left fornix removal: A case report. *International Journal of Neuroscience*, *12*, 201.

Charness, M. E. (1993). Brain lesions in alcoholics. *Alcohol: Clinical and Experimental Research*, *17*, 2–11.

Charness, M. E., & DeLaPaz, R. L. (1987). Mamillary body atrophy in Wernicke's encephalopathy: Antemortem identification using magnetic resonance imaging. *Annals of Neurology*, *22*, 595–600.

Cohen, N. J., Ryan, J., Hunt, C., Romine, L., Wszalek, T., & Nash, C. (1999). Hippocampal system and declarative (relational) memory: Summarizing the data from functional neuroimaging studies. *Hippocampus*, *9*, 83–98.

Cole, M., Winkelman, M. D., Morris, J. C., Simon, J. E., & Boyd, T. A. (1992). Thalamic amnesia: Korsakoff syndrome due to left thalamic infarction. *Journal of Neurological Science*, *110*, 62–67.

Corbetta, M., Miezin, F. M., Dobmeyer, S., Shulman, G. L., & Petersen, S. E. (1991). Selective and divided attention during visual discriminations of shape, color and speed: Functional anatomy by positron emission tomography. *Journal of Neuroscience*, *11*, 2383–2402.

Corkin, S. (1965). Tactually-guided maze learning in man: Effects of unilateral cortical excisions and bilateral hippocampal lesions. *Neuropsychologia*, *3*, 339–351.

Corkin, S., Amaral, D. G., Gonzalez, R. G., Johnson, K. A., & Hyman, B. T. (1997). H. M.'s medial temporal lobe lesion: Findings from magnetic resonance imaging. *Journal of Neuroscience*, *17*, 3964–3979.

Cramon, D. Y. von, Hebel, N., & Ebeling, U. (1990). Anatomical considerations on memory and learning deficits due to focal cerebral lesions in man. In L. R. Squire & E. Lindenlaub (Eds.), *The biology of memory* (pp. 527–540). Stuttgart: F. K. Schattauer.

Cramon, D. Y. von, Hebel, N., & Schuri, U. (1985). A contribution to the anatomical basis of thalamic amnesia. *Brain*, *108*, 993–1008.

Cramon, D. Y. von, & Schuri, U. (1992). The septo-hippocampal pathways and their relevance to human memory: A case report. *Cortex*, *28*, 411–422.

Cummings, J. L. (1993). Frontal-subcortical circuits and human behavior. *Archives of Neurology*, *50*, 873–880.

Cummings, J. L., Tomiyasu, U., Read, S., & Benson, D. F. (1984). Amnesia with hippocampal lesions after cardiopulmonary arrest. *Neurology*, *42*, 263–271.

Damasio, A. R. (1989). Time-locked multiregional retroactivation: A systems-level proposal for the neural substrates of recall and recognition. *Cognition*, *33*, 25–62.

Damasio, A. R., Graff-Radford, N. R., Eslinger, P. J., Damasio, H., & Kassell, N. (1985). Amnesia following basal forebrain lesions. *Archives of Neurology*, *42*, 263–271.

Daum, I., & Ackermann, H. (1994). Frontal-type memory impairment associated with thalamic damage. *International Journal of Neuroscience*, *77*, 187–198.

Davila, M. D., Shear, P. K., Lane, B., Sullivan, E. V., & Pfefferbaum, A. (1994). Mamillary body and cerebellar shrinkage in chronic alcoholics: An MRI and neuropsychological study. *Neuropsychology, 8,* 433–444.

de Leon, M. J., George, A. E., Golomb, J., Tarshish, C., Convit, A., Kluger, A., De Santi, S., McRae, T., Ferris, S. H., Reisberg, B., Ince, C., Rusinek, H., Bobinski, M., Quinn, B., Miller, D. C., & Wisniewski, H. M. (1997). Frequency of hippocampus atrophy in normal elderly and Alzheimer's disease patients. *Neurobiology of Aging, 18,* 1–11.

de Leon, M. J., Golomb, J., George, A. E., Convit, A., Tarshish, C. Y., McRae, T., De Santi, S., Smith, G., Ferris, S. H., Noz, M., & Rusinek, H. (1993). The radiologic prediction of Alzheimer disease: The atrophic hippocampal formation. *American Journal of Neuroradiology, 14,* 897–906.

Demb, J. B., Desmond, J. E., Wagner, A. D., Vaidya, C. J., Glover, G. H., & Gabrieli, J. D. E. (1995). Semantic encoding and retrieval in the left inferior prefrontal cortex. *Journal of Neuroscience, 15,* 5870–5878.

Desmond, J. E., Gabrieli, J. D. E., & Glover, G. H. (1998). Dissociation of frontal and cerebellar activity in a cognitive task: Evidence for a distinction between selection and search. *Neuroimage, 7,* 368–376.

D'Esposito, M., Verfaellie, M., Alexander, M. P., & Katz, D. I. (1995). Amnesia following traumatic bilateral fornix transection. *Neurology, 45,* 1546–1550.

Dolan, R., & Fletcher, P. (1997). Dissociating prefrontal and hippocampal function in episodic memory encoding. *Nature, 388,* 582–585.

Dott, N. M. (1938). Surgical aspects of the hypothalamus. In W. E. L. Clark, J. Beattie, G. Riddoch, & N. M. Dott (Eds.), *The hypothalamus: morphological, functional, clinical and surgical aspects* (pp. 131–185). Edinburgh: Oliver and Boyd.

Eichenbaum, H., Otto, T., & Cohen, N. J. (1994). Two functional components of the hippocampal memory system. *Behavioral Brain Science, 17,* 449–518.

Estruch, R., Bono, G., Laine, P., Antunez, E., Petrucci, A., Morocutti, C., & Hilbom, M. (1998). Brain imaging in alcoholism. *European Journal of Neurology, 5,* 119–135.

Fiez, J. (1997). Phonology, semantics, and the role of the left inferior prefrontal cortex. *Human Brain Mapping, 5,* 79–83.

Fillenbaum, G. G., Beekly, D., Edland, S. D., Hughes, J. P., Heyman, A., & van Belle, G. (1997). Consortium to establish a registry for Alzheimer's disease: Development, database structure, and selected findings. *Topics in Health Information Management, 18,* 47–58.

Fink, G. R. (1996). Cerebral representation of one's own past: Neural networks involved in autobiographical memory. *Journal of Neuroscience, 16,* 4275–4282.

Fletcher, P. C., Firth, C. D., Grasby, P. M., Shallice, T., Frackowiak, R. S. J., & Dolan, R. J. (1995). Brain systems for encoding and retrieval of auditory-verbal memory. An *in vivo* study in humans. *Brain, 118,* 401–416.

Fletcher, P. C., Shallice, T., & Dolan, R. J. (1998). The functional roles of prefrontal cortex in episodic memory. *Brain, 121,* 1239–1248.

Foerster, O., & Gagel, O. (1933). Ein fall von ependymcyste des III ventrikels. Ein beitrag zur frage der beziehungen psychischer störungen zum hirnstamm. *Zeitschrift für die Gesamte Neurologie und Psychiatrie, 149,* 312–344.

Folstein, M. F., Folstein, S, E., & McHugh, P. R. (1975). "Mini-mental state": A practical method for grading the mental state of patients for the clinician. *Journal of Psychiatry Research, 12,* 189–198.

Freedman, D. P., Murray, E. A., O'Neili, J. B., & Mishkin, M. (1986). Cortical connections of the somatosensory fields of the lateral sulcus of macaques: Evidence for a corticolimbic pathway for touch. *Journal of Comparative Neurology, 252,* 323–347.

Frith, C. D., Friston, K., Liddle, P. F., & Frackowiak, R. S. J. (1991). Willed action and the prefrontal cortex in man: A study with PET. *Proceedings of the Royal Society of London, Ser. B 244,* 241–246.

Fujii, T., Okuda, J., Kawashima, R., Yamadori, A., Fukatsu, R., Suzuki, K., Ito, M., Goto, R., & Fukuda, H. (1997). Different roles of the left and right parahippocampal regions in verbal recognition: A PET study. *NeuroReport, 8,* 1113–1117.

Gabrieli, J. D. E. (1998). Cognitive neuroscience y of human memory, *Annual Review of Psychology, 49,* 87–115.

Gabrieli, J. D. E. (2001). Functional neuroimaging of episodic memory. In R. Cabezad A. Kingstone. (Eds.) *Handbook of Functional Neuroimaging of Cognition* (pp. 253–291). Cambridge, MA: MIT Press.

Gabrieli, J. D. E., Brewer, J. B., Desmond, J. E., & Glover, G. H. (1997). Separate neural bases of two fundamental memory processes in the human medial temporal lobe. *Science, 276,* 264–266.

Gabrieli, J. D. E., Desmond, J. E., Demb, J. B., Wagner, A. D., Stone, M. V., Vaidya, C. J., & Glover, G. H. (1996). Functional magnetic resonance imaging of semantic-memory processes in the frontal lobes. *Psychological Science, 7*, 278–283.

Gaffan, D. (1994a). Dissociated effects of perirhinal cortex ablation, fornix transection and amygdalectomy: Evidence for multiple memory systems in the primate temporal lobe. *Experimental Brain Research, 99*, 411–422.

Gaffan, D. (1994b). Scene-specific memory for objects: A model of episodic memory impairment in monkeys with fornix transection. *Journal of Cognitive Neuroscience, 6*, 305–320.

Gaffan, D., & Gaffan, E. A. (1991). Amnesia in man following transection of the fornix. *Brain, 114*, 2611–2618.

Gaffan, D., & Parker, A. (2000). Mediodorsal thalamic function in scene memory in rhesus monkeys. *Brain, 123*, 816–827.

Garcia-Bengochea, F., De La Torre, O., Esquivel, O., Vieta, R., & Fernandec, C. (1954). The section of the fornix in the surgical treatment of certain epilepsies: A preliminary report. *Transactions of the American Neurological Association, 79*, 176–178.

Garcia-Bengochea, F., & Friedman, W. A. (1987). Persistent memory loss following section of the anterior fornix in humans. *Surgical Neurology, 27*, 361–364.

Gardiner, J. M., & Parkin, A. J. (1990). Attention and recollective experience in recognition memory. *Memory and Cognition, 18*, 579–583.

Gentilini, M., DeRenzi, E., & Crisi, G. (1987). Bilateral paramedian thalamic artery infarcts: Report of eight cases. *Journal of Neurology, Neurosurgery and Psychiatry, 50*, 900–909.

Ghaem, O., Mellet, E., Crivello, F., Tzourio, N., Mazoyer, B., Berthoz, A., & Denis, M. (1997). Mental navigation along memorized routes activates the hippocampus, precuneus, and insula. *NeuroReport, 8*, 739–744.

Gonzalo-Ruiz, A., Morte, L., & Lieberman, A. R. (1997). Evidence for collateral projections to the retrosplenial granular cortex and thalamic reticular nucleus from glutamate and/or aspartate-containing neurons of the anterior thalamic nuclei in the rat. *Experimental Brain Research, 116*, 63–72.

Graff-Radford, N. R., Tranel, D., Van Hoesen, G. W., & Brandt, J. P. (1990). Diencephalic amnesia. *Brain, 113*, 1–25.

Grafman, J., Salazar, A. M., Weingartner, J., Vance, S. C., & Ludlow, C. (1985). Isolated impairment of memory following a penetrating lesion of the fornix cerebri. *Archives of Neurology, 42*, 1162–1168.

Grasby, P. M., Frith, C. D., Friston, K. J., Bench, C., Frackowiak, R. S. J., & Dolan, R. J. (1993). Functional mapping of brain areas implicated in auditory-verbal memory function. *Brain, 116*, 1–20.

Grünthal, E. (1939). Ueber das corpus mamillare und den korsakowschen symptomenkomplex. *Confinia Neurologica, 2*, 64–95.

Harding, A., Halliday, G., Caine, D., & Kril, J. (2000). Degeneration of anterior thalamic nuclei differentiates alcoholics with amnesia. *Brain, 123*, 141–154.

Hassler, R., & Riechert, T. (1957). Über einen fall von doppelseitiger fornicotomie bei sogenannter temporaler epilepsie. *Acta Neurochirurgica, 5*, 330–340.

Haxby, J. V., Ungerleider, L. G., Horwitz, B., Maisog, J. M., Rapoport, S. I., & Grady, C. L. (1996). Face encoding and recognition in the human brain. *Proceedings of the National Academy of Sciences U.S.A., 93*, 922–927.

Haxby, J. V., Ungerleider, L. G., Horwitz, B., Rapoport, S. I., & Grady, C. L. (1995). Hemispheric differences in neural systems for face working memory: A PET rCBF study. *Human Brain Mapping, 3*, 68–82.

Heilman, K. M., & Sypert, G. W. (1977). Korsakoff's syndrome resulting from bilateral fornix lesions. *Neurology, 27*, 490–493.

Henke, K., Buck, A., Weber, B., & Wieser, H. G. (1997). Human hippocampus establishes associations in memory. *Hippocampus, 7*, 249–256.

Henson, R. N. A., Rugg, M. D., Shallice, T., Josephs, O., & Dolan, R. J. (1999). Recollection and familiarity in recognition memory: An event-related functional magnetic resonance imaging study. *Journal of Neuroscience, 19*, 3962–3972.

Horel, J. A. (1978). The neuroanatomy of amnesia. A critique of the hippocampal memory hypothesis. *Brain, 101*, 403–445.

Horton, D. L., Pavlick, T. J., & Moulin-Julian, M. W. (1993). Retrieval-based and familiarity-based recognition and the quality of information in episodic memory. *Journal of Memory Language, 32*, 39–55.

Ikeda, M., Mori, E., Hirono, N., Imamura, T., Shimomura, T., Ikejiri, Y., & Yamashita, H. (1998). Amnestic people with Alzheimer's disease who remembered the Kobe earthquake. *British Journal of Psychiatry*, *172*, 425–428.

Ilinsky, I. A., Jouandet, M. L., & Goldman-Rakic, P. S. (1985). Organization of the nigrothalamocortical system in the rhesus monkey. *Journal of Comparative Neurology*, *236*, 315–330.

Insausti, R., Amaral, D. G., & Cowan, W. M. (1987). The entorhinal cortex of the monkey: II. Cortical afferents. *Journal of Comparative Neurology*, *264*, 356–395.

Jones, A. K. P., Brown, W. D., Friston, K. J., Qi, L. Y., & Frackowiak, R. S. J. (1991). Cortical and subcortical localization of response to pain in man using positron emission tomography. *Proceeding of the Royal Society of London, Ser. B*, *244*, 39–44.

Jones-Gotman, M., & Milner, B. (1977). Design fluency: The invention of nonsense drawings after focal cortical lesions. *Neuropsychologia*, *15*, 653–674.

Kaplan, E., Goodglass, H., & Weintraub, S. (1984). *The Boston naming test*. Philadelphia: Lea & Febiger.

Kapur, N., Friston, K. J., Young, A., Frith, C. D., & Frackowiak, R. S. J. (1995a). Activation of human hippocampal formation during memory for faces: A PET study. *Cortex*, *31*, 99–108.

Kapur, S., Craik, F. I. M., Jones, C., Brown, G. M., Houle, S., & Tulving, E. (1995b). Functional role of the prefrontal cortex in memory retrieval: A PET study. *Neuroreport*, *6*, 1880–1884.

Kapur, S., Tulving, E., Cabeza, R., McIntosh, A. R., Houle, S., & Craik, F. I. M. (1996). The neural correlates of intentional learning of verbal materials: A PET study in humans. *Brain Research. Cognitive Brain Research*, *4*, 243–249.

Kelley, W. M., Miezin, F. M., McDermott, K. B., Buckner, R. L., Raichle, M. E., Cohen, N. J., Ollinger, J. M., Akbudak, E., Conturo, T. E., Snyder, A. Z., & Peterson, S. E. (1998). Hemispheric specialization in human dorsal frontal cortex and medial temporal lobe for verbal and nonverbal memory encoding. *Neuron*, *20*, 927–936.

Klingberg, T., & Roland, P. E. (1998). Right prefrontal activation during encoding, but not during retrieval, in a non-verbal paired associates task. *Cerebral Cortex*, *8*, 73–79.

Knowlton, B. J., & Fanselow, M. S. (1998). The hippocampus, consolidation and on-line memory. *Current Opinion in Neurobiology*, *8*, 293–296.

Kopelman, M. D. (1995). The Korsakoff syndrome. *British Journal of Psychiatry*, *166*, 154–173.

Kopelman, M., Stevens, T., Foli, S., & Grasby, P. (1998). PET activation of the medial temporal lobe in learning. *Brain*, *121*, 875–887.

Korsakoff, S. S. (1889). Etude medico-psychologique sur une forme des maladies de la memoire. *Revue Philosophique*, *28*, 501–530.

Kritchevsky, M., Graff-Radford, N. R., & Damasio, A. R. (1987). Normal memory after damage to medial thalamus. *Archives of Neurology*, *44*, 959–962.

Kuroda, M., Yokofujita, J., & Murakami, K. (1998). An ultrastructural study of the neural circuit between the prefrontal cortex and the mediodorsal nucleus of the thalamus. *Progress in Neurobiology*, *54*, 417–458.

Leonard, B. W., Amaral, D. G., Squire, L. R., & Zola-Morgan, S. (1995). Transient memory impairment in monkeys with bilateral lesions of the entorhinal cortex. *Journal of Neuroscience*, *15*, 5637–5659.

Lepage, M., Habib, R., & Tulving, E. (1998). Hippocampal PET activations of memory encoding and retrieval: The HIPER model. *Hippocampus*, *8*, 313–322.

Lewis, P. R., & Shute, C. C. D. (1967). The cholinergic limbic system: projections of the hippocampal formation, medial cortex, nuclei of the ascending cholinergic reticular system, and the subfornical organ and supra-optic crest. *Brain*, *90*, 521–540.

Lhermitte, J., Doussinet, & de Ajuriaguerra, J. (1937). Une observation de la forme Korsakoweinne des tumuers de 3ᵉ ventricule. *Revue Neurologique (Paris)*, *68*, 709–711.

Lindqvist, G., & Norlen, G. (1966). Korsakoff's syndrome after operation on ruptured aneurysm of the anterior communicating artery. *Acta Psychiatria Scandinavia*, *42*, 24–34.

Lugaresi, E., Tobler, I., Gambetti, P., & Montagna, P. (1998). The pathophysiology of fatal familial insomnia. *Brain Pathology*, *8*, 521–526.

MacLean, P. D. (1949). Psychosomatic disease and the "visceral brain." Recent developments bearing on the Papez theory of emotion. *Psychosomatic Medicine*, *11*, 338–353.

Maguire, E., Burgess, N., Donnett J., Frackowiak, R., Frith, C., & O'Keefe, J. (1998). Knowing where and getting there: A human navigation network. *Science*, *280*, 921–924.

Maguire, E., Frackowiak, R., & Frith, C. (1996). Learning to find your way: A role for the human hippocampal formation. *Proceedings of the Royal Society of London, Ser. B*, *263*, 1745–1750.

Mahut, H., Zola-Morgan, S., & Moss, M. (1982). Hippocampal resections impair associative learning and recognition memory in the monkey. *Journal of Neuroscience, 2*, 1214–1220.

Mair, W. G., Warrington, E. K., & Weiskrantz, L. (1979). Memory disorder in Korsakoff's psychosis: A neuropathological and neuropsychological investigation of two cases. *Brain, 102*, 749–783.

Malamut, B. L., Graff-Radford, N., Chawluk, J., Grossman, R. I., & Gur, R. C. (1992). Memory in case of bilateral thalamic infarction. *Neurology, 42*, 163–169.

Mandler, G. (1980). Recognizing: The judgment of previous occurrence. *Psychological Review, 87*, 252–271.

Markowitsch, H. J. (1995). Which brain regions are critically involved in the retrieval of old episodic memory? *Brain Research Review, 21*, 117–127.

Mayes, A. R., Meudell, P. R. M., D., & Pickering, A. (1988). Location of lesions in Korsakoff's syndrome: Neuropsychological and neuropathological data on two patients. *Cortex, 24*, 367–388.

McDermott, K, B., Buckner, R. L., Petersen, S. E., Kelley, W. M., & Sanders, A. L. (1999). Set-specific and code-specific activation in frontal cortex: An fMRI study of encoding and retrieval of faces and words. *Journal of Cognitive Neuroscience, 11*, 631–640.

McDowell, J. R., & LeBlanc, H. J. (1984). Computed tomographic findings in Wernicke-Korsakoff syndrome. *Archives of Neurology, 41*, 453–454.

McMackin, D., Cockburn, J., Anslow, P., & Gaffan, D. (1995). Correlation of fornix damage with memory impairment in six cases of colloid cyst removal. *Acta Neurochirurgica, 135*, 12–18.

Mega, M. S., & Cummings, J. L. (1997). The cingulate and cingulate syndromes. In M. R. Trimble & J. L. Cummings (Eds.), *Contemporary behavioral neurology* (pp. 189–214). Boston: Butterworth-Heinemann.

Mega, M, S., Cummings, J. L., Salloway, S., & Malloy, P. (1997). The limbic system: An anatomic, phylogenetic, and clinical perspective. *Journal of Neuropsychiatry and Clinical Neuroscience, 9*, 315–330.

Mesulam, M.-M., & Mufson, E. J. (1985). The insula of Reil in man and monkey: Architectonics, connectivity, and function. In E. G. Jones & A. A. Peters (Eds.), *Cerebral cortex* (pp. 179–226). New York: Plenum.

Mesulam, M.-M., Mufson, E. J., Levey, A. I., & Wainer, B. H. (1983). Cholinergic innervation of cortex by the basal forebrain: Cytochemistry and cortical connections of the septal area, diagonal band nuclei, nucleus basalis (substantia innominata), and hypothalamus in the rhesus monkey. *Journal of Comparative Neurology, 214*, 170–197.

Mesulam, M.-M., & Mulson, E. J. (1982). Insula of the old world monkey. I. Architectonics in the insulo-orbito-temporal component of the paralimbic brain. *Journal of Comparative Neurology, 212*, 1–22.

Meunier, M., Bachevalier, J., Mishkin, M., & Murray, E. A. (1993). Effects on visual recognition of combined and separate ablations of the entorhinal and perirhinal cortex in rhesus monkeys. *Journal of Neuroscience, 13*, 5418–5432.

Mishkin, M., & Murray, E. A. (1994). Stimulus recognition. *Current Opinion in Neurobiology, 4*, 200–206.

Molchan, S. E., Sunderland, T., McIntosh, A. R., Herscovitch, P., & Schreurs, B. G. (1994). A functional anatomical study of associative learning in humans. *Proceedings of the National Academy of Sciences U.S.A., 91*, 8122–8126.

Morecraft, R. J., Geula, C., & Mesulam, M.-M. (1993). Architecture of connectivity within a cingulfronto-parietal neurocognitive network. *Archives of Neurology, 50*, 279–284.

Morecraft, R. J., & Van Hoesen, G. W. (1991). A comparison of frontal lobe afferents to the primary, supplementary and cingulate cortices in the rhesus monkey. *Society of Neuroscience Abstracts, 17*, 1019.

Mori, E., Ikeda, M., Hirono, N., Kitagaki, H., Imamura, T., & Shimomura, T. (1999). Amygdalar volume and emotional memory in Alzheimer's disease. *American Journal of Psychiatry, 156*, 216–222.

Morris, M. K., Bowers, D., Chatterjee, A., & Heilman, K. M. (1992). Amnesia following a discrete basal forebrain lesion. *Brain, 115*, 1827–1847.

Moscovitch, M., Kapur, S., Kohler, S., & Houle, S. (1995). Distinct neural correlates of visual long-term memory for spatial location and object identity: A positron emission tomography (PET) study in humans. *Proceedings of the National Academy of Sciences U.S.A., 92*, 3721–3725.

Murray, E. A. (1991). Contributions of the amygdalar complex to behavior in macaque monkeys. *Progress in Brain Research, 87*, 167–180.

Neave, N., Nagle, S., & Aggleton, J. P. (1997). Evidence for the involvement of the mamillary bodies and cingulum bundle in allocentric spatial processing by rats. *European Journal of Neuroscience, 9*, 941–955.

Nolde, S. F., Johnson, M. K., & D'Esposito, M. (1998a). Left prefrontal activation during episodic remembering: An event-related fMRI study. *NeuroReport, 9*, 3509–3514.

Nolde, S. F., Johnson, M. K., & Raye, C. L. (1998b). The role of the prefrontal cortex during tests of episodic memory. *Trends in Cognitive Science, 2*, 399–406.

Nyberg, L., Tulving, E., Habib, R., Nilsson, L., Kapur, S., Houle, S., Cabeza, R., & McIntosh, A. R. (1995). Functional brain maps of retrieval mode and recovery of episodic information. *NeuroReport, 7*, 249–252.

Osterrieth, P. A. (1944). Le test decopie d'une figure complexe. *Archives de Psychologie, 30*, 206–256.

Owen, A. M., Milner, B., Petrides, M., & Evans, A, C. (1996). Memory for object features versus memory for object location: A positron-emission tomography study of encoding and retrieval processes. *Proceedings of the National Academy of Sciences U.S.A., 93*, 9212–9217.

Pandya, D. N., & Yeterian, E. H. (1985). Architecture and connections of cortical association areas. In A. Peters & E. G. Jones (Eds.), *Cerebral cortex* (pp. 3–55). New York: Plenum.

Papez, J. W. (1937). A proposed mechanism of emotion. *Archives of Neurology and Psychiatry, 38*, 725–733.

Pardo, J. V., Pardo, P. J., Haner, K. W., & Raichle, M. E. (1990). The anterior cingulate cortex mediates processing selection in the Stroop attentional conflict, paradigm. *Proceedings of the National Academy of Sciences U.S.A., 87*, 256–259.

Parker, A., Eacott, M. J., & Gaffan, D. (1997). The recognition memory deficit caused by mediodorsal thalamic lesion in non-human primates: A comparison with rhinal cortex lesion. *European Journal of Neuroscience, 9*, 2423–2431.

Parker, A., & Gaffan, D. (1997a). The effect of anterior thalamic and cingulate cortex lesions on object-in-place memory in monkeys. *Neuropsychologia, 35*, 1093–1102.

Parker, A., & Gaffan, D. (1997b). Mamillary body lesions in monkeys impair object-in-place memory: Functional unity of the fornix-mamillary system. *Journal of cognitive Neuroscience, 9*, 512–521.

Penfield, W., & Mathieson, G. (1974). Memory: Autopsy findings and comments on the role of the hippocampus in experimental recall. *Archives of Neurology, 31*, 145–154.

Penfield, W., & Milner, B. (1958). Memory deficit produced by bilateral lesions in the hippocampal zone. *Archives of Neurology and Psychiatry, 79*, 475–497.

Peru, A., & Fabbro, F. (1997). Thalamic amnesia following venous infarction: Evidence from a single case study. *Brain Cognition, 33*, 278–294.

Petersen, R. C., Smith, G. E., Waring, S. C., Ivnik, R. J., Tangalos, E. G., & Kokmen, E. (1999). Mild cognitive impairment: Clinical characterization and outcome. *Archives of Neurology, 56*, 303–308.

Petersen, S. E., Fox, P. T., Posner, M. I., Mintun, M., & Raichle, M. E. (1988). Positron emission tomographic studies of the cortical anatomy of single word processing. *Nature, 331*, 585–589.

Petersen, S. E., Fox, P. T., Posner, M. I., Mintun, M., & Raichle, M. E. (1989). Positron emission tomographic studies of the processing of single words. *Journal of Cognitive Neuroscience, 1*, 153–170.

Petrides, M., Alivasatos, B., & Evans, A. C. (1995). Functional activation of the human ventrolateral frontal cortex during mnemonic retrieval of verbal information. *Proceedings of the National Academy of Sciences U.S.A., 92*, 5803–5807.

Poldrack, R. A., Wagner, A. D., Prull, M. W., Desmond, J. E., Glover, G. H., & Gabrieli, J. D. E. (1999). Functional specialization for semantic and phonological processing in the left inferior prefrontal cortex. *Neuroimage, 10*, 15–35.

Price, J. L. (1999). Prefrontal cortical networks related to visceral function and mood. *Annals of the New York Academy of Science, 877*, 383–396.

Raichle, M. E., Fiez, J. A., Videen, T. O., MacLeod, A.-M. K., Pardo, J. V., Fox, P. T., & Petersen, S. E. (1994). Practice-related changes in human brain functional anatomy during nonmotor learning. *Cerebral Cortex, 4*, 8–26.

Rempel-Clower, N. L., Zola, S. M., Squire, L. R., & Amaral, D. G. (1996). Three cases of enduring memory impairment after bilateral damage limited to the hippocampal formation. *Journal of Neuroscience, 15*, 5233–5255.

Rey, A. (1941). L'examen psychologique dans les cas d'encephalopathie traumatique. *Archives de Psychologie, 28*, 286–340.

Roland, P., & Gulyas, B. (1995). Visual memory, visual imagery, and visual recognition of large field patterns by the human brain: Functional anatomy by positron emission tomography. *Cerebral Cortex, 1*, 79–93.

Rombouts, S., Machielsen, W., Witter, M., Barkhof, F., Lindeboom, J., & Scheltens, P. (1997). Visual association encoding activates the medial temporal lobe: A functional magnetic resonance imaging study. *Hippocampus, 7,* 594–601.

Rudge, P., & Warrington, E. K. (1991). Selective impairment of memory and visual perception in splenial tumours. *Brain, 114,* 349–360.

Rugg, M. D., Fletcher, P. C., Frith, C. D., Frackowiak, R. S. J., & Dolan, R. J. (1996). Differential activation of the prefrontal cortex in successful and unsuccessful memory retrieval. *Brain, 119,* 2073–2083.

Rugg, M. D., Fletcher, P. C., Frith, C. D., Frackowiak, R. S. J., & Dolan, R. J. (1997). Brain regions supporting intentional and incidental memory: A PET study. *Neuroreport, 8,* 1283–1287.

Russchen, F. T., Amaral, D. G., & Price, J. L. (1987). The afferent input to the magnocellular division of the mediodorsal thalamic nucleus in the monkey, *Macaca fascicularis. Journal of Comparatives Neurology, 256,* 175–210.

Schacter, D. L., Alpert, N. M., Savage, C. R., Ranch, S. L., & Albert, M. S. (1996a). Conscious recollection and the human hippocampal formation: Evidence from positron emission tomography. *Proceedings of the National Academy of Sciences U.S.A., 91,* 321–325.

Schacter, D. L., Buckner, R. L., Koutstaal, W., Dale, A. M., & Rosen, B. R. (1997a). Late onset of anterior prefrontal activity during true and false recognition: An event-related fMRI study. *Neuroimage, 6,* 259–269.

Schacter, D. L., Curran, T., Galluccio, L., Milberg, W. P., & Bates, J. F. (1996b). False recognition and the right frontal lobe: A case study. *Neuropsychologia, 34,* 793–808.

Schacter, D. L., Reiman, E., Uecker, A., Polster, M. R., Yung, L. S., & Cooper, L. A. (1995). Brain regions associated with retrieval of structurally coherent visual information. *Nature, 368,* 633–635.

Schacter, D. L., Savage, C. R., Alpert, N. M., Rauch, S. L., & Albert, M. S. (1996c). The role of hippocampus and frontal cortex in age-related memory changes: A PET study. *NeuroReport, 7,* 1165–1169.

Schacter, D. L., Uecker, A., Reiman, E., Youn, L. S., Brandy, D., Chen, K., Cooper, L. A., & Curran, T. (1997b). Effects of size and orientation change on hippocampal activation during episodic recognition: A PET study. *NeuroReport, 8,* 3993–3998.

Schacter, D. L., & Wagner, A. D. (1999). Medial temporal lobe activations in fMRI and PET studies of episodic encoding and retrieval. *Hippocampus, 9,* 7–24.

Schnider, A., Gutbrod, K., Hess, C. W., & Schroth, G. (1996). Memory without context: Amnesia with confabulations after infarction of the right capsular genu. *Journal of Neurology, Neurosurgery and Psychiatry, 61,* 186–193.

Scoville, W. B., & Milner, B. (1957). Loss of recent memory after bilateral hippocampal lesions. *Journal of Neurology, Neurosurgery and Psychiatry, 20,* 11–21.

Selemon, L. D., & Goldman-Rakic, P. S. (1985). Longitudinal topography and interdigitation of corticostriatal projections in the rhesus monkey. *Journal of Neuroscience, 5,* 776–794

Shallice, T., Fletcher, P., Firth, C. D., Grasby, P., Frackowiak, R. S. J., & Dolan, R. J. (1994). Brain regions associated with acquisition and retrieval of verbal episodic memory. *Nature, 368,* 633–635.

Shear, P. K., Sullivan, E. V., Lane, B., & Pfefferbaum, A. (1996). Mamillary body and cerebellar shrinkage in chronic alcoholics with and without amnesia. *Alcohol: Clinical and Experimental Research, 20,* 1489–1495.

Shimamura, A. P., Jernigan, T. L., & Squire, L. R. (1988). Korsakoff's syndrome: Radiological (CT) findings and neuropsychological correlates. *Journal of Neuroscience, 8,* 4400–4410.

Shipley, M. T., & Sørensen, K. E. (1975). Evidence for an ipsilateral projection from the subiculum to the deep layers of the presubicular and entorhinal cortices. *Experimental Brain Research, 23,* 190.

Shuren, J. E., Jacobs, D. H., & Heilman, K. M. (1997). Diencephalic temporal order amnesia. *Journal of Neurology, Neurosurgery and Psychiatry, 62,* 163–168.

Sprofkin, B. E., & Sciarra, D. (1952). Korsakoff's psychosis associated with cerebral tumors. *Neurology, 2,* 427–434.

Squire, L. R., & Alvarez, P. (1995). Retrograde amnesia and memory consolidation: A neurobiological perspective. *Current Opinion in Neurobiology, 5,* 169–177.

Squire, L. R., Amaral, D. G., Zola-Morgan, S., Kritchevsky, M., & Press, G. (1989). Description of brain injury in the amnesia patient N. A. based on magnetic resonance imaging. *Experimental Neurology, 105,* 23–35.

Squire, L. R., & Moore, R. Y. (1979). Dorsal thalamic lesion in a noted case of chronic memory dysfunction. *Annals of Neurology, 6,* 503–506.

Squire, L. R., Ojemann, J. G., Miezin, F. M., Petersen, S. E., Videen, T. O., & Raichle, M. E. (1992). Activation of the hippocampus in normal humans: A functional anatomical study of memory. *Proceedings of the National Academy of Sciences U.S.A., 89*, 1837–1841.

Squire, L. R., & Shimamura, A. P. (1986). Characterizing amnesic patients for neurobehavioral study. *Behavioral Neuroscience, 100*, 866–877.

Stern, C., Corkin, S., Gonzalez, R., Guimares, A., Baker, J., Jennings, P., Carr, C., Sugiura, R., Vedantham, V., & Rosen, B. (1996). The hippocampal formation participates in novel picture encoding: Evidence from functional magnetic resonance imaging. *Proceedings of the National Academy of Sciences U.S.A., 93*, 8660–8665.

Sutherland, R. J., & Hoesing, J. M. (1993). Posterior cingulate cortex and spatial memory; A microlimnology analysis. In B. A. Vogt & M. Gabriel (Eds.), *Neurobiology of cingulate cortex and limbic thalamus: A comprehensive handbook* (pp. 461–477). Boston: Birkhäuser.

Suzuki, W. A., & Amaral, D. G. (1994). Perirhinal and parahippocampal cortices of the macaque monkey: Cortical afferents. *Journal of Comparative Neurology, 350*, 497–533.

Suzuki, W. A., Zola-Morgan, S., Squire, L. R., & Amaral, D. G. (1993). Lesions of the perirhinal and parahippocampal cortices in the monkey produce long-lasting memory impairment in the visual and tactual modalities. *Journal of Neuroscience, 13*, 2430–2451.

Sweet, W. H., Talland, G. A., & Ervin, F. R. (1959). Loss of recent memory following section of fornix. *Transactions of the American Neurological Association, 84*, 76–82.

Sziklas, V., & Petrides, M. (1997). Memory and the region of the mamillary bodies. *Progress in Neurobiology, 54*, 55–70.

Talbot, J. D., Marrett, S., Evans, A. C., Meyer, E., Bushnell, M. C., & Duncan, G. H. (1991). Multiple representations of pain in human cerebral cortex. *Science, 251*, 1355–1358.

Talland, G. A., Sweet, W. H., & Ballantine, H. T. (1967). Amnesic syndrome with anterior communicating aneurysm. *Journal of Nervous and Mental Disease, 145*, 179–192.

Teng, E., & Squire, L. R. (1999). Memory for places learned long ago is intact after hippocampal damage. *Nature, 400*, 675–677.

Teuber, H. L., Milner, B., & Vaughan, H. G. (1968). Persistent, anterograde amnesia after stab wound to the basal brain. *Neuropsychologia, 6*, 267–282.

Teyler, T. J., & DiScenna, P. (1986). The hippocampal memory indexing theory. *Behavioral Neuroscience, 100*, 147–154.

Thompson-Schill, S. L., D'Esposito, M., Aguirre, G. K., & Farah, M. J. (1997). Role of the left inferior prefrontal cortex in retrieval of semantic knowledge: A reevaluation. *Proceedings of the National Academy of Sciences U.S.A., 94*, 14792–14797.

Torvik, A. (1985). Two types of brain lesions in Wernicke's encephalopathy. *Neuropathology Applied Neurobiology, 11*, 179–190.

Torvik, A. (1987). Topographic distribution and severity of brain lesions in Wernicke's encephalopathy. *Clinical Neuropathology, 6*, 25–29.

Tranel, D., Brady, D. R., Van Hoesen, G. W., & Damasio, A. R. (1988). Parahippocampal projections to posterior auditory association cortex (area Tpt) in old-world monkeys. *Experimental Brain Research, 70*, 406–416.

Tucker, D. M., Roeltgen, D. P., Tully, R., Hartmann, J., & Boxell, C. (1988). Memory dysfunction following unilateral transection of the fornix: A hippocampal disconnection syndrome. *Cortex, 24*, 465–472.

Tulving, E., Kapur, S., Craik, F. I. M., Moscovitch, M., & Houle, S. (1994a). Hemispheric encoding/retrieval asymmetry in episodic memory: Positron emission tomography findings. *Proceedings of the National Academy of Sciences U.S.A., 91*, 2016–2020.

Tulving, E., Kapur, S., Markowitsch, H. J., Craik, F. I., Habib, R., & Houle, S. (1994b). Neuroanatomical correlates of retrieval in episodic memory: Auditory sentence recognition. *Proceedings of the National Academy of Sciences U.S.A., 91*, 2012–2015.

Tulving, E., Markowitsch, H. J., Craik, F. I. M., Habib, R., & Houle, S. (1996). Novelty and familiarity activations in PET studies of memory encoding and retrieval. *Cerebral Cortex, 6*, 71–79.

Ungerleider, L. G. (1995). Functional brain imaging studies of cortical mechanisms for memory. *Science, 270*, 769–775.

Valenstein, E., Bowers, D., Verfaellie, M., Heilman, K. M., Day, A., & Watson, R, T. (1987). Retrosplenial amnesia. *Brain, 110*, 1631–1646.

Van Hoesen, G. W. (1982). The parahippocampal gyrus: New observations regarding its cortical connections in the monkey. *Trends in Neurosciences, 5*, 345–350.

Vandenberghe, R., Price, C., Wise, R., Josephs, O., & Frackowiak, R. S. J. (1996). Functional anatomy of a common semantic system for words and pictures. *Nature, 383*, 254–256.

Vargha-Khadem, F., Gadian, D. G., Watkins, K. E., Connelly, A., Van Paesschen, W., & Mishkin, M. (1997).

Differential effects of early hippocampal pathology on episodic and semantic memory. *Science*, *277*, 376–380.

Victor, M., Adams, R. D., & Collins, G. H. (1971). *The Wernicke-Korsakoff syndrome*. Philadelphia: F. A. Davis.

Vogt, B. A., & Pandya, D. N. (1987). Cingulate cortex of the rhesus monkey: II. Cortical afferents. *Journal of Comparative Neurology*, *262*, 271–289.

Wagner, A. D., Desmond, J. E., Glover, G. H., & Gabrieli, J. D. E. (1998a). Prefrontal cortex and recognition memory: fMRI evidence for context-dependent retrieval processes. *Brain*, *121*, 1985–2002.

Wagner, A. D., Poldrack, R. A., Eldridge, L. E., Desmond, J. E., Glover, G. H., & Gabrieli, J. D. E. (1998b). Material-specific lateralization of prefrontal activation during episodic encoding and retrieval. *NeuroReport*, *9*, 3711–3717.

Wagner, A. D., Schacter, D. L., Rotte, M., Koustaal, W., Maril, A., Dale, A. M., Rosen, B. R., & Buckner, R. L. (1998c). Building memories: Remembering and forgetting verbal experiences as predicted by brain activity. *Science*, *281*, 1188–1191.

Warrington, E. K. (1984). *The recognition memory test*. Windsor, UK: NFER-Nelson.

Webster, M. J., Ungerleider, L. G., & Bachevalier, J. (1991). Connections of inferior temporal areas TE and TEO with medial temporal-lobe structures in infant and adult monkeys. *Neuroscience*, *191*, 255–281.

Wechsler, D. (1945). A standardized memory scale for clinical use. *Journal of Psychology*, *19*, 87–95.

Wechsler, D. (1955). *Wechsler adult intelligence scale*. New York: Psychological Corp.

Williams, M., & Pennybacker, J. (1954). Memory disturbances in third ventricle tumours. *Journal of Neurology, Neurosurgery and Psychiatry*, *17*, 115–123.

Winocur, G., Oxbury, S., Roberts, R., Agnetti, V., & Davis, C. (1984). Amnesia in a patient with bilateral lesions to the thalamus. *Neuropsychologia*, *22*, 123–143.

Witter, M. P., & Amaral, D. G. (1991). Entorhinal cortex of the monkey. V. Projections to the dentate gyrus, hippocampus, and subicular complex. *Journal of Comparative Neurology*, *307*, 437–459.

Woolsey, R. M., & Nelson, J. S. (1975). Asymptomatic destruction of the fornix in man. *Archives of Neurology*, *32*, 566–568.

Xuereb, J. H., Perry, R. H., Candy, J. M., Perry, E. K., Marshall, E., & Bonham, J. R. (1991). Nerve cell loss in the thalamus in Alzheimer's disease and Parkinson's disease. *Brain*, *114*, 1363–1379.

Yasuda, Y., Watanabe, T., Tanaka, H., Tadashi, I., & Akiguchi, I. (1997). Amnesia following infarction in the right retrosplenial region. *Clinical Neurology and Neurosurgery*, *99*, 102–105.

Yeterian, E. H., & Pandya, D. N. (1993). Striatal connections of the parietal association cortices in rhesus monkeys. *Journal of Comparative Neurology*, *332*, 175–197.

Zatorre, R. J., Meyer, E., Gjedde, A., & Evans, A. (1996). PET studies of phonetic processing of speech: Review, replication, and reanalysis. *Cerebral Cortex*, *6*, 21–30.

Zola-Morgan, S., Squire, L. R., & Amaral, D. G. (1986). Human amnesia and the medial temporal region: Enduring memory impairment following a bilateral lesion limited to field CA1 of the hippocampus, *Journal of Neuroscience*, *6*, 2950–2967.

Zola-Morgan, S., Squire, L. R., & Amaral, D. G. (1989a). Lesions of the amygdala that spare adjacent cortical regions do not impair memory or exacerbate the impairment following lesions of the hippocampal formation. *Journal of Neuroscience*, *9*, 1922–1936.

Zola-Morgan, S., Squire, L. R., & Amaral, D. G. (1989b). Lesions of the hippocampal formation but not lesions of the fornix or the mamillary nuclei produce long-lasting memory impairment in monkeys. *Journal of Neuroscience*, *9*, 898–913.

Zola-Morgan, S., Squire, L. R., Amaral, D. G., & Suzuki, W. A. (1989c). Lesions of perirhinal and parahippocampal cortex that spare the amygdala and hippocampal formation produce severe memory impairment. *Journal of Neuroscience*, *9*, 4355–4370.

Zola-Morgan, S., Squire, L. R., Clower, R. P., & Rempel, N. L. (1993). Damage to the perirhinal cortex exacerbates memory impairment following lesions to the hippocampal formation. *Journal of Neuroscience*, *13*, 251–265.

Zola-Morgan, S., Squire, L. R., & Ramus, S. (1994). Severity of memory impairment in monkeys as a function of locus and extent of damage within the medial temporal lobe memory system. *Hippocampus*, *4*, 483–495.

Zola-Morgan, S., Squire, L. R., Rempel, N. L., Clower, R. P., & Amaral, D. G. (1992). Enduring memory impairment in monkeys after ischemic damage to the hippocampus. *Journal of Neuroscience*, *12*, 2582–2596.

4 Semantic Dementia: A Disorder of Semantic Memory

John R. Hodges

Memory, in its broadest sense, refers to the storage and retrieval of any form of information, but when considered as an aspect of human cognition, it clearly does not describe a unitary function. Memorizing a new telephone number, recalling the details of a past holiday, acquiring the facts necessary to practice medicine, learning a new language, or knowing how to drive a car, are all tasks that depend on memory, but proficiency in one does not guarantee competence in the other. More important, these abilities may break down differentially in patients with brain disease. There is as yet no universally accepted classification of subcomponents of memory, but virtually all contemporary cognitive models distinguish between working (immediate) and longer term memory, and within the latter, recognize both explicit and implicit types.

Of the examples given here, the ability to repeat a telephone number reflects working memory. The acquisition of motor skills such as driving a car requires implicit procedural memory. Within explicit long-term memory, an influential distinction is that between episodic and semantic memory. The former refers to our personal store of temporally specific experiences (or episodes), the recall of which requires "mental time travel." In contrast, semantic memory refers to our database of knowledge about things in the world and their interrelationship; these include words, objects, places, and people (Garrard, Perry, & Hodges, 1997; Hodges & Patterson, 1997).

Semantic memory is, therefore, the most central of all cognitive processes and is fundamental to language production and comprehension, reading and writing, object and face perception, etc. Despite the central role of semantic memory, its study is relatively recent, and in the modern era begins in 1975 with Warrington's seminal observation of selective impairment of semantic memory, now referred to as *semantic dementia* (Warrington, 1975), followed a few years later by Warrington and Shallice's finding of category-specific semantic impairment (Warrington & Shallice, 1984).

A breakdown of semantic memory occurs in a number of conditions, most notably after herpes simplex encephalitis (Pietrini et al., 1988; Warrington & Shallice, 1984), in Alzheimer's disease (Hodges & Patterson, 1995), and in semantic dementia (Hodges, Patterson, Oxbury, & Funnell, 1992a). In the former two conditions, the semantic deficit is almost always accompanied by other major cognitive deficits. For this reason, the study of patients with semantic dementia, who have a progressive, yet selective and often profound breakdown of semantic memory, provides unparalleled insights into the organization of semantic memory and the impact of semantic disintegration on other cognitive processes.

Following the description of a typical case, the rest of this chapter consists of an overview of our work on semantic dementia over the past decade (Hodges, Garrard, & Patterson, 1998; Patterson & Hodges, 1994), with particular emphasis on what can be learned about normal semantic memory processes in the human brain from the study of patients with semantic dementia.

Case Report

The following case history of a patient who has been studied longitudinally over the past 5 years illustrates the pattern of cognitive deficits commonly seen in the disorder (see also Graham & Hodges, 1997; Hodges & Patterson, 1996; Knott, Patterson, & Hodges, 1997).

A.M. presented in April 1994 at age 64 with a history of loss of memory for words that had progressed slowly over the past 2 years. His wife also noted a decline in his comprehension ability that initially affected less common words. Despite these problems, he still played golf (to a high standard) and tennis. The patient was still driving and able to find his way to various golf clubs alone and without difficulty. Day-to-day memory was also good and when seen in the clinic A.M. was able to relate, albeit anomically, the details of their holiday in Australia and his recent golfing achievements. There had been only a slight change in personality at that time, with mild disinhibition and a tendency to stick to fixed routines.

The following transcription illustrates that A.M.'s speech was fluent and without phonological or syntactic errors, but was strikingly devoid of content. It also shows his recall of undergoing a brain scan some 6 months before.

Examiner: "Can you tell me about a last time you were in hospital?"

A.M.: "That was January, February, March, April, yes April last year, that was the first time, and eh, on the Monday, for example, they were checking all my whatsit, and that was the first time when my brain was, eh, shown, you know, you know that bit of the brain [*indicates left*], not that one, the other one was okay, but that was lousy, so they did that, and then like this [*indicates scanning by moving his hands over his head*] and probably I was a bit better than I am just now."

Formal neuropsychological testing in April 1994 revealed that A.M. was severely impaired in tests of picture naming. In the category fluency test, in which subjects are asked to generate exemplars from a range of semantic categories within a set time, he was able to generate a few high-frequency animal names (cat, dog, horse), but no exemplars from more restricted categories such as birds or breeds of dog. He was only able to name three out of forty-eight black-and-white line drawings of highly familiar objects and animals from the Hodges and Patterson semantic battery (Hodges & Patterson, 1995). Most responses were vague circumlocutions such as "thing you use," but he also produced some category coordinate errors, such as saying "horse" for "elephant."

On a word-picture matching test, based on the same forty-eight items, in which A.M. had to point out a picture from eight other exemplars (e.g., zebra from eight other foreign animals), he scored 36/48 (twenty-five age-matched controls score on average 47.4 ± 1.1). When asked to provide descriptions of the forty-eight items in the battery, from their names, he produced very few details; most were vague or generic responses containing the superordinate category only ("a musical instrument," "in the sea," etc.). A number of examples are shown in table 4.1. On the picture version of the Pyramid and Palm Trees Test, a test of associative semantic knowledge in which the subject has to decide which of two pictures (a fir tree or a palm tree) goes best with a target picture, a pyramid (Howard & Patterson, 1992), A.M. scored 39/52 when he first presented. Control subjects typically score close to ceiling on this test.

On tests of reading, A.M. showed the typical pattern of surface dyslexia (Patterson & Hodges, 1992): a normal ability to read aloud words with regular spelling-to-sound correspondence, but errors when reading aloud irregular words (pint, island, leopard, etc.)

By contrast, on nonsemantic tasks (such as copying the Rey Complex Figure, figure 4.1) A.M.'s performance was faultless. When asked to reproduce the Rey Complex Figure after a 45-minute delay, A.M. scored well within the normal range (12.5 versus a control mean = 15.2 ± 7.4). On nonverbal tests of problem solving, such as Raven's Colored Matrices, a multiple-choice test of visual pattern matching that requires the subject to conceptualize spatial relationships, A.M. was also remarkably unimpaired. Auditory-verbal short-term memory was also spared, as judged by a digit span of six forward and four backward.

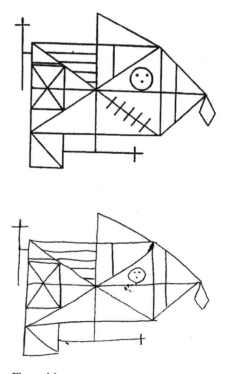

Figure 4.1
Patient A.M.'s copy (*bottom*) of the Rey Complex Figure (*top*).

Table 4.1
Examples of definitions provided by patient A.M. from reading the word

Crocodile	I can't remember it at all . . . not in the sea is it?
Swan	Is it a duck, it's a bird . . . can't recall anything else.
Ostrich	Is it an animal, don't know what kind . . . I never see it in Sainsbury's [a super market].
Zebra	I've no idea what it is.
Lion	A very violent animal, it's a lion in Africa, got a very big mouth, eat lots of animals and humans. They bite on the back of the neck etc.
Deer	They're owned by farmers, in the fields of course, we shave their fur off . . . or is it a sheep? Do we do that too, with deer? I'm not sure.
Frog	I think I've seen them on the ground, they're very small, I think they might be a bit in the water too, I couldn't describe them.
Seahorse	I didn't know they had horses in the sea.
Harp	I don't know what a harp is, not a kind of musical instrument is it?
Trumpet	Yes, I do seem to remember the word trumpet. If only I had a dictionary I could tell you what it is.
Toaster	We put bread in the toaster to make toast for breakfast. It heats the bread up, makes it a bit dark, then it ejects the bread up to the top etc.
Sledge	A sledge? . . . A sledge we use in the snow. You slide on the snow in a sledge.
Aeroplane	It has wings and takes off at the airport into the sky. I know I've been in an aeroplane. It has wings and a jet etc.

A.M. was tested approximately every 6 months over the next 3 years. He was so profoundly anomic when he first presented that there was little room for further decline. On tests of comprehension, by contrast, there was a relentless decline; for instance, on the word-picture matching test, A.M.'s score fell from 36 to 5/48 in November 1996 (controls = 47.4 ± 1.1). Likewise on the pictorial version of the Pyramid and Palm Trees Test, his score fell progressively from 39/52 to chance.

Despite this rapid loss of semantic knowledge, A.M. showed no significant decline on tests of nonverbal problem solving or visuospatial ability over the same time period. For instance, on Raven's Colored Matrices, he still scored perfectly in November 1996.

A.M.'s impairment in semantic knowledge had a considerable impact on his everyday activities. On various occasions he misused objects (e.g., he placed a closed umbrella horizontally over his head during a rainstorm), selected an inappropriate item (e.g., bringing his wife, who was cleaning in the upstairs bathroom, the lawnmower instead of a ladder), and mistook various food items (e.g.,

on different occasions, A.M. put sugar into a glass of wine, orange juice on his lasagne, and ate a raw defrosting salmon steak with yoghurt). Activities that used to be commonplace acquired a new and frightening quality to him: on a plane trip early in 1996 he became clearly distressed at his suitcase being X-rayed and refused to wear a seatbelt in the plane.

After 1996, the behavioral changes became more prominent, with increasing social withdrawal, apathy, and disinhibition. Like another patient described by Hodges, Graham, and Patterson (1995), A.M. showed a fascinating mixture of "preserved and disturbed cognition." Hodges et al.'s patient, J.L., would set the house clocks and his watch forward in his impatience to get to a favorite restaurant, not realizing the relationship between clock and actual time.

A.M. made similar apparently "insightful" attempts to get his own way. For example, his wife reported that she secretly removed his car keys from his key ring to stop him from taking the car for a drive. At this point, A.M. was obsessed with driving and very quickly noticed the missing keys. He solved the problem by taking his wife's car keys off her key ring without her knowledge and going to the locksmiths, successfully, to get a new set cut. At no point did A.M. realize his wife had taken the keys from his key ring. Despite virtually no language output and profound comprehension difficulties, he still retained some skills; for example, he continued to play sports (particularly golf) regularly each week, remembering correctly when he was to be picked up by his friends, until 1998, when he entered permanent nursing care.

Figure 4.2 shows three coronal magnetic resonance images (MRIs) through A.M.'s temporal lobes that were obtained in 1995. The striking asymmetric atrophy of the anterior temporal lobes is clearly visible, involving particularly the temporal pole and fusiform gyrus and inferolateral region, but with relative sparing of the hippocampus.

In summary, A.M.'s case history illustrates a number of the characteristic features of semantic dementia: (1) selective impairment of semantic memory, causing severe anomia, impaired single-word comprehension, reduced generation of exemplars on category fluency tests, and an impoverished fund of general knowledge; (2) surface dyslexia; (3) relative sparing of syntactic and phonological aspects of language; (4) normal perceptual skills and nonverbal problem-solving abilities; (5) relatively preserved recent autobiographical and day-to-day (episodic) memory; (6) anterolateral temporal lobe atrophy.

A Historical Perspective on Semantic Dementia

The last decades of the nineteenth century and the early twentieth century were a golden age for neurologists interested in higher cognitive function. During this period most of the classic syndromes of behavioral neurology were first clearly defined. One of the stars of this era was Arnold Pick, a neurologist, psychiatrist, and linguist. In a remarkable series of papers (now available in translation; Pick, 1892, in Girling & Berrios, 1994; Pick, 1901, in Girling & Markova, 1995; Pick, 1904, in Girling & Berrios, 1997), he described patients who presented with unusually severe fluent aphasia in the context of a dementia and at postmortem had marked atrophy of the cortical gyri of the left temporal lobe.

Pick wanted to call attention to the fact that progressive brain atrophy can lead to focal symptoms

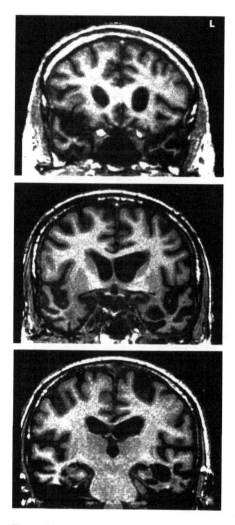

Figure 4.2
Coronal T1-weighted MRI images showing profound atrophy of the temporal pole (left > right) and inferolateral cortex, with relative sparing of the hippocampus.

through local accentuation of the disease process. He also made specific and highly perceptive predictions regarding the role of the midtemporal region of the left hemisphere in the representation of word meaning. Unfortunately Pick's contributions to understanding the neural basis of meaning systems in the brain were largely forgotten and his name became associated with his later discoveries related to focal degeneration of the frontal lobes. As we will see later, patients with focal anterior temporal and frontal degeneration are part of the same spectrum that is often referred to as Pick's disease or more recently, frontotemporal dementia.

Following a dark age of dementia studies, a renaissance of interest—particularly in the syndromes associated with focal lobar atrophy—occurred in the 1970s and 1980s. This revival occurred almost simultaneously in the fields of cognitive neuropsychology and behavioral neurology, but only some time later were the two strands united.

Elizabeth Warrington (1975) was the first to clearly delineate the syndrome of selective semantic memory impairment. She reported three patients, two of whom were subsequently shown to have the histological changes of Pick's disease at autopsy (Cummings & Duchen, 1981 and personal communication from E. Warrington). Drawing on the work of Tulving (1972, 1983), Warrington recognized that the progressive anomia in her patients was not simply a linguistic deficit, but reflected a fundamental loss of semantic memory (or knowledge) about items, which thereby affected naming, word comprehension, and object recognition. Such patients would previously have been described as having a combination of "amnesic, or transcortical sensory, aphasia" and "associative agnosia."

A very similar syndrome was reported by Schwartz, Marin, and Saffran (1979), who observed a profound loss of knowledge for the meaning of a word with preservation of phonological and syntactic aspects of language in a patient, W.L.P., who could also read aloud words that he no longer comprehended. These findings had a profound impact on contemporary models of reading processes (Patterson & Lambon Ralph, 1999).

The major contribution in neurology came from Marsel Mesulam, who in 1982 reported on six patients with a long history of insidiously worsening aphasia in the absence of signs of more generalized cognitive failure. Over the next 15 years it became clear that within the broad category of primary progressive aphasia, two distinct syndromes could be identified: progressive nonfluent aphasia and progressive fluent aphasia (for a review see Hodges & Patterson, 1996; Mesulam & Weintraub, 1992; Snowden, Griffiths, & Neary, 1996a).

In the nonfluent form, speech is faltering and distorted, with frequent phonological substitutions and grammatical errors, but the semantic aspects of language remain intact. The latter syndrome presents in many ways the mirror image: speech remains fluent, grammatically correct, and well articulated, but becomes progressively devoid of content words, with semantic errors and substitution of generic superordinate terms (animal, thing, etc.). As illustrated earlier, the deficit involves word production and comprehension, but is not confined to word meaning (performance on nonverbal tests of semantic knowledge, such as the Pyramid and Palm Trees Test, is invariably affected). To reflect this fundamental breakdown in the knowledge system underlying the use of language, Snowden, Goulding, and Neary (1989) coined the term *semantic dementia* which we have adopted in our studies of the syndrome (Hodges & Patterson, 1996; Hodges et al., 1992a; Hodges et al., 1999a; Hodges, Spatt, & Patterson, 1999b).

There are a number of compelling reasons to consider semantic dementia as part of a spectrum that includes dementia of the frontal type, collectively now most often referred to as *frontotemporal dementia*. The first is pathological; of the fourteen clinicopathological studies of cases fulfilling criteria for semantic dementia, all had either classic Pick's disease (i.e., Pick bodies and/or Pick cells) or a nonspecific spongiform change of the type found in the majority of cases with other forms of frontotemporal dementia (Hodges et al., 1998). The second is the evolution of the pattern of cognitive and behavioral changes over time. As illustrated earlier, semantic dementia patients present with progressive anomia and other linguistic deficits, but on follow-up, the behavioral changes characteristic of orbitobasal frontal lobe dysfunction invariably emerge (Edwards-Lee et al., 1997; Hodges & Patterson, 1996). Third is the fact that modern neuroimaging techniques demonstrate subtle involvement of the orbitofrontal cortex in the majority of cases presenting prominent temporal atrophy and semantic dementia (Mummery et al., 2000; Mummery et al., 1999).

Structural and Functional Imaging Studies in Semantic Dementia

The most striking, and consistent, finding in semantic dementia is focal, and often severe, atrophy of the anterior portion of the temporal lobe (see A.M.'s MRI, figure 4.2). Early studies based upon visual inspection suggested involvement of the polar and inferolateral regions, with relative sparing of the superior temporal gyrus and the hippocampal formation (Hodges & Patterson, 1996; Hodges et al., 1992a). All cases involved the left side, but some had bilateral atrophy. Functional position emission tomography (PET) activation studies in normal subjects, which typically employed paradigms similar to the Pyramids and Palm Trees Test, also pointed to a key role for the left temporal lobe in both verbal and visual semantic knowledge (Martin, Wiggs, Ungerleider, & Haxby, 1996; Mummery, Patterson, Hodges, & Wise, 1996; Vandenberghe, Price, Wise, Josephs, & Frackowiak, 1996). It appeared, therefore, that despite a large body of work on split-brain subjects and normal controls using tachisoscopic techniques, knowledge systems in the brain are surprisingly lateralized.

More recent findings cast doubt on this simple conclusion. We have recently employed methods of quantification (both automated voxel-based morphometry and manual volumetry of defined anatomical structures) of brain atrophy. These studies confirm the profound involvement of the temporal pole, the fusiform gyrus, and the inferolateral cortex, but have shown that in virtually all cases these changes are bilateral and in a number of them the right side is more severely affected than the left (Galton et al., 2001; Mummery et al., 2000).

The status of the hippocampus and parahippocampal structures (notably the entorhinal and perirhinal cortices) has also become less certain. Despite previous reports of relative sparing of the hippocampus, a recent volumetric analysis of ten cases of semantic dementia (including that of A.M.) has shown asymmetric atrophy of the hippocampus, which on the left was actually more marked than in a group of ten Alzheimer's disease patients, matched for disease duration, but was equivalent in severity on the right side. The appearance of the "relative" preservation of medial temporal structures is due to the profound atrophy of surrounding structures compared with the hippocampus. The average volume loss of the temporal pole, fusiform, and inferolateral gyri was 50%, and in some cases up to 80% compared with an average 20% loss of hippocampal volume. In Alzheimer's disease the 20% loss of the hippocampi stands out against the normal polar and inferolateral structures (Galton et al., 2001).

There was also considerable variability among semantic dementia cases. The entorhinal cortex, which constitutes a major component of the parahippocampal gyrus, is also severely affected in semantic dementia. The perirhinal cortex has a complex anatomy in humans, occupying the banks of the collateral sulcus and the medial aspect of the temporal lobe (Corkin, Amaral, Gonzalez, Johnson, & Hyman, 1997). The rostral part is almost certainly affected in semantic dementia, although the caudal part might be partially spared (Simons, Graham, & Hodges, 1999).

Functional imaging in semantic dementia and other disorders is in its infancy, in part owing to the still only partially resolved problems of analyzing and normalizing brains with significant lesions. It is, however, clear that functional imaging will form an essential and increasingly prominent research tool in our attempts to understand functional–anatomical relationships. As argued by Price (1998), functional imaging studies of normal participants can yield vital information about the various brain regions activated during the performance of some cognitive task, but these studies cannot on their own identify which of multiple activations constitute the sine qua non of that cognitive function. Structural lesion data have typically been thought to provide evidence of this nature. However, even greater advances should be possible if we can also identify structurally intact regions of the patient's brain that—presumably because of reduced input from the damaged areas to which they are normally connected—no longer function adequately.

The first activation study of semantic dementia (Mummery et al., 1999) used a combination of structural MRI and PET. The behavioral activation task required associative semantic judgments about triplets of pictures of common objects or printed words corresponding to the names of the pictures. Four patients at early to middle stages of semantic decline were able to perform this task at rates that, although impaired relative to controls, were significantly above chance. For the normal participants, the semantic task (compared with a visual judgment baseline) activated the expected network of left temporal, temporoparietal, and frontal regions previously demonstrated by Vandenberghe et al. (1996).

This distributed set of regions included the left anterior and middle temporal areas that reveal consistent atrophy in semantically impaired patients. A logical conclusion—and indeed one that we endorse—is therefore that this territory is somehow the core, the sine qua non, of the semantic processing required by this task. There was, however, an unexpected PET result: significant hypometabolism (lack of activation), for all four patients relative to normal controls, in a more posterior temporal region, Brodmaum area (BA) 37, the posterior inferior temporal gyrus on the left.

Morphometric analysis of MR images from the same four patients revealed no significant atrophy in BA 37. This is therefore a functional abnormality, not a structural one, but it raises at least the possibility that the patients' semantic deficit is related to this functional posterior-temporal lesion. A somewhat different interpretation, supported by a substantial number of PET results from normal individuals (for a review see Price, 1998) is that BA 37 is critical for translating semantic (and other)

representations into a phonological code. Although the task employed in this study did not require overt naming, it is plausible that the normal subjects automatically generated internal phonological codes for the stimulus items. Since patients with semantic dementia are significantly anomic, their lack of activation in BA 37 might reflect a malfunction of the procedure for computing the phonological code of a stimulus (see Foundas, Daniels, & Vasterling, 1998, for evidence of anomia arising from a focal vascular lesion in left BA 37). This is our preferred interpretation of the PET result for semantic dementia, because of the consistent findings of semantic deficits in conjunction with anterior temporal damage, plus the absence of reports (at least that we have seen) of any notable semantic impairments following selective posterior temporal lesions.

Insights from Behavioral Studies of Semantic Dementia

Our behavioral studies of semantic dementia can be divided into those dealing with spared versus affected cognitive abilities. These studies have provided valuable insights into both the modularity of cognitive processes and the organization of semantic memory.

Cognitive Abilities That Are Relatively Independent of Semantic Memory

The spared abilities can be divided into three domains: (1) memory systems other than semantic memory, (2) aspects of language processing other than those that are necessarily disrupted by a semantic impairment, and (3) cognitive abilities outside the domains of memory and language.

Working Memory

There is good evidence for normal operation of working memory in semantic dementia. For example, it is clear from clinical observations, beginning with Warrington (1975), that these patients do not forget what they or others have just done or said. In terms of formal measures of short-term memory, patients with semantic dementia demonstrate completely normal digit span (e.g., Knott et al., 1997; Patterson, Graham, & Hodges, 1994), as in our patient A.M., at least until very late in the course of decline, and also demonstrate normal performance on the nonverbal Corsi span (Lauro-Grotto, Piccini, & Shallice, 1997).

Episodic Memory

Initial clinical descriptions of patients with semantic dementia suggested that this syndrome provided compelling evidence for a dissociation between preserved episodic and impaired semantic memory. Patients are well oriented and can relate the details, albeit anomically, of recent life events. They also retain broad facts about their own life, such as past occupation, whether they are married, and numbers of children and grandchildren (Hodges, Salmon, & Butters, 1992b). More detailed exploration reveals, however, a major confound of time of memory acquisition. While patients with the amnesic syndrome, as a result of hippocampal damage (following anoxic brain damage or in the early stags of Alzheimer's disease), typically show preservation of autobiographical memory for their early life compared with the more recent past (Greene, Hodges, & Baddeley, 1995; for a review see Hodges, 1995), patients with semantic dementia show the opposite pattern, that is to say, a reversal of the usual temporal gradient effect, with memory for remote events the most vulnerable (Graham & Hodges, 1997; Hodges & Graham, 1998; Snowden, Griffiths, & Neary, 1996b).

This phenomenon of reversal of the usual temporal gradient was explored in a detailed case study of A.M. (described earlier) using the so-called Crovitz technique (Crovitz & Shiffman, 1974) in which subjects are asked to recount specific episodes in response to cue words, such as boat or baby, from particular life periods (Graham & Hodges, 1997). The richness of each memory was then scored by two independent assessors blind to

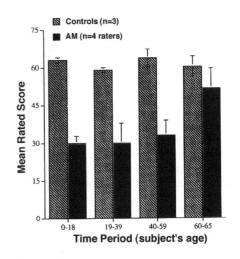

Figure 4.3
Performance of patient A.M. and three age- and education-matched controls on the Crovitz test (Crovitz, Diaco, Apter, 1992) over four different life periods.

the hypothesis under investigation. A.M. was able to produce fairly specific episodes from the past 5 years, but his early life memories were all vague generic descriptions (figure 4.3). This finding explains the ability of patients with semantic dementia to relate recent life events and reveals the shortcomings of clinical observations.

We have demonstrated, therefore, that patients with semantic dementia show impairment on both semantic and autobiographical memory when the age of acquisition of the memories is equated. Tests of semantic memory typically tap knowledge about things learned in early life, and patients' autobiographical memory from this era is poor. One simple interpretation of these findings is that old episodic and semantic memories are essentially the same type of memory. A number of theorists have argued that repeatedly rehearsed episodes have the state of semantic knowledge and that general semantic information is merely the residue of numerous episodes (Baddeley, 1976; Cermak, 1984; McClelland, McNaughton, & O'Reilly, 1995). It should be pointed out, however, that patients with semantic dementia have a *profound* loss of knowledge; for example, they typically call all animals "dog" or "cat" (the equivalent of the knowledge level of a 2-year-old) and, while it is true that their autobiographical memory is impoverished, they retain a considerable amount of personal information.

We conclude, therefore, that although distant episodic memory is affected, it is less severely impaired than semantic memory. By contrast, patients with diffuse brain damage—for instance, patient J.M., who sustained patchy cerebral damage from cerebral vasculitis (Evans, Breen, Antoun, & Hodges, 1996)—show the opposite pattern, i.e., preserved semantic memory and severe autobiographical amnesia.

To explain these patterns, we have suggested that while semantic memory is segregated to particular brain regions (particularly the inferolateral temporal lobes), autobiographical memories are multimodal and distributed (Kitchener & Hodges, 1999). Patients with semantic dementia can compensate while damage remains confined to one temporal lobe, but suffer from severe loss of autobiographical memory when the damage extends to multiple or bilateral brain regions. This also explains why autobiographical memory is devastated fairly early in the course of Alzheimer's disease, which affects the medial and lateral temporal lobes bilaterally (Greene et al., 1995). A similar hypothesis was proposed by Eslinger, who found impaired autobiographical memory following herpes simplex encephalitis only in those patients with bilateral damage (Eslinger, 1998).

The relatively preserved recent autobiographical memory clearly suggests that the mechanisms for encoding new episodic memories may be functioning adequately in semantic dementia. If true, this would run counter to Tulving's (1983, 1995) influential theory of long-term memory organization, which asserts that episodic memory is essentially a subsystem of semantic memory, and that new episodic learning is dependent upon semantic knowledge of the items and concepts to be remembered. Until recently, this claim that episodic memory is dependent upon semantic memory and

that patients should not be able to establish normal episodic memory for stimuli they fail to comprehend had not been addressed. Our recent studies of anterograde memory function in semantic dementia have begun to explore the relationship between semantic and episodic memory in more detail.

Performance on tests of verbal anterograde memory, such as logical memory (story recall) and word-list learning tests, is uniformly poor, which we have interpreted in the context of the patient's poor semantic knowledge of the words to be encoded. By contrast, patients, like A.M., often score within the normal range on nonverbal memory tests such as recall of the Rey Complex Figure (Hodges et al., 1999a). They also show excellent recognition memory when color pictures are used as the stimuli, although recently it has been demonstrated that they rely heavily upon perceptual information. Graham, Simons, Pratt, Patterson, and Hodges (2000a) compared recognition memory for "known" and "unknown" items (known items were pictures that subjects were able to name or correctly identify and vice versa) in two different conditions. In one, the item was perceptually identical at study and test (e.g., it was the same telephone), while in the other condition a different exemplar was presented at study and test (e.g., a different telephone). Patients with semantic dementia showed near-perfect recognition memory for both known and unknown items in the former, perceptually identical condition, but in the latter (perceptually different) condition, recognition memory for the unknown items was very impaired. Together with the findings of the studies described earlier, these data suggest that episodic memory is *not* solely reliant upon the integrity of semantic knowledge and that perceptual information regarding events plays a complementary role in providing a basis for recognition memory.

Turning to the anatomical basis for the preservation of recent autobiographical memory and of anterograde memory in semantic dementia, our initial explanation for this phenomenon—in terms of the apparent sparing of the hippocampal complex (Graham & Hodges, 1997)—also requires some revision in light of the recent anatomical finding of asymmetric hippocampal atrophy in at least a portion of patients with semantic dementia (see earlier discussion).

Most theories of long-term memory posit a time-limited role for the hippocampus (Graham & Hodges, 1997; McClelland et al., 1995). According to such theories, the hippocampal complex provides vital support for recent but not for old memory. "Recent" in this context still means long-term memory, over periods of weeks or months. Over this period, the hippocampus is vital for linking pieces of sensory information in the cortex, but with repeated rehearsals, connections develop in the cortex—a process referred to as *long-term consolidation*—and gradually the memory trace becomes independent of the hippocampus. We had explained the preservation of recent autobiography and anterograde memory in terms of hippocampal sparing in semantic dementia, but as we will see later, there is now evidence that the hippocampus is involved in this disorder. It may be that although the hippocampus is affected, the cellular pathology is distinct and less disruptive than that found in Alzheimer's disease. There is also considerable variability in the extent of hippocampal atrophy, and the asymmetrical involvement (typically the left is greater than the right) might be an important factor. Current studies are pursuing these aspects.

Language

As indicated earlier, two prominent symptoms of semantic dementia are degraded expressive and receptive vocabulary; this is only to be expected since, of all aspects of language processing, the abilities to produce and to comprehend content words rely most obviously on activation of semantic representations. Apart from the semantic system, the two other major components of language—phonology and syntax—seem to function reasonably well in semantic dementia.

Phonology   There is a striking absence of phonological errors in the patients' spontaneous speech or in their performance of more controlled tasks of speech output such as naming objects, repeating single words, and reading aloud. Virtually all aphasic stroke patients, whatever their classification in schemes of aphasic syndromes (e.g., Broca's, Wernicke's, conduction, anomic aphasia), make some errors in naming objects that are phonological approximations to the correct name; the same is true of patients with nonfluent progressive aphasia (Croot, Patterson, & Hodges, 1998; Snowden et al., 1996a). In contrast, anomic errors in patients with semantic dementia take the form of single-word semantic errors (category coordinates or superordinates), circumlocutions (often with very impoverished content), and omissions ("I don't know"), but these patients almost never make phonological errors (Hodges & Patterson, 1996; Snowden et al., 1996a). The speech-production deficit in semantic dementia is therefore probably the result of the patient having insufficient semantic information to activate the correct, or often any, phonological representation, rather than a disruption of the phonological system itself.

The skills of reading aloud and writing to dictation are well preserved for stimuli consisting of high-frequency words and/or words with typical correspondences between spelling and pronunciation. The great majority of patients, however, show a striking pattern of surface dyslexia and surface dysgraphia, making "regularization" errors to lower-frequency words with an unpredictable relationship between spelling and sound; this has been frequently reported in English-speaking patients (e.g., Knott et al., 1997; Patterson & Hodges, 1992), but also in other languages that are characterized by a variety of levels and degrees of consistency in spelling-sound correspondences (see for example, Lauro-Grotto et al., 1997, for Italian; Diesfeldt, 1992, for Dutch; Patterson, Suzuki, Wydell, & Sasanuma, 1995, for Japanese kanji). We have attributed these "surface" patterns of reading and spelling disorders to the reduction in normal semantic constraints on deriving the correct pronunciation or spelling of previously known words

(Graham, Hodges, & Patterson, 1994; Graham, Patterson, & Hodges, 2000b).

Syntax Comprehension of the syntactic aspects of language is also well preserved, at least until late in the course of semantic dementia (Hodges & Patterson, 1996). On a test of sentence–picture matching designed to assess the processing of various syntactic structures (the Test for the Reception of Grammar; Bishop, 1989), patients typically score within the normal range; and where the number of errors exceeds normal limits, the errors are often lexical rather than syntactic in nature (Hodges et al., 1992a).

On the expressive side, the grammatical accuracy of aphasic patients' spontaneous speech is really rather difficult to judge (except in the case of flagrant impairments, as in the syndrome of agrammatism); this is mainly because normal speakers' spontaneous speech is often grammatically ill formed, full of starts and stops and repairs that largely go unnoticed by the listener because the comprehension process is so automatic and so forgiving. On the basis of other researchers' reports (e.g., Snowden et al., 1996a) and our own experience of listening to patients with this disorder over the past decade, the striking abnormality of speech is always word-finding difficulty and almost never any major syntactic anomaly. As the condition worsens and the vocabulary deterioration becomes very marked, speech output not surprisingly becomes reduced in quantity and often rather stereotyped in quality. Even the stock phrases that tend to emerge, however—such as the distressingly accurate ones used by P.P. (Hodges, Patterson, & Tyler, 1994): "I don't understand at all" or M.C. (Hodges et al., 1992a): "I wish I knew what you meant"—are usually well-formed utterances.

Visuospatial Abilities and Nonverbal Problem Solving

Patients score within the normal range on tests of visuospatial function such as Judgment of Line Orientation, the Rey Complex Figure test, and object matching (the latter test requires a decision about which of two photographs shows the same object, but viewed from a different angle, as a target photograph) (Hodges & Patterson, 1996). As described earlier, when asked to copy the Rey figure, these patients produce excellent reproductions (Hodges et al., 1992a), indicating not only good visuospatial skills but also competent planning and organization. Scores on the Raven's Matrices are almost always normal (Hodges et al., 1992a; Snowden et al., 1996a; Waltz et al., 1999), demonstrating that problem solving is unimpaired as long as it does not require knowledge of specific concepts. Waltz and Colleagues (1999) have also recently shown that unlike patients with frontal dementia, semantic dementia patients are able to solve complex deductive and inductive reasoning puzzles.

Insights into the Organization of Semantic Memory

The following sections deal with our studies of semantic breakdown in semantic dementia. The first section addresses the overall architecture of knowledge and whether the evidence from patients suggests a hierarchical (knowledge tree) or distributed (network) model. The following sections then turn to the internal structure and whether knowledge is organized according to semantic categories, modalities of input (words versus pictures), or output (language versus action).

Pruning the Semantic Tree or Holes in the Semantic Net?

The pattern of naming responses made by patients with semantic dementia shows a characteristic evolution with progression of the condition (Hodges et al., 1995). In the early stages, their responses (e.g., "elephant" for "hippopotamus") indicate an inability to distinguish between individual members of a category, but indicate preservation of broad category-level information. Later in the course of

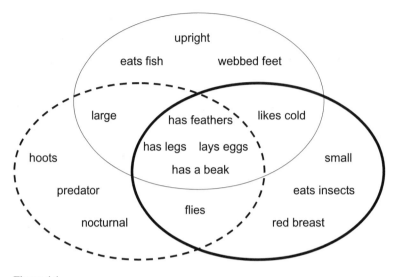

Figure 4.4
Distributed representation (microfeature) model illustrating penguin (thin line), owl (dashed line), and robin (thick line).

the disease, they produce prototypical (e.g., "horse" for "hippopotamus" and for any other large animal) or superordinate responses ("animal"), but only in very advanced cases are cross-category errors produced.

This characteristic progression appears most readily interpretable in terms of a hierarchically structured semantic system, in which specific information is represented at the extremities of a branching "tree of knowledge." More fundamental distinctions, such as the division of animate beings into land animals, water creatures, and birds, are thought to be represented closer to the origin of the putative hierarchy, with living versus nonliving things at the very top. The defining characteristics of higher levels are inherited by all lower points (Collins & Quillian, 1969). Such a model has intuitive appeal and the deficits of semantic dementia can be seen as a progressive pruning back of the semantic tree (Warrington, 1975).

An alternative account, which we favor, is based on the concept of microfeatures in a distributed connectionist network (McClelland et al., 1995;

McClelland & Rumelhart, 1985). The basic idea is illustrated in figure 4.4. An advantage of such a model is that the low-level "features" of individual concepts need only be represented once, while a hierarchical model requires distinctive features to be represented separately for every concept for which they are true (e.g., "has a mane" for both lion and horse). Category membership is then understood as an emergent property of the sharing of elements of these patterns between concepts and thus becomes a matter of degree—another intuitively appealing property. A distributed feature network could predict preservation of superordinate at the expense of finer-grained knowledge, as seen in semantic dementia, because even in a network that had lost the representations of many individual attributes, category coordinates would continue to possess common elements, allowing judgments about category membership to be supported long after more fine-grained distinctions had become impossible.

Do Patients with Semantic Dementia Show Category-Specific Loss of Knowledge?

Living versus Nonliving Things

Semantic memory impairment that selectively affects some categories of knowledge and spares others has been most extensively documented in patients with herpes simplex virus encephalitis, who typically demonstrate a memory advantage for nonliving over living and natural things (animals, fruit, etc.) (Pietrini et al., 1988; Warrington & Shallice, 1984). The complementary dissociation, which effectively rules out any explanation based exclusively on either lower familiarity or a greater degree of visual similarity among the exemplars of living categories, has also been described, typically in patients who have suffered ischemic strokes in the territory of the left middle cerebral artery (for a review see Caramazza, 1998; Gainotti, Silveri, Daniele, & Giustolisi, 1995).

The simplest interpretation of this phenomenon would be that the neural representations of different categories are located in separate cortical regions (Caramazza, 1998; Caramazza & Shelton, 1998). An alternative hypothesis is, however, that the attributes critical to the identification of items within these two broad domains differ in kind. According to this view, one group of items, dominated by living things, depends more strongly on perceptual attributes, while another, mostly artifacts, depends on their functional properties (Warrington & Shallice, 1984). Support for the sensory–functional dichotomy as a basis for category specificity came initially from a group study of patients showing this phenomenon. In these patients the impaired categories did not always respect the living versus manmade distinction (Warrington & McCarthy, 1987). In particular, body parts were found to segregate with nonliving things while fabrics, precious stones, and musical instruments behaved more like living things. The division of knowledge into these fundamental subtypes has been supported by positron emission tomography activation studies of normal volunteers (Martin et al., 1996; Mummery et al., 1999), but studies examining the status of perceptual and functional knowledge in patients with category-specific impairments have provided only limited endorsement of the hypothesis (DeRenzi & Lucchelli, 1994; Silveri & Gainotti, 1988).

The picture in semantic dementia presents a similar inconsistency. When asked to provide definitions of common concepts, these patients volunteer very little visuoperceptual information. For instance, when asked to describe a horse, they typically produce phrases such as "you ride them," "they race them," and "you see them in fields," but only rarely comment on their size, shape, color, or constituent parts (Lambon Ralph, Graham, Patterson, & Hodges, 1999). In view of the striking temporal lobe involvement, the sensory–functional theory might be confidently expected to predict a significant advantage for artifact categories on tests of naming or comprehension. When considered as a group, the expected pattern does emerge in these patients (albeit to a rather modest degree), but a striking category effect is only rarely seen in individual cases (Garrard, Lambon Ralph, & Hodges, 2002).

It seems, therefore, that lesion location and type of information are not the sole determinants of category specificity. Whether the additional factors relate mainly to brain region (it has been hypothesized, for instance, that involvement of medial temporal structures may be important) (Barbarotto, Capitani, Spinnler, & Trivelli, 1995; Pietrini et al., 1988) or to some unidentified aspect of cognitive organization, is as yet unclear.

Knowledge of People versus Objects: The Role of Right and Left Temporal Lobes

A number of earlier authors had suggested an association between right temporal atrophy and the selective loss of knowledge of persons (DeRenzi, 1986; Tyrrell, Warrington, Frackowiak, & Rossor, 1990), but the first fully documented case, V.H., was reported by our group in 1995 (Evans, Heggs, Antoun, & Hodges, 1995). Initially, V.H. appeared to have the classic features of modality-specific prosopagnosia, i.e., a severe inability to identify familiar people from their faces, but much better performance on names and voices. With time, however, it became clear that the deficit was one of a loss of knowledge about people affecting all modalities of access to knowledge. V.H. was unable to identify a photograph of Margaret Thatcher (the patient was English) or to provide any information when presented with the name, yet general semantic and autobiographical memory remained intact (Kitchener & Hodges, 1999). We hypothesized a special role for the right temporal lobe in the representation of knowledge about people (Evans et al., 1995). As with most clear predictions, subsequent studies have produced rather conflicting data. While further patients with predominantly right-sided atrophy have all shown a severe loss of knowledge of persons, we have also observed significant (though not selective) impairments of such knowledge in patients with a predominantly left-sided abnormality, suggesting that knowledge of people is especially vulnerable to temporal atrophy on either side (Hodges & Graham, 1998).

With regard to familiar objects rather than people, our working hypothesis is that conceptual knowledge is represented as a distributed network across both the left and right temporal neocortex. This conclusion is supported by some, but not all, sources of relevant evidence. For example, PET results with normal participants would lead one to believe that essentially all of the semantic action occurs in the left hemisphere (Mummery et al., 1999; Vandenberghe et al., 1996). Our tentative claim for bilateral representation of general conceptual knowledge is based on evidence from semantic dementia. Deficits in semantic tests (such as naming objects, matching words and pictures, sorting, or making associative semantic judgments) are seen not only in patients with predominantly left temporal atrophy (e.g., Breedin, Saffran, & Coslett, 1994; Hodges et al., 1994; Lauro-Grotto et al., 1997; Mummery et al., 1999; Snowden, Griffiths, & Neary, 1994; Tyler & Moss, 1998; Vandenberghe et al., 1996) but also in those with mainly right-

sided damage (e.g., Barbarotto et al., 1995; Hodges et al., 1995; Knott et al., 1997).

V.H., the patient just described whose unilateral anterior right temporal atrophy produced a selective deficit for recognition and knowledge of people (Evans et al., 1995), went on to develop a more generalized semantic deficit in conjunction with the spread of atrophy to the left temporal region (Kitchener & Hodges, 1999). The opposite scenario has occurred in two patients whose semantic dementia began with a phase of unilateral left anterior temporal changes in association with only minimal semantic abnormality. Both cases were shown to have a progressive anomia and developed more pervasive semantic breakdown only when the pathology spread to involve both temporal lobes.

The most dramatic cognitive difference that has emerged from our analyses of patients with greater left than right atrophy (L > R), in contrast to those with greater abnormality on the right (R > L), is not in the extent or pattern of the semantic impairment per se, but rather in its relationship to anomia. This relationship was explored in a combined cross-sectional and longitudinal analysis in which we plotted the patient's picture-naming score for the forty-eight concrete concepts in our semantic battery as a function of the corresponding level of semantic deficit—defined for this purpose as the patient's score on a word-picture matching test for the same forty-eight items. This analysis reveals that for a given level of semantic impairment, the L > R patients are substantially more anomic on average than the R > L cases. The nature of the naming errors is also different in the two subgroups; although all patients make some of each of the three main naming-error types seen in semantic dementia (which, as noted earlier, are single-word semantic errors, circumlocutions, and omissions), there are relatively more semantic errors in the R > L patients and relatively more failures to respond at all in the L > R group.

Our account of this pattern is that semantic representations of concrete concepts are distributed across left and right temporal regions, but because speech production is so strongly lateralized to the left hemisphere, the semantic elements on the left side are much more strongly connected to the phonological representations required to name the concepts. This explains how a patient in the early stages of semantic dementia with atrophy exclusively on the left side can be significantly anomic, with only minor deficits on semantic tasks that do not require naming (Lambon Ralph et al., 1999).

Modalities of Input and Output

One of the continuing debates in the field has related to the issue of whether knowledge is divided according to the modality of input or output. Put simply, when you hear or see the word "asparagus," is the semantic representation activated by this input the same as or different from the conceptual knowledge tapped by seeing or tasting it? Likewise, when you speak about or name a hammer, is the conceptual representation that drives speech production the same as or different from the semantic knowledge that guides your behavior when pick up and use a hammer? The latter kind of knowledge is often referred to, by theorists who hold that it is a separate system, as *action semantics* (Buxbaum, Schwartz, & Carew, 1997; Lauro-Grotto et al., 1997; Rothi, Ochipa, & Heilman, 1991).

Our hypothesis, based upon work in semantic dementia, is that central semantic representations are modality free. We tend to side with the theorists arguing for one central semantic system (e.g., Caramazza, Hillis, Rapp, & Romani, 1990; Howard & Patterson, 1992), rather than those proposing separate modality-specific semantic systems (e.g., Lauro-Grotto et al., 1997; McCarthy & Warrington, 1988; Rothi et al., 1991; Shallice & Kartsounis, 1993). This view has been formed mainly by the fact that none of the cases of semantic dementia that we have studied have demonstrated a striking dissociation between different modalities of input or output and the following studies.

Are There Two Separate Systems for Words and Objects?

To address this question, we recently (Lambon Ralph et al., 1999) evaluated definitions of concrete concepts provided by nine patients with semantic dementia (including A.M.) (table 4.1). The stimulus materials consisted of the forty-eight items from the semantic battery described earlier (Hodges & Patterson, 1995). Each patient was asked, on different occasions, to define each concept both in response to a picture of it and in response to its spoken name. The definitions were scored in a variety of ways, including an assessment of whether the patient's definition achieved the status of "core concept": that is, the responses provided sufficient information for another person to identify the concept from the definition.

The view that there are separate verbal and visual semantic systems predicts no striking item-specific similarities across the two conditions. In keeping with our alternative expectation, however, there was a highly significant concordance between definition success (core concept) and words and pictures referring to or depicting the same item. The number of definitions containing no appropriate semantic information was significantly larger for words than for the corresponding pictures. This difference might be taken by theorists preferring a multiple-systems view as indicating the relative preservation of visual semantics, but we argue that it is open to the following alternative account: The mapping between an object (or a picture of it) and its conceptual representation is inherently different from the mapping between a word and its central concept. Although not everything about objects can be inferred from their physical characteristics, there is a systematic relationship between many of the sensory features of an object or picture and its meaning. This relationship is totally lacking for words; phonological forms bear a purely arbitrary relationship to meaning. Expressed another way, real objects or pictures afford certain properties (Gibson, 1977); words have no affordances. Unless one is familiar with Turkish, there is no way of knowing whether *piliç* describes a chicken, an aubergine, or a fish (actually it is a chicken). When conceptual knowledge is degraded, it therefore seems understandable that there should be a number of instances where a patient would be able to provide some information, even though it is impoverished, in response to a picture, but would draw a complete blank in response to the object's name.

When the nine patients were analyzed as individual cases and definitions were scored for the number of appropriate features that they contained, seven patients achieved either equivalent scores for the two stimulus conditions or better performance for pictures than words, but the remaining two patients in fact scored more highly in response to words than to pictures. Furthermore, these latter two were the only two cases whose bilateral atrophy on MRI was clearly more severe in the right temporal lobe than on the left.

This outcome might be thought to provide even stronger support for separable verbal and visual semantic systems, with verbal representations more reliant on left hemisphere structures, and visual representations based more on a right hemisphere semantic system. Once again, this was not our interpretation. In any picture–word dissociation, one must consider the possibility that the patient has a presemantic deficit in processing the stimulus type, yielding poorer performance. For the two patients who provided more concept attributes for words than pictures, their clear central semantic impairment (indicated by severely subnormal definitions for words as well as pictures) was combined with abnormal presemantic visuoperceptual processing. For example, both had low scores on matching the same object across different views; and one of the cases (also reported in Knott et al., 1997) was considerably more successful in naming real objects (21/30) than line drawings of the same items (2/30), reflecting difficulty in extracting the necessary information for naming from the somewhat sparse visual representation of a line drawing. We have concluded that none of our results require an interpretation in terms of separate

semantic representations activated by words and objects.

Is There a Separate Action Semantic System?

Our recent investigations addressing this general issue were motivated by the claim (e.g., Buxbaum et al., 1997; Lauro-Grotto et al., 1997; Rothi et al., 1991) that there is a separate "action semantic" system that can be spared when there is insufficient knowledge to drive other forms of response—not only naming, but even nonverbal kinds of responding such as sorting, word–picture matching, or associative matching of pictures or words. This view is promoted by frequent anecdotal reports that patients with semantic dementia, who fail a whole range of laboratory-based tasks of the latter kind, function normally in everyday life (e.g., Snowden, Griffiths, & Neary, 1995). We too have observed many instances of such correct object use in patients, although there are also a number of counterexamples (see A.M. above). Nevertheless, the documented successes in object use by patients with severe semantic degradation require explanation. We have recently tried to acquire some evidence on this issue (Hodges, Bozeat, Lambon Ralph, Patterson, & Spatt, 2000; Hodges et al., 1999b).

The ability of six patients with semantic dementia to demonstrate the use of twenty everyday objects such as a bottle opener, a potato peeler, or a box of matches was assessed. The patients also performed a series of other semantic tasks involving these same objects, including naming them, matching a picture of the object with a picture of the location in which it is typically found (a potato peeler with a picture of a kitchen rather than a garden) or to the normal recipient of the object's action (a potato peeler with a potato rather than an egg). In addition, the patients performed the novel tool test designed by Goldenberg and Hagmann (1998) in which successful performance must rely on problem solving and general visual affordances of the tools and their recipients, since none of these correspond to real, familiar objects.

The results of these experiments can be summarized in terms of the questions that we framed. (1) Are patients with semantic dementia generally much more successful in using real objects than would be expected from their general semantic performance? No. (2) If a patient's success in object use varies across different items, can this usually be predicted on the basis of his or her success in other, nonusage semantic tasks for the same objects? On the whole, yes. (3) Where there is evidence for correct use of objects for which a patient's knowledge is clearly impaired, can this dissociation be explained by preservation of general mechanical problem-solving skills combined with real-object affordances, rather than requiring an interpretation of retained object-specific action semantics? Yes. In other words, we have obtained no convincing evidence for a separate action semantic system that is preserved in semantic dementia.

The patient successes appear to be explicable in terms of two main factors. The first is that the patients have good problem-solving skills and that many objects give good clues to their function. The second is that success with objects is significantly modulated by factors of exemplar-specific familiarity and context. As demonstrated by the ingenious experiments of Snowden et al. (1994), a patient who knows how to use her own familiar teakettle in the kitchen may fail to recognize and use both the experimenter's (equally kettlelike but unfamiliar) teakettle in the kitchen and her own teakettle when it is encountered out of a familiar context (e.g., in the bedroom). Our experimental assessments of object use involved standard examples of everyday objects, but these were not exemplars previously used by and known to the patients, and moreover they were presented in a laboratory setting, not in their normal contexts.

Conclusions and Future Directions

Clearly, a great deal has been learned about the neural basis of semantic memory, and the relationship between semantic and other cognitive processes, from the study of patients with semantic dementia. Despite this, much remains to be done. In particular, there is a dearth of clinicopathological studies that combine good in vivo neuropsychological and imaging data with postmortem brain analysis. The role of left and right temporal lobe structures in specific aspects of semantic memory remains controversial, but can be addressed by the longitudinal analysis of rare cases who present with predominant left over right temporal lobe atrophy. The recent finding of asymmetrical medial temporal (hippocampal and/or entorhinal) atrophy despite good episodic memory processing in early semantic dementia also raises a number of important issues for future study.

Until very recently, the study of memory in nonhuman primates has focused almost exclusively on working memory and paradigms thought to mirror human episodic memory. It is now believed that some object-based tasks (e.g., delayed matching and nonmatching-to-sample) more closely resemble human semantic memory tests, and that animals failing such tasks after perirhinal ablation have deficits in object recognition and/or high-level perceptual function (see Murray & Bussey, 1999; Simons et al., 1999). This radical departure has stimulated interest in the role of the human perirhinal cortex in semantic memory and the relationship between perception and knowledge in humans. A number of projects exploring parallels between monkey and human semantic memory are already under way and promise to provide further exciting insights over the next few years.

Acknowledgment

This chapter is dedicated to my neuropsychology colleague and friend, Karalyn Patterson, who has inspired much of the work described in this chapter; and to the research assistants, graduate students, and postdoctoral researchers who have made the work possible. We have been supported by the Medical Research Council, the Wellcome Trust, and the Medlock Trust.

References

Baddeley, A. D. (1976). *The Psychology of memory.* New York: Basic Books.

Barbarotto, R., Capitani, E., Spinnler, H., & Trivelli, C. (1995). Slowly progressive semantic impairment with category specificity. *Neurocase, 1,* 107–119.

Bishop, D. V. M. (1989). *Test for the reception of grammar* (2nd ed.), London: Medical Research Council.

Breedin, S. D., Saffran, E. M., & Coslett, H. B. (1994). Reversal of the concreteness effect in a patient with semantic dementia. *Cognitive Neuropsychology, 11,* 617–660.

Buxbaum, L. J., Schwartz, M. F., & Carew, T. G. (1997). The role of semantic memory in object use. *Cognitive Neuropsychology, 14,* 219–254.

Caramazza, A. (1998). The interpretation of semantic category-specific deficits: What do they reveal about the organization of conceptual knowledge in the brain? Introduction. *Neurocase, 4,* 265–272.

Caramazza, A., Hillis, A. E., Rapp, B. C., & Romani, C. (1990). The multiple semantics hypothesis: Multiple confusions. *Cognitive Neuropsychology, 7,* 161–189.

Caramazza, A., & Shelton, J. R. (1998). Domain-specific knowledge systems in the brain: The animate-inanimate distinction. *Journal of Cognitive Neuroscience, 10,* 1–34.

Cermak, L. S. (1984). The episodic/semantic distinction in amnesia. In L. R. Squire & N. Butters (Eds.), *The neuropsychology of memory* (pp. 52–62). New York: Guilford Press.

Collins, A. M., & Quillian, M. R. (1969). Retrieval time from semantic memory. *Journal of Verbal Learning and Verbal Behaviour, 8,* 240–247.

Corkin, S., Amaral, D. G., Gonzalez, R. G., Johnson, K. A., & Hyman, B. T. (1997). H.M.'s medial temporal lobe lesion: Findings from magnetic resonance imaging. *Journal of Neuroscience, 17,* 3964–3979.

Croot, K., Patterson, K., & Hodges, J. R. (1998). Single word production in non-fluent progressive aphasia. *Brain and Language, 61,* 226–273.

Crovitz, H. F., & Schiffman, H. (1974). Frequency of episodic memories as a function of their age. *Bulletin of the Psychonomic Society, 4,* 517–518.

Cummings, J. L., & Duchen, L. W. (1981). Kluver-Bucy syndrome in Pick's disease: Clinical and pathological correlations. *Neurology, 31,* 1415–1422.

DeRenzi, E. (1986). Prosopagnosia in two patients with CT scan evidence of damage confined to the right hemisphere. *Neuropsychologia, 24,* 385–389.

DeRenzi, E., & Lucchelli, F. (1994). Are semantic systems separately represented in the brain? The case of living category impairment. *Cortex, 30,* 3–25.

Diesfeldt, H. F. A. (1992). Impaired and preserved semantic memory functions in dementia. In L. Backman (Ed.), *Memory functioning in dementia* (pp. 227–263). Amsterdam: Elsevier.

Edwards-Lee, T., Miller, B., Benson, F., Cummings, J. L., Russell, G. L., Boone, K., & Mena, I. (1997). The temporal variant of frontotemporal dementia. *Brain, 120,* 1027–1040.

Eslinger, P. J. (1998). Autobiographical memory after temporal and frontal lobe lesions. *Neurocase, 4,* 481–495.

Evans, J. J., Breen, E. K., Antoun, N., & Hodges, J. R. (1996). Focal retrograde amnesia for autobiographical events following cerebral vasculitis: A connectionist account. *Neurocase, 2*(1), 1–12.

Evans, J. J., Heggs, A. J., Antoun, N., & Hodges, J. R. (1995). Progressive prosopagnosia associated with selective right temporal lobe atrophy: A new syndrome? *Brain, 118,* 1–13.

Foundas, A. L., Daniels, S. K., & Vasterling, J. J. (1998). Anomia: Case studies with lesion localization. *Neurocase, 4,* 35–43.

Gainotti, G., Silveri, M. C., Daniele, A., & Giustolisi, L. (1995). Neuroanatomical correlates of category-specific semantic disorders: A critical survey. *Memory, 3,* 247–264.

Galton, C. J., Patterson, K., Graham, K., Lambon Ralph, M. A., Williams, G., Antoun, N., Sahakian, B. J., & Hodges, J. R. (2001). Differing patterns of temporal atrophy in Alzheimer's disease and semantic dementia. *Neurology, 57,* 216–225.

Garrard, P., Lambon Ralph, M. A., & Hodges, J. R. (2002). Semantic dementia: A category-specific paradox. In E. M. E. Forde & G. W. Humphreys (Eds.), *Category specificity in brain and mind.* East Sussex: Psychology Press.

Garrard, P., Perry, R., & Hodges, J. R. (1997). Disorders of semantic memory. *Journal of Neurology, Neurosurgery and Psychiatry, 62*(5), 431–435.

Gibson, J. J. (1977). The theory of affordances. In R. Shaw, J. Bransford, (Eds.), *Perceiving, acting and knowing: Toward an ecological psychology.* Hillsdale, NY: Lawrence Erlbaum Associates.

Girling, D. M., & Berrios, G. E. (1994). On the relationship between senile cerebral atrophy and aphasia. (Translation of A. Pick, Über die beziehungen der senilen hirnatrophie zur aphasie. *Prager Medicinische Wochenschrift* 1892, *17*, 165–167.) *History of Psychiatry, 8*, 542–547.

Girling, D. M., & Berrios, G. E. (1997). On the symptomatology of left-sided temporal lobe atrophy. (Translation of Zur symptomatologie der linksseitigen schäfenlappenatrophie. *Monatschrift für Psychiatrie und Neurologie*, 1904, *16*, 378–388.) *History of Psychiatry, 8*, 149–159.

Girling, D. M., & Markova, I. S. (1995). Senile atrophy as the basis for focal symptoms. (Translation of A. Pick, Senile hirnatrophie als grundlage von herdereseinungen. *Wiener klinische Wochenschrift* 1901, *14*, 403–404.) *History of Psychiatry, 6*, 533–537.

Goldenberg, G., & Hagmann, S. (1998). Tool use and mechanical problem solving in patients with apraxia. *Neuropsychologia, 36*, 581–589.

Graham, K. S., & Hodges, J. R. (1997). Differentiating the roles of the hippocampal complex and the neocortex in long-term memory storage; evidence from the study of semantic dementia and Alzheimer's disease. *Neuropsychology, 11*, 77–89.

Graham, K. S., Hodges, J. R., & Patterson, K. (1994). The relationship between comprehension and oral reading in progressive fluent aphasia. *Neuropsychologia, 32*, 299–316.

Graham, K. S., Simons, J. S., Pratt, K. H., Patterson, K., & Hodges, J. R. (2000a). Insights from semantic dementia on the relationship between episodic and semantic memory. *Neuropsychologia, 38*, 313–324.

Graham, N. L., Patterson, K., & Hodges, J. R. (2000b). The impact of semantic memory impairment on spelling: Evidence from semantic dementia. *Neuropsychologia, 38*, 143–163.

Greene, J. D. W., Hodges, J. R., & Baddeley, A. D. (1995). Autobiographical memory and executive function in early dementia of Alzheimer type. *Neuropsychologia, 33*, 1647–1670.

Hodges, J. R. (1995). Retrograde amnesia. In A. D. Baddeley, B. A. Wilson, & F. N. Watts (Eds.), *Handbook of memory disorders* (pp. 81–109). Chichester, UK: Wiley.

Hodges, J. R. (2000). Pick's disease: Its relationship to semantic dementia, progressive aphasia and frontotemporal dementia. In J. O'Brien, D. Ames, & A. Burns (Eds.), *Dementia*, 2nd Edition (pp. 747–758). London: Hodder Headline.

Hodges, J. R., Bozeat, S., Lambon Ralph, M. A., Patterson, K., & Spatt, J. (2000). The role of conceptual knowledge in object use: Evidence from semantic dementia. *Brain, 123*, 1913–1925.

Hodges, J. R., Garrard, P., & Patterson, K. (1998). Semantic dementia. In A. Kertesz & D. G. Munoz (Eds.), *Pick's disease and Pick complex* (pp. 83–104). New York: Wiley-Liss.

Hodges, J. R., & Graham, K. S. (1998). A reversal of the temporal gradient for famous person knowledge in semantic dementia: Implications for the neural organisation of long-term memory. *Neuropsychologia, 36*(8), 803–825.

Hodges, J. R., Graham, N., & Patterson, K. (1995). Charting the progression in semantic dementia: Implications for the organisation of semantic memory. *Memory, 3*, 463–495.

Hodges, J. R., & Patterson, K. (1995). Is semantic memory consistently impaired early in the course of Alzheimer's disease? Neuroanatomical and diagnostic implications. *Neuropsychologia, 33*(4), 441–459.

Hodges, J. R., & Patterson, K. (1996). Nonfluent progressive aphasia and semantic dementia: A comparative neuropsychological study. *Journal of the International Neuropsychological Society, 2*, 511–524.

Hodges, J. R., & Patterson, K. E. (1997). Semantic memory disorders. *Trends in Cognitive Science, 1*, 67–72.

Hodges, J. R., Patterson, K., Oxbury, S., & Funnell, E. (1992a). Semantic dementia: Progressive fluent aphasia with temporal lobe atrophy. *Brain, 115*, 1783–1806.

Hodges, J. R., Patterson, K., & Tyler, L. K. (1994). Loss of semantic memory: Implications for the modularity of mind. *Cognitive Neuropsychology, 11*, 505–542.

Hodges, J. R., Patterson, K., Ward, R., Garrard, P., Bak, T., Perry, R., & Gregory, C. (1999a). The differentiation of semantic dementia and frontal lobe dementia (temporal and frontal variants of frontotemporal dementia) from early Alzheimer's disease: A comparative neuropsychological study. *Neuropsychology, 13*, 31–40.

Hodges, J. R., Salmon, D. P., & Butters, N. (1992b). Semantic memory impairment in Alzheimer's disease: Failure of access or degraded knowledge? *Neuropsychologia, 30*, 301–314.

Hodges, J. R., Spatt, J., & Patterson, K. (1999b). What and How: Evidence for the dissociation of object knowledge and mechanical problem-solving skills in the human brain. *Proceedings of the National Academy of Sciences U.S.A., 96*, 9444–9448.

Howard, D., & Patterson, K. (1992). *Pyramids and palm trees: A test of semantic access from pictures and words.* Bury St. Edmunds, UK: Thames Valley Test Company.

Kitchener, E., & Hodges, J. R. (1999). Impaired knowledge of famous people and events and intact autobiographical knowledge in a case of progressive right temporal lobe degeneration: Implications for the organization of remote memory. *Cognitive Neuropsychology, 16*, 589–607.

Knott, R., Patterson, K., & Hodges, J. R. (1997). Lexical and semantic binding effects in short-term memory: Evidence from semantic memory. *Cognitive Neuropsychology, 14*, 1165–1218.

Lambon Ralph, M., Graham, K. S., Patterson, K., & Hodges, J. R. (1999). Is a picture worth a thousand words? Evidence from concept definitions by patients with semantic dementia. *Brain and Language, 70*, 309–335.

Lauro-Grotto, R., Piccini, C., & Shallice, T. (1997). Modality-specific operations in semantic dementia. *Cortex, 33*, 593–622.

Martin, A., Wiggs, C. L., Ungerleider, L. G., & Haxby, J. V. (1996). Neural correlates of category-specific knowledge. *Nature, 379*, 649–652.

McCarthy, R. A., & Warrington, E. K. (1988). Evidence for modality-specific meaning systems in the brain. *Nature, 334*, 428–430.

McClelland, J. L., McNaughton, B. L., & O'Reilly, R. C. (1995). Why there are complementary learning systems in the hippocampus and neocortex: Insights from the successes and failures of connectionist models of learning and memory. *Psychological Review, 102*, 419–457.

McClelland, J. L., & Rumelhart, D. E. (1985). Distributed memory and the representation of general and specific information. *Journal of Experimental Psychology, 114*(2), 159–188.

Mesulam, M. M., & Weintraub, S. (1992). Primary progressive aphasia. In F. Boller (Ed.), *Heterogeneity of Alzheimer's disease* (pp. 43–66). Berlin: Springer-Verlag.

Mummery, C. J., Patterson, K. E., Hodges, J. R., & Wise, R. J. S. (1996). Generating "Tiger" as an animal name and a word beginning with T: Differential brain activation. *Proceeedings of the Royal Society of London, Ser. B, 263*, 989–995.

Mummery, C. J., Patterson, K., Price, C. J., Ashburner, J., Frackowiak, R. S. J., & Hodges, J. R. (2000). A voxel-based morphometry study of semantic dementia: The relationship between temporal lobe atrophy and semantic dementia. *Annals of Neurology, 47*, 36–45.

Mummery, C. J., Patterson, K., Wise, R. J. S., Vandenbergh, R., Price, C. J., & Hodges, J. R. (1999). Disrupted temporal lobe connections in semantic dementia. *Brain, 122*, 61–73.

Murray, E. A., & Bussey, T. J. (1999). Perceptual-mnemonic functions of the perirhinal cortex. *Trends in Cognitive Science, 3*, 142–151.

Patterson, K., Graham, N., & Hodges, J. R. (1994). The impact of semantic memory loss on phonological representations. *Journal of Cognitive Neuroscience, 6*, 57–69.

Patterson, K., & Hodges, J. R. (1992). Deterioration of word meaning: Implications for reading. *Neuropsychologia, 30*, 1025–1040.

Patterson, K. E., & Hodges, J. R. (1994). Disorders of semantic memory. In A. D. Baddeley, B. A. Wilson, & F. N. Watts (Eds.), *Handbook of memory disorders* (pp. 167–187). Chichester, UK: Wiley.

Patterson, K., & Lambon Ralph, M. A. (1999). Selective disorders of reading? *Current Opinion in Neurobiology, 9*, 235–239.

Patterson, K., Suzuki, T., Wydell, T., & Sasanuma, S. (1995). Progressive aphasia and surface alexia in Japanese. *Neurocase, 1*(2), 155–166.

Pietrini, V., Nertempi, P., Vaglia, A., Revello, M. G., Pinna, V., & Ferro-Milone, F. (1988). Recovery from herpes simplex encephalitis: Selective impairment of specific semantic categories with neuroradiological correlation. *Journal of Neurology, Neurosurgery and Psychiatry, 51*, 1284–1293.

Price, C. J. (1998). The functional anatomy of word comprehension and production. *Trends in Cognitive Science, 2*, 281–288.

Rothi, L. J. G., Ochipa, C., & Heilman, K. M. (1991). A cognitive neuropsychological model of limb praxis. *Cognitive Neuropsychology, 8*, 443–458.

Schwartz, M. F., Marin, O. S. M., & Saffran, E. M. (1979). Dissociations of language function in dementia: A case study. *Brain and Language, 7*, 277–306.

Shallice, T., & Kartsounis, L. D. (1993). Selective impairment of retrieving people's names: A category-specific disorder? *Cortex, 29*, 281–291.

Silveri, M. C., & Gainotti, G. (1988). Interaction between vision and language in category-specific semantic impairment. *Cognitive Neuropsychology, 3*, 677–709.

Simons, J. S., Graham, K. S., & Hodges, J. R. (1999). What does semantic dementia reveal about the functional role of the perirhinal cortex? *Trends in Cognitive Sciences, 3*, 248–249.

Snowden, J. S., Goulding, P. J., & Neary, D. (1989). Semantic dementia: A form of circumscribed cerebral atrophy. *Behavioural Neurology, 2*, 167–182.

Snowden, J. S., Griffiths, H. L., & Neary, D. (1994). Semantic dementia: Autobiographical contribution to preservation of meaning. *Cognitive Neuropsychology, 11*, 265–288.

Snowden, J. S., Griffiths, H. L., & Neary, D. (1995). Autobiographical experience and word meaning. *Memory, 3*, 225–246.

Snowden, J. S., Griffiths, H. L., & Neary, D. (1996a). Progressive language disorder associated with frontal lobe degeneration. *Neurocase, 2*, 429–440.

Snowden, J. S., Griffiths, H. L., & Neary, D. (1996b). Semantic-episodic memory interactions in semantic dementia: Implications for retrograde memory function. *Cognitive Neuropsychology, 13*, 1101–1137.

Tulving, E. (1972). Episodic and semantic memory. In E. Tulving & W. Donaldson (Eds.), *Organisation of memory* (pp. 381–403). New York: Academic Press.

Tulving, E. (1983). *Elements of episodic memory*. Oxford: Clarendon Press.

Tulving, E. (1995). Organization of memory: Quo vadis. In M. S. Gazzaniga (Ed.), *The cognitive neurosciences* (pp. 839–847). Cambridge, MA: MIT Press.

Tyler, L. K., & Moss, H. E. (1998). Going, going, gone . . . ? Implicit and explicit tests of conceptual knowledge in a longitudinal study of semantic dementia. *Neuropsychologia, 36*, 1313–1323.

Tyrrell, P. J., Warrington, E. K., Frackowiak, R. S. J., & Rossor, M. N. (1990). Progressive degeneration of the right temporal lobe studied with positron emission tomography. *Journal of Neurology, Neurosurgery and Psychiatry, 53*, 1046–1050.

Vandenberghe, R., Price, C., Wise, R., Josephs, O., & Frackowiak, R. S. J. (1996). Functional anatomy of a common semantic system for words and pictures. *Nature, 383*, 254–256.

Waltz, J. A., Knowlton, B. J., Holyoak, K. J., Boone, K. B., Mishkin, F. S., de Menezes Santos, M., Thomas, C. R., & Miller, B. L. (1999). A system for relational reasoning in human prefrontal cortex. *Psychological Science, 10*, 119–125.

Warrington, E. K. (1975). Selective impairment of semantic memory. *Quarterly Journal of Experimental Psychology, 27*, 635–657.

Warrington, E. K., & McCarthy, R. A. (1987). Categories of knowledge: Further fractionation and an attempted integration. *Brain, 110*, 1273–1296.

Warrington, E. K., & Shallice, T. (1984). Category-specific semantic impairments. *Brain, 107*, 829–854.

5 Topographical Disorientation: A Disorder of Way-Finding Ability

Geoffrey K. Aguirre

Topographical disorientation (hereafter, TD) refers to the selective loss of way-finding ability within the locomotor environment. Despite sharing this general impairment and a diagnostic label, patients with TD present in a rather heterogeneous manner, with considerable variability in the precise nature of their cognitive deficit and lesion site. This variability in clinical presentation might be expected, given the tremendous complexity of way-finding and the multifaceted solutions that are brought to bear on the challenge. It should further be clear that many general impairments, which have little to do with representation of environmental information per se (e.g., blindness, global amnesia, paralysis) might prevent a person from successfully traveling from their home to a well-known destination. Historically, the treatment of TD as a neurological disorder has been a bit of a muddle, with considerable debate regarding the singular, "essential nature" of the disorder and confusion regarding the terminology used to describe the cases. (For a historical review see Barrash, 1998, or Aguirre and D'Esposito, 1999.)

Despite these challenges, the complexities of TD yield to an understanding of the behavioral elements of way-finding and an appreciation of the parcellation of cognitive function within the cortex. I consider here a framework that can be used to categorize cases of TD based upon the behavioral impairment and the location of the responsible lesion. I begin with four cases of TD, which provide a sense of the range of disabilities seen. Next, I consider the cognitive processes involved in way-finding and the interpretation of clinical tests of disoriented patients. The cases presented initially are then revisited in greater detail, and a four-part "taxonomy" of TD explored. Finally, I discuss the results of recent neuropsychological and functional neuroimaging studies of environmental representation.

Case Reports

Case 1: A patient reported by Levine and colleagues (Levine, Warach, & Farah, 1985) presented with severe spatial disorientation following development of intracerebral hemorrhages. He would become lost in his own house and was unable to travel outside without a companion because he was completely unable to judge which direction he needed to travel. The patient demonstrated a right homonymous hemianopia, but had intact visual acuity and no evidence of prosopagnosia, object agnosia, or achromatopsia. His disabilities were most strikingly spatial. He had difficulty fixating on individual items within an array, demonstrated right-left confusion for both external space and his own limbs, and could not judge relative distance. He became grossly disoriented in previously familiar places; was unable to learn his way around even simple environments; and provided bizarre descriptions of routes. A computed tomography (CT) scan revealed bilateral posterior parietal lesions extending into the posterior occipital lobe on the left.

Case 2: Patient T.Y. (Suzuki, Yamadori, Hayakawa, & Fujii, 1998) presented with severe difficulties in finding her way to her doctor's office, a route which she had routinely walked over the previous 10 years. Although T.Y. initially demonstrated unilateral spatial neglect and constructional apraxia, these resolved over the following weeks. She did have a stable, incomplete, left lower quadrantanopia. She was without object agnosia or prosopagnosia, and had intact visual and spatial memory as measured by standard table-top tests. Despite an intact ability to recognize her house and famous buildings, T.Y. was unable to state the position from which the photographs of these structures were taken. She was also utterly unable to judge her direction of heading on a map while performing a way-finding task through a college campus. In contrast to these deficits, T.Y. was able to draw accurate maps and provide verbal directions to places familiar to her prior to her disability. A magnetic resonance imaging (MRI) scan revealed a subcortical hemorrhage involving primarily the right posterior cingulate.

Case 3: Patient A.H. (Pallis, 1955) woke one morning to find that he could not recognize his bedroom and became lost trying to return from the toilet to his room. In addition to a central scotoma, he developed achromatopsia and marked prosopagnosia. He was without neglect, left-right confusion, or apraxia. His primary and most distressing complaint was his inability to recognize places. While he could intuit his location within his hometown from the turns he had taken and the small details he might notice (i.e., the color of a particular park bench), he was unable to distinguish one building from another, for example, mistaking the post office for his pub. His trouble extended to new places as well as previously familiar locales. Vertebral angiography revealed defective filling of the right posterior cerebral artery.

Case 4: Patient G.R. (Epstein, DeYoe, Press, Rosen, & Kanwisher, 2001) developed profound difficulties learning his way around new places following cardiac surgery. In addition to his way-finding complaints, G.R. demonstrated a left hemianopsia, right upper quadrantanopsia, and dyschromatopsia. He had no evidence of neglect, left-right confusion, or apraxia, and no prosopagnosia or object agnosia. G.R. did have subtle memory impairments on formal testing, with greater disability for visual than verbal material. Despite being able to follow routes marked on maps, G.R. was totally unable to learn new topographical information, including the appearance of environmental features and exocentric spatial relationships. He was unimpaired in navigating through environments familiar to him prior to the onset of his symptoms. An MRI scan revealed bilateral damage to the parahippocampal gyri, with extension of the right lesion posteriorly to involve the inferior lingual gyrus, medial fusiform gyrus, and occipital lobe.

Normative Way-Finding and Clinical Tests

People employ a variety of strategies and representations when solving way-finding tasks. These variations have been attributed to subject variables (e.g., gender, age, length of residence), differences in environmental characteristics (e.g., density of landmarks, regularity of street arrangements), and differences in knowledge acquisition (e.g., navigation versus map learning). One basic tenet of environmental psychology studies is that these differences are largely the result of differences in representation; a subject not only improves his or her knowledge of the environment with increasing familiarity, for example, but comes to represent that knowledge in qualitatively different ways with experience (Appleyard, 1969; Piaget, Inhelder, & Szeminska, 1960; Siegel, Kirasic, & Kail, 1978; Siegel & White, 1975). This shift in representation in turn supports the ability to produce more accurate, flexible, and abstract spatial judgments. Specifically, a distinction has frequently been drawn between representations of the environment that are route based and those that are more "maplike." This gross division has appeared under many labels (i.e., taxon versus locale, O'Keefe & Nadel, 1978; procedural versus survey, Thorndyke & Hayes, 1982; route versus configural, Siegel & White, 1975; network versus vector map, Byrne, 1982), but they generally possess the same basic structure.

Most environmental representation is predicated on the ability to recognize specific locations where navigational decisions are executed. This perceptual ability is called "landmark (or place) recognition" and is thought to be the first "topographic" ability acquired in developing infants (Piaget et al., 1960). Subjects improve in their ability to successfully identify environmental features with developmental age and there is considerable between-subject agreement as to what constitutes a useful landmark (Allen, Kirasic, Siegel, & Norman, 1979). For example, buildings located at street intersections seem to provide primary anchor points for real-world navigational learning (Presson, 1987).

Route knowledge describes the information that encodes a sequential record of steps that lead from a starting point, through landmarks, and finally to a destination. This representation is essentially linear, in that each landmark is coupled to a given instruction (i.e., go right at the old church), which leads to another landmark and another instruction, repeated until the goal is reached. Indeed, the learning of landmark-instruction paths has been likened to the learning of stimulus-response pairs (Thorndyke, 1981). While more information can be stored along with a learned route—for example, distances, the angles of turns and features along the route

(Thorndyke & Hayes, 1982)—there is evidence that subjects often encode only the minimal necessary representation (Byrne, 1982).

Descriptions of route learning also emphasize its grounding in an egocentric coordinate frame. It is assumed that a set of transformations take place by which the retinal position of an image is combined with information regarding the position of the eyes in the orbits and the position of the head upon the neck in order to represent the location of an object with reference to the body. This is called an "ego-centric (or body-centered) space" and is the domain of spatial concepts such as left and right. Orientation is maintained within a learned route by representing an egocentric position with respect to a landmark (i.e., pass to the left of the grocery store, then turn right). A final, and crucial, aspect of route knowledge is its presumed inflexibility. Because a route encodes only a series of linear instructions, the representation is fragile in that changes in crucial landmarks or detours render the learned path useless.

Whereas route learning is conducted within egocentric space, maplike representations are located within the domain of *exocentric* space, in which spatial relations between objects within the environment, including the observer, are emphasized (Taylor & Tversky, 1992). A developmental dissociation between egocentric and exocentric spatial representation has been demonstrated in a series of experiments by Acredolo (1977), indicating that these two coordinate frames are represented by adult subjects. In order to generate a representation of exocentric space, egocentric spatial decisions must be combined with an integrated measure of one's motion in the environment. While a tree may be to my right now, if I walk forward ten paces and turn around, the tree will now be to my left. Though the egocentric position of the landmark has changed, I am aware that the tree has not moved; the exocentric position has remained invariant. A representation of this invariance is made available by combining the egocentric spatial judgments with a measure of the vector motion that was undertaken.

An important lesson from this cursory review is that the particular type of representation that a subject generates of his or her environment can be dependent upon (1) the subject's developmental age, (2) the duration of a subject's experience with a particular environment, (3) the manner in which the subject was introduced to the environment (i.e., self-guided exploration, map reading), (4) the level of differentiation (detail) of the environment, and (5) the tasks that the subject is called upon to perform within the space. The multiplicity and redundancy of strategies that may be brought to bear upon way-finding challenges make the interpretation of standard clinical tests of topographical orientation problematic. For example, asking a patient to describe a route in his or her town is not guaranteed to evoke the same cognitive processes for different routes, let alone different subjects. Since these commonly employed tests of topographical orientation (i.e., describing a route, drawing a map) are poorly defined with regard to the cognitive processes they require, it is always possible to provide a post hoc explanation for any particular deficit observed.

This inferential complication is further confounded by the ability of patients to store a particular representation in any one of several forms. Consider, for example, the frequently employed bedside test of producing a sketch map. Patients are asked to draw a simple map of a place (e.g., their home, their town, the hospital) with the intention of revealing intact or impaired exocentric (i.e., maplike) representations of space. It is possible however, to produce a sketch map of a place without possessing an exocentric representation (Pick, 1993). For example, complete route knowledge of a place, combined with some notion of the relative path lengths composing the route segments, is sufficient to allow the construction of an accurate sketch map. Thus, while a subject may be able to produce a sketch map of a place, this does not necessarily indicate that the subject ever possessed or considered an exocentric representation of that place prior to the administration of the test (Byrne,

1982). Alternatively, it is possible that considerable experience with map representations of a place would lead a subject to develop a "picturelike" representation. If, for example, a subject has had the opportunity to consult or draw maps of his home or hometown several times previously, then he might be able to draw a map of that place in the same manner that he might draw a picture of an object.

In a similar manner, impairments in one area of topographical representation might lead to poor performance on tests that ostensibly probe a different area of competence. For example, if a patient is asked to describe a route through a well-known place, it is frequently assumed that the patient is relying only upon intact egocentric spatial knowledge. However, it is entirely possible that if producing a verbal description of a route is not a well-practiced behavior, the subjects engage in an imaginal walk along the route to produce the description (Farrell, 1996). In this case, deficits in the ability to represent and manipulate information about the appearance of landmarks would also impair performance. Thus, given that subjects might have to generate maplike representations only at the time of testing, and given that this process can be dependent upon route representations which themselves may require intact representations of environmental landmarks, it is conceivable that tertiary impairments in producing a sketch map might be produced by primary impairments in landmark recognition!

How then are we to proceed in interpreting the clinical tests given to patients with TD? The only possible means of gaining inferential knowledge of these disorders is to obtain additional information regarding the nature of the impairment. One simple approach is to attach credence to the patient's description of their disability. As will be examined later, some categories of TD give rise to rather consistent primary complaints across patients. When these reports are sufficiently clear and consonant, they provide a reasonable basis for theorizing. Naturally, there are limitations to this approach as well. Patient reports might simply be wrong (Farrell, 1996); the case reported by DeRenzi and Faglioni

(1962) offers an example in which the patient's claim of intact recognition for buildings and environmental features was at odds with his actual performance.

Additional clinical tests, with more transparent interpretations, may also be used to help interpret topographical impairments. Demonstrations of stimulus-specific deficits in visual memory and impairments of egocentric spatial representation have been particularly helpful. For example, Whiteley and Warrington (1978) introduced tests of visual recognition and matching of landmarks, which have led to a deeper understanding of one type of TD. Of course, such tests themselves require careful interpretation and monitoring. As has been demonstrated for general object agnosia, patients can maintain intact performance on such tasks by using markedly altered strategies (Farah, 1990).

While more complex clinical tests have been employed, these frequently are as subject to various interpretations as the original patient deficit. For example, the stylus-maze task (Milner, 1965), in which the subject must learn an invisible path through an array of identical bolt heads, has been widely applied. Despite the vague similarity of maze learning and real-world navigation, it is conceivable that failure to successfully complete the task might be due to a number of cognitive impairments that are unrelated to way-finding; indeed, neuropsychological studies that have employed this test have noted that many patients who are impaired on the stylus maze task have no real-world orientation difficulties whatsoever (Newcombe & Ritchie, 1969) and vice versa (Habib & Sirigu, 1987). Other tests that have been applied with varying degrees of success include the Semmes Extrapersonal Orientation Test, which requires retention and updating of right-left orientation, and tests of geographical knowledge (i.e., is Cincinnati east or west of Chicago?), which seem to bear no relationship to TD per se.

The ability of patients to compensate for their deficits and the techniques that they use are also informative. For example, it has long been noted that some patients navigate by reference to an extensive body of minute environmental features, such as distinctive doorknobs, mailboxes, and park benches (Meyer, 1900). As discussed later, this compensatory strategy speaks both to the nature of the impairment and to the intact cognitive abilities of the patient.

Finally, the traditional sketch map production and route description tests can provide useful information in some situations. Consider the case of a patient who is able to generate accurate sketch maps of places that were unfamiliar prior to sustaining the lesion and that the patient has only experienced through direct exploratory contact. In this situation, the patient must have an intact ability to represent spatial relationships (either egocentric or exocentric) to have been able to generate this representation. In a similar vein, the demonstration of intact representational skills using these "anecdotal" clinical measures may be interpreted with slightly more confidence than impairments.

Neuropsychological Studies of Way-Finding

While the early neurological literature regarding TD contains almost exclusively case studies, the 1950s and 1960s witnessed the publication of a number of group and neuropsychological studies. The research from this era has been ably reviewed and evaluated by Barrash (1998). Essentially, these studies emphasized that lesions of the "minor hemisphere" (right) were most frequently associated with topographical difficulties and the studies initiated the process of distinguishing types of disorientation. The modern era of neuropsychological investigation of TD began with Maguire and colleagues' (Maguire, Burke, Phillips, & Staunton, 1996a) study of the performance of patients with medial temporal lesions on a standardized test of real-world wayfinding. One valuable contribution of this study was to emphasize the importance of evaluating TD within the actual, locomotor environment, as opposed to the use of table-top tests.

Twenty patients who had undergone medial temporal lobectomy (half on either side) were tested on a videotaped route-learning task. While these patients denied frank TD and did not have any measurable general memory impairments, they were impaired relative to controls on tests of route-learning and judgment of exocentric position. It is interesting that patients with left or right excisions had roughly equivalent impairments.

Another report (Bohbot et al., 1998) also examined the involvement of the hippocampal formation in topographical learning. Fourteen patients with well-defined thermocoagulation lesions of the medial temporal lobes were tested on a human analog of the Morris (Morris, Garrud, Rawlins, & O'Keefe, 1982) water maze task. Patients with lesions confined to the right parahippocampal cortex were impaired more than those with lesions of the left parahippocampal cortex, right or left hippocampus, and epileptic controls.

The focus on the medial temporal lobes in general (and the hippocampus in particular) in these studies derives from the compelling finding in rodents of "place cells" within the hippocampus. Considered in more detail later, these neurons are "tuned" to fire maximally when the rodent is within a particular position within an exocentric space. The existence of these neurons led to the proposal that the hippocampus is the anatomical site of the "cognitive map" of exocentric space emphasized by O'Keefe and Nadel (1978). As we will see, the role of the hippocampus and its adjacent structures in human navigation is still rather uncertain, but the studies of Maguire (1996a) and Bohbot (1998) demonstrated that lesions within the medial temporal lobes could impair real-world navigation.

The neuropsychological study by Barrash and colleagues (Barrash, Damasio, Adolphs, & Tranel, 2000) is notable for its comprehensive examination of patients with lesions distributed throughout the cortex on a real-world route-finding test. One hundred and twenty-seven patients with stable, focal lesions were asked to learn a complex, one-third-mile route through a hospital. The primary finding was that lesions to several discrete areas of the right hemisphere were frequently associated (>75% of the time) with impaired performance on the route-learning test. The identified area extended from the inferior medial occipital lobe (lingual and fusiform gyri) to the parahippocampal and hippocampal cortices, and also included the intraparietal sulcus and white matter of the superior parietal lobule. A much smaller region of the medial occipital lobe and parahippocampus on the left was also identified. This study is valuable in that it identifies the full extent of cortical areas that are necessary in some sense for the acquisition of new topographical knowledge.

There are two important caveats, however, which were well recognized and discussed by the authors of the study. First, the patients were studied using a comprehensive navigation task. As has been discussed, there are many different underlying cognitive impairments that might lead to the final common pathway of route-learning deficits. Therefore, the various regions identified as being necessary for intact route learning might each be involved in the task in a very different way. Second, because the patients have "natural" as opposed to experimentally induced lesions, the identification of the necessary cortical regions cannot be accepted uncritically. For example, while lesions of the right hippocampus were associated with impaired performance, a high proportion of patients with hippocampal damage also have parahippocampal damage because of the distribution of the vascular territories. If so, it is possible that damage to the parahippocampus alone is sufficient, and that the finding of an association between hippocampal lesions and impaired performance is the erroneous result of an anatomical confound.

Both of these objections can be addressed by using alternative approaches. By studying the precise cognitive deficits present in patients with localized lesions, the cognitive, way-finding responsibility of each identified region can be more precisely defined. In addition, functional neuroimaging studies in humans (although strictly providing for different kinds of inference) can be used to refine anatomical identifications without reliance upon the capricious distributions of stroke lesions. We discuss this in greater detail later.

A Taxonomy of Topographical Disorientation

Now armed with the distribution of cortical lesion sites known to be associated with route-learning impairments and with an understanding of the behavioral basis of way-finding, we can return to the cases presented originally. As we will see, these four cases each serve as an archetype for a particular variety of TD. These four varieties of TD are summarized in table 5.1, and the lesion site primarily responsible for each disorder is illustrated in figure 5.1.

Egocentric Disorientation (Case 1)

The patient described by Levine, Warach, and Farah (1985) demonstrated profound way-finding difficulties within his own home and new places following bilateral damage to the posterior parietal cortex. While he (and a number of similar patients: M.N.N., Kase, Troncoso, Court, & Tapia, 1977; Mr. Smith, Hanley, & Davies, 1995; G.W., Stark, Coslett, & Saffran, 1996; and the cases of Holmes & Horax, 1919) has been described as topographically disoriented, it is clear that his impairments extended far beyond the sphere of extended, locomotor space. To quote Levine and Farah:

[His] most striking abnormalities were visual and spatial. . . . He could not reach accurately for visual objects, even those he had identified, whether they were presented in central or peripheral visual fields. When shown two objects, he made frequent errors in stating which was nearer or farther, above or below, or to the right or left. . . .

He could not find his way about. At 4 months after the hemorrhages, he frequently got lost in his own house and never went out without a companion. . . . Spatial imagery was severely impaired. He could not say how to get from his house to the corner grocery store, a trip he had made several times a week for more than 5 years. In contrast, he could describe the store and its proprietor. His descriptions of the route were frequently bizarre: "I live a block away. I walk direct to the front door." When asked which direction he would turn on walking out of his front door, he said, "It's on the right or left, either way." . . . When,

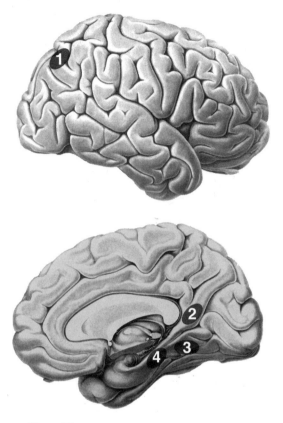

Figure 5.1
Locations of lesions responsible for varieties of topographical disorientation: (1) the posterior parietal cortex, associated with egocentric disorientation; (2) the posterior cingulate gyrus, associated with heading disorientation; (3) the lingual gyrus, associated with landmark agnosia; and (4) the parahippocampus, associated with anterograde disorientation. These sites are illustrated in the right hemisphere since the great majority of cases of topographical disorientation follow damage to right-sided cortical structures.

seated in his room, he was blindfolded and asked to point to various objects named by the examiner, he responded [very poorly]. (Levine, Warach, & Farah, 1985, p. 1013)

These patients, as a group, had severe deficits in representing the relative location of objects with respect to the self. While they were able to gesture toward objects they could see, for example, this ability was completely lost when their eyes were closed. Performance was impaired on a wide range of visual-spatial tasks, including mental rotation and spatial span tasks. It thus seems appropriate to locate the disorder within the egocentric spatial frame. Indeed, Stark and colleagues (1996) have suggested that one of these patients (G.W.) had sustained damage to a spatial map that represents information within an egocentric coordinate system. It is interesting that these cases suggest that neural systems capable of providing immediate information on egocentric position can operate independently of systems that store this information (Stark et al., 1996).

These patients were uniformly impaired in wayfinding tasks in both familiar and novel environments. Most remained confined to the hospital or home, willing to venture out only with a companion (Kase et al., 1977; Levine et al., 1985). Route descriptions were impoverished and inaccurate (Levine et al., 1985; Stark et al., 1996) and sketch map production disordered (Hanley & Davies, 1995). In contrast to these impairments, visual-object recognition was informally noted to be intact. Patient M.N.N. was able to name objects correctly without hesitation, showing an absence of agnosic features in the visual sphere. Patient G.W. had no difficulty in recognizing people or objects and case 2 of Levine et al. (1985) was able to identify common objects, pictures of objects or animals, familiar faces, or photographs of the faces of family members and celebrities.

Unfortunately, these patients were not specifically tested on visual recognition tasks employing landmark stimuli. As noted earlier, Levine and colleagues reported that their case 2 was able to describe a grocery store and its proprietor, but this

Table 5.1
A four-part taxonomy of topographical disorientation

Lesion site	Disorder label	Proposed impairment	Model case
Posterior parietal	Egocentric disorientation	Unable to represent the location of objects with respect to self	G.W. (Stark, Coslett, Saff, 1996)
Posterior cingulate gyrus	Heading disorientation	Unable to represent direction of orientation with respect to external environment	T.Y. (Suzuki, Yamador, Hayakawa, Fujii, 1998)
Lingual gyrus	Landmark agnosia	Unable to represent the appearance of salient environmental stimuli (landmarks)	· A.H. (Pallis, 1955)
Parahippocampus	Anterograde disorientation	Unable to create new representations of environmental information	G.R. (Epstein, Deyoe, Press, Rosen, Kanwisher 2001)

does not constitute a rigorous test. It is possible that despite demonstrating intact object and face recognition abilities, patients with egocentric disorientation will be impaired on recognition tasks that employ topographically relevant stimuli. Thus, until these tests are conducted, we can offer only the possibility that these patients are selectively impaired within the spatial sphere.

It seems plausible that the way-finding deficits that these patients display are a result of their profound disorientation in egocentric space. As noted earlier, route-based representations of large-scale space are formed within the egocentric spatial domain. This property of spatial representation was well illustrated by Bisiach, Brouchon, Poncet, & Rusconi's 1993 study of route descriptions in a patient with unilateral neglect. Regardless of the direction that the subject was instructed to imagine traveling, turns on the left-hand side tended to be ignored. Thus, the egocentric disorientation that these patients display seems sufficient to account for their topographical disorders. In this sense, it is perhaps inappropriate to refer to these patients as selectively topographically disoriented—their disability includes forms of spatial representation that are clearly not unique to the representation of large-scale, environmental space.

Barrash (1998) has emphasized the variable duration of the symptoms of TD. In particular, many patients who demonstrate egocentric disorientation in the days and weeks following their lesion gradually recover near-normal function. Following this initial period, patients can demonstrate a pattern of deficits described by Passini, Rainville, & Habib (2000) as being confined to "micro" as opposed to "macroscopic" space. Their distinction is perhaps more subtle than the egocentric versus exocentric classification made here, because the recovered patients may demonstrate impairments in the manipulation of technically nonegocentric spatial information (e.g., mental rotation), but do not show gross way-finding difficulties.

Those egocentrically disoriented patients for whom lesion data are available all have either bilateral or unilateral right lesions of the posterior parietal lobe, commonly involving the superior parietal lobule. Studies in animals (both lesion and electrophysiology based) support the notion that neurons in these areas are responsible for the representation of spatial information in a primarily egocentric spatial frame. Homologous cortical areas in monkeys contain cells with firing properties that represent the position of stimuli in both retinotopic and head-centered coordinate spaces simultaneously (i.e., planar gain fields; Anderson, Snyder, Li, & Stricanne, 1993). Notably, cells with exocentric firing properties have not been identified in the rodent parietal cortex, although cells responsive to complex conjunctions of stimulus egocentric position and egomotion have been reported (McNaughton et al., 1994).

Heading Disorientation (Case 2)

While the previous group of patients evidenced a global spatial disorientation, rooted in a fundamental disturbance of egocentric space, a second group of patients raises the intriguing possibility that exocentric spatial representations can be selectively damaged. These are patients who are both able to recognize salient landmarks and who do not have the dramatic egocentric disorientation described earlier. Instead, they seem unable to derive directional information from landmarks that they do recognize. They have lost a sense of exocentric direction, or "heading" within their environment.

Patient T.Y. (Suzuki et al., 1998) presented with great difficulty in way-finding following a lesion of the posterior cingulate gyrus. She showed no evidence of aphasia, acalculia, or right-left disorientation, object agnosia, prosopagnosia, or achromatopsia. She also had intact verbal and visual memory as assessed by the Wechsler Memory Scale, intact digit span, and normal performance on Raven's Progressive Matrices. Her spatial learning was intact, as demonstrated by good performance on a supraspan block test and the Porteus Maze test. In contrast to these intact abilities, T.Y. was unable to state the position from which photographs of familiar buildings were taken. Or judge her direction of heading on a map while performing a way-finding task through a college campus.

Three similar patients have been reported by Takahashi and colleagues (Takahashi, Kawamura, Shiota, Kasahata, & Hirayama, 1997). Like patient T.Y., they were unable to derive directional information from the prominent landmarks that they recognized. The patients were able to discriminate

among buildings when several photographs were displayed and were able to recognize photographs of familiar buildings and landscapes near their homes. The basic representation of egocentric space, both at immediate testing and after a 5-minute delay, was also demonstrated to be preserved. In contrast to these preserved abilities, Takahashi et al.'s patients were unable to describe routes between familiar locations and could not describe the positional (directional) relationship between one well-known place and another. In addition, the three patients were unable to draw a sketch map of their hospital floor. A patient (M.B.) reported by Cammalleri et al. (1996) had similar deficits.

Takahashi and colleagues suggested that their patients had lost the sense of direction that allows one to recall the positional relationships between one's current location and a destination within a space that cannot be fully surveyed in one glance. This can also be described as a sense of heading, in which the orientation of the body with respect to external landmarks is represented. Such a representation would be essential for both route-following and the manipulation of maplike representations of place. The possibility of isolated deficits in the representation of spatial heading is an intriguing one. These patients have a different constellation of deficits from those classified as egocentrically disoriented, and the existence of these cases suggests that separate cortical areas mediate different frames of spatial representation.

Patient T.Y., Takahashi's three patients, and patient M.B. had lesions located within the right retrosplenial (posterior cingulate) gyrus. Figure 5.2 shows the lesion site in patient T.Y. It is interesting that this area of the cortex in the rodent has been implicated in way-finding ability. Studies in rodents (Chen, Lin, Green, Barnes, & McNaughton, 1994) have identified a small population of cells within this area that fire only when the rat is maintaining a certain heading, or orientation within the environment. These cells have been dubbed "head-direction" cells (Taube, Goodridge, Golob, Dudchenko, & Stackman, 1996), and most likely

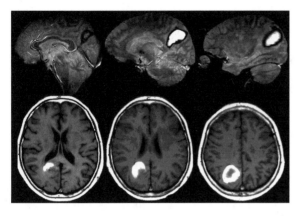

Figure 5.2
MRI scan of patient T.Y., revealing a right-sided, posterior cingulate gyrus lesion. (Images courtesy of Dr. K. Suzuki.)

generate their signals based upon a combination of landmark, vestibular, and idiothetic (self-motion) cues. Representation of the orientation of the body within a larger spatial scheme is a form of spatial representation that might be expected to be drawn upon for both route-based and map-based navigation. Neuroimaging studies in humans (considered later) have also added to this account.

Landmark Agnosia (Case 3)

The third class of topographically disoriented patient can be described as *landmark agnosic*, in that the primary component of their impairment is an inability to use prominent, salient environmental features for orientation. The patients in this category of disorientation are the most numerous and best studied.

Patient A.H. described by C. A. Pallis in 1955, woke to find that he could not recognize his bedroom and became lost trying to return from the toilet to his room. He also noted a central "blind spot," an inability to see color, and that all faces seemed alike. He quickly became lost upon leaving his house, and was totally unable to recognize what had previously been very familiar surroundings.

Upon admission, the patient was found to have visual field deficits consistent with two adjacent, upper quadrantic scotomata, each with its apex at the fixation point. A.H. had no evidence of neglect, was able to localize objects accurately in both the left and right hemifields and had intact stereognostic perception, proprioception, and graphaesthetic sense. There was no left-right confusion, acalculia, or apraxia. General memory was reported as completely intact. A.H.'s digit span was eight forward and six backward, and he repeated the Babcock sentence correctly on his first try.

The patient had evident difficulty recognizing faces. He was unable to recognize his medical attendants, wife, or daughter, and failed to identify pictures of famous, contemporary faces. He had similar difficulty identifying pictures of animals, although a strategy of scrutinizing the photos for a critical detail that would allow him to intuit the identity of the image was more successful here than for the pictures of human faces. For example, he was able to identify a picture of a cat by the whiskers.

His primary and most distressing complaint was his inability to recognize places:

In my mind's eye I know exactly where places are, what they look like. I can visualize T . . . square without difficulty, and the streets that come into it. . . . I can draw you a plan of the roads from Cardiff to the Rhondda Valley. . . . It's when I'm out that the trouble starts. My reason tells me I must be in a certain place and yet I don't recognize it. It all has to be worked out each time. . . . For instance, one night, having taken the wrong turning, I was going to call for my drink at the Post Office. . . . I have to keep the idea of the route in my head the whole time, and count the turnings, as if I were following instructions that had been memorized. (Pallis, 1955, p. 219)

His difficulty extended to new places as well as previously familiar locales: "It's not only the places I knew before all this happened that I can't remember. Take me to a new place now and tomorrow I couldn't get there myself" (Pallis, 1955, p. 219). Despite these evident problems with way-finding, the patient was still able to describe and draw maps of the places that were familiar to him prior to his illness, including the layout of the mineshafts in which he worked as an engineer.

Patient A.H. is joined in the literature by a number of well-studied cases, including patients J.C. (Whiteley & Warrington, 1978), A.R. (Hécaen, Tzortzis, & Rondot, 1980), S.E. (McCarthy, Evans, & Hodges, 1996), and M.S. (Rocchetta, Cipolotti, & Warrington, 1996); several of the cases reported by Landis, Cummings, Benson, & Palmer (1986); and the cases reported by Takahashi, Kawamura, Hirayama, & Tagawa (1989); Funakawa, Mukai, Terao, Kawashima, & Mori (1994), and Suzuki, Yamadori, Takase, Nagamine, & Itoyama (1996). These patients have several features in common: (1) disorientation in previously familiar and novel places, (2) intact manipulation of spatial information, and (3) an inability to identify specific buildings. In other words, despite a preserved ability to provide spatial information about a familiar environment, the patient is unable to find his or her way because of the inability to recognize prominent landmarks.

This loss of landmark recognition, and its relative specificity, has been formally tested by several authors, usually by asking the subject to identify pictures of famous buildings. Patient S.E. (McCarthy et al., 1996) was found to be markedly impaired at recalling the name or information about

pictures of famous landmarks and buildings compared with the performance of control subjects and his own performance recalling information about famous people.

Patient M.S. (Rocchetta et al., 1996) performed at chance level on three different delayed-recognition memory tests that used pictures of (1) complex city scenes, (2) previously unfamiliar buildings, and (3) country scenes. M.S. was also found to be impaired at recognizing London landmarks that were familiar before his illness. Takahashi and colleagues (1989) obtained seventeen pictures of the patient's home and neighborhood. The patient was unable to recognize any of these, but he could describe from memory the trees planted in the garden, the pattern printed on his fence, the shape of his mailbox and windows, and was able to produce an accurate map of his house and hometown.

In contrast, tests of spatial representation have generally shown intact abilities in these patients. Patients S.E., M.S., and J.C. were all found to have normal performance on a battery of spatial learning and perceptual tasks that included Corsi span, Corsi supraspan, and "stepping-stone" mazes (Milner, 1965). (Patient A.R., however, was found to be impaired on the last of these tests.) In general, the ability to describe routes and produce sketch maps of familiar places is intact in these patients. As discussed previously, these more anecdotal measures of intact spatial representation should be treated with some caution because there is considerable ambiguity as to the specific nature of the cognitive requirements of these tasks. Nonetheless, the perfectly preserved ability of patients A.R. and A.H. to provide detailed route descriptions, and the detailed and accurate maps produced by S.E., A.H., and Takahashi's patient (Takahashi et al., 1989), are suggestive of intact spatial representations of some kind. (Patient M.S., however, was noted to have poor route description abilities.) Particularly compelling, moreover, are reports of patients producing accurate maps of places that were not familiar prior to the lesion event (Cole & Perez-Cruet, 1964; Whiteley & Warrington, 1978). In this case, the patient can only be drawing upon preserved spatial representational abilities to successfully transform navigational experiences into an exocentric representation.

Several neuropsychological deficits have been noted to co-occur with landmark agnosia, specifically, prosopagnosia (Cole & Perez-Cruet, 1964; Landis et al., 1986; McCarthy et al., 1996; Pallis, 1955; Takahashi et al., 1989) and achromatopsia (Landis et al., 1986; Pallis, 1955), along with some degree of visual field deficit. These impairments do not invariably accompany landmark agnosia (e.g., Hécaen et al., 1980), however, and are known to occur without accompanying TD (e.g., Tohgi et al., 1994). Thus it is unlikely that these ancillary impairments are actually the causative factor of TD. More likely, the lesion site that produces landmark agnosia is close to, but distinct from, the lesion sites responsible for prosopagnosia and achromatopsia.

There is also evidence that landmark agnosics have altered perception of environmental features, in addition to the loss of familiarity (as is the case with general-object agnosics and prosopagnosics; Farah, 1990). For example, Hécaen's patient A.R. was able to perform a "cathedral matching" task accurately, but "he [AR] spontaneously indicated that he was looking only for specific details 'a window, a doorway . . . but not the whole.' . . . Places were identified by a laborious process of elimination based on small details" (Hécaen et al., 1980, p. 531).

An additional hallmark feature of landmark agnosia is the compensatory strategy employed by these patients. The description of patient J.C. is typical:

He relies heavily on street names, station names, and house numbers. For example, he knows that to get to the shops he has to turn right at the traffic lights and then left at the Cinema. . . . When he changes his place of work he draws a plan of the route to work and a plan of the interior of the "new" building. He relies on these maps and plans. . . . He recognizes his own house by the number or by his car when parked at the door. (Whiteley & Warrington, 1978, pp. 575–576)

This reliance upon small environmental details, called variously "signs," "symbols," and "landmarks" by the different authors, is common to all of the landmark agnosia cases described here and provides some insight into the cognitive nature of the impairment. First, it is clear that these patients are capable of representing the strictly spatial aspect of their position in the environment. In order to make use of these minute environmental details for wayfinding, the patient must be able to associate spatial information (if only left or right turns) with particular waypoints. This is again suggestive evidence of intact spatial abilities. Second, although these patients are termed "landmark agnosics," it is not the case that they are unable to make use of any environmental object with orienting value. Instead, they seem specifically impaired in the use of high-salience environmental features, such as buildings, and the arrangement of natural and artificial stimuli into scenes. Indeed, these patients become disoriented within buildings, suggesting that they are no longer able to represent a configuration of stimuli that allows them to easily differentiate one place from another. It thus seems that careful study of landmark agnosics may provide considerable insight into the normative process of selection and utilization of landmarks.

The parallels between prosopagnosia and landmark agnosia (which we might refer to as *synoragnosia*, from the Greek for landmark) are striking. Prosopagnosic patients are aware that they are viewing a face, but do not have access to the effortless perception of facial identity that characterizes normal performance. They also develop compensatory strategies that focus on the individual parts of the face, often distinguishing one person from another by careful study of the particular shape of the hairline, for example.

The lesion sites reported to produce landmark agnosia are fairly well clustered. Except for patient J.C. (who suffered a closed head injury and for whom no imaging data are available) and patient M.S. (who suffered diffuse small-vessel ischemic disease), the cases of landmark agnosia reviewed here all had lesions either bilaterally or on the right side of the medial aspect of the occipital lobe, involving the lingual gyrus and sometimes the parahippocampal gyrus. The most common mechanism of injury is an infarction of the right posterior cerebral artery.

The type of visual information that is represented in this critical area of the lingual gyrus is an open question. Is this a region involved in the representation of all landmark information, or simply certain object classes that happen to be used as landmarks? How would such a region come to exist? One account of the "lingual landmark area" (Aguirre, Zarahn, & D'Esposito, 1998a) posits the existence of a cortical region predisposed to the representation of the visual information employed in wayfinding. Through experience, this area comes to represent environmental features and visual configurations that have landmark value (i.e., that tend to aid navigation). We might imagine that such a spatially segregated, specialized area would develop because of the natural correlation of some landmark features with other landmark features (Polk & Farah, 1995). Furthermore, such a region might occupy a consistent area of cortex from person to person as a result of the connection of the area with other visual areas (e.g., connections to areas with large receptive fields or to areas that process "optic flow").

We have a sense from environmental psychology studies of the types of visual features that would come to be represented in such an area: large, immobile things located at critical, navigational choice points in the environment. Certainly buildings fit the bill for western, urban dwellers. We might suspect that in other human populations that navigate through entirely different environments, different kinds of visual information would be represented. In either case, lesions to this area would produce the pattern of deficits seen in the reported cases of landmark agnosia. Evidence for such an account has been provided by neuroimaging studies in intact human subjects, which are considered below.

Anterograde Disorientation and the Medial Temporal Lobes (Case 4)

Our discussion so far has focused on varieties of TD that follow damage to neocortical structures. The posterior parietal cortex, the posterior cingulate gyrus, and areas of the medial fusiform gyrus have all been associated with distinct forms of navigational impairments. Despite this, much of the extant TD literature has been concerned with an area of the paleocortex: the medial temporal lobes. As mentioned previously, this focus on the medial temporal lobes derives from the compelling neurophysiological finding that hippocampal cells in the rodent fire selectively when the freely moving animal is in certain locations within the environment. The existence of these place cells is the basis for theories that offer the hippocampus as a repository of information about exocentric spatial relationships (O'Keefe & Nadel, 1978). Additional evidence regarding the importance of the hippocampus in animal spatial learning was provided by Morris and colleagues (1982), who reported that rats with hippocampal lesions were impaired on a test of place learning, the water maze task. The specificity of the role played by the hippocampus (i.e., Ammon's horn, the dentate gyrus, and the subiculum) in spatial representation has subsequently been debated at length (e.g., Cohen & Eichenbaum, 1993).

At the very least, it is clear that selective (neurotoxic), bilateral lesions of this structure in the rodent greatly impair performance in place learning tasks such as the water maze (Jarrard, 1993; Morris, Schenk, Tweedie, & Jarrard, 1990). The central role of the hippocampus in theories of spatial learning in animals has influenced the neurological literature on TD to some extent. For example, many case reports of topographically disoriented patients with neocortical damage are at pains to relate the lesion location to some kind of disruption of hippocampal function (e.g., through disconnection or loss of input).

In recent decades, the "cognitive map" theory has come to be contrasted with models of medial temporal lobe function in the realm of long-term memory. In this account, which is supported primarily through lesion studies in human patients, the hippocampus is responsible for the initial formation and maintenance of "declarative" memories, which over a period of months are subsequently consolidated within the neocortex and become independent of hippocampal function.

What of the impact of medial temporal lesions upon navigational ability? It is clear that unilateral lesions of the hippocampus do not produce any appreciable real-world way-finding impairments in humans (DeRenzi, 1982). While one study (Vargha-Khadem et al., 1997) has reported anterograde way-finding deficits in the setting of general anterograde amnesia following bilateral damage restricted to the hippocampus, this obviously cannot be considered a selective loss. Other studies of patients with bilateral hippocampal damage have not commented upon anterograde way-finding ability (Rempel-Clower, Zola, Squire, & Amaral, 1996; Scoville & Milner, 1957; Zola-Morgan, Squire, & Amaral, 1986). Retrograde loss of way-finding knowledge in

these patients is not apparently disproportionate to losses in other areas (Rempel-Clower et al., 1996) and this knowledge can be preserved (Milner, Corkin, & Teuber, 1968; Teng & Squire, 1999).

Cases have been reported, however, of topographical impairment that is primarily confined to novel environments, although it is not associated with lesions to the hippocampus per se. It is interesting that this anterograde TD, described in two patients by Ross (1980), one patient by Pai (1997), the patient of Luzzi, Pucci, Di Bella, & Piccirilli (2000), and the first two cases of Habib and Sirigu (1987), appears to affect both landmark and spatial spheres. By far the most comprehensive study has been provided by Epstein and colleagues (2001) in their examination of patients G.R. and C.G.

At the time of testing, G.R. was a well-educated, 60-year-old man who had suffered right and left occipital-temporal strokes 2 years previously. Figure 5.3 shows the lesion site in this patient. These strokes had left him with a left hemianopsia and right upper quadrantanopsia and dyschromatopsia. He had no evidence of neglect, left-right

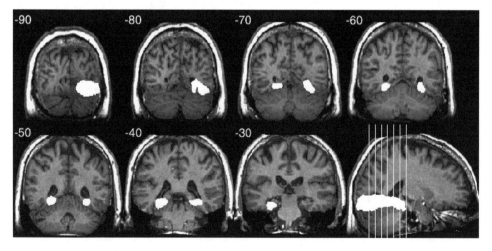

Figure 5.3
MRI scan of patient G.R., revealing bilateral damage to the parahippocampal gyri, with extension of the right lesion posteriorly to involve the inferior lingual gyrus, medial fusiform gyrus, and occipital lobe. (Images courtesy of Dr. R. Epstein.)

confusion or apraxia, and no prosopagnosia or object agnosia. His primary disability was a dramatic inability to orient himself in new places:

According to both GR and his wife, this inability to learn new topographical information was typical of his experience since his strokes, as he frequently gets lost in his daily life. Soon after his injury, he moved to a neighborhood with many similar-looking houses. He reported that in order to find his new house after a walk to a market 6–7 blocks away, he had to rely on street signs to guide him to the correct block, and then examine each house on the block in detail until he could recognize some feature that uniquely distinguished his home. Subsequently, GR and his wife moved to a different house in a different country. He reported that for the first six months after the move, his new home was like a "haunted house" for him insofar as he was unable to learn his way around it. (Epstein et al., 2001, p. 5)

Epstein noted the inability of the patient to learn his way about the laboratory testing area despite repeat visits, and described the results of a landmark learning test in which the subject performed rather poorly. In contrast, G.R. was able to successfully follow a route marked on a map, indicating intact, basic spatial representation. In addition, G.R. was able to draw accurate sketch maps of places known to him prior to his stroke and performed the same as age-matched controls on a recognition test of famous landmarks. These findings suggest that G.R. had intact representation of previously learned spatial and landmark topographical information. Epstein and colleagues report the results of additional tests that suggest that G.R.'s primary deficit was in the encoding of novel information on the appearance of spatially extended scenes.

The patients reported by Habib and Sirigu (1987) and those of Ross (1980) had similar impairments. All four patients displayed preserved way-finding in environments known at least 6 months before their lesion. Ross's patient 1 was able to draw a very accurate map of his parent's home. Both case 1 and case 2 of Habib and Sirigu reported that following an initial period of general impairment, no orientation difficulties were encountered in familiar parts of town.

The lesion site in common among these cases is the posterior aspect of the right parahippocampus. Figure 5.3 shows the lesion site in patient G.R. This finding is in keeping with the results of the group neuropsychological studies reported earlier. Both Bohbot and Barrash found that lesions of the right parahippocampus were highly associated with deficits in real-world topographical ability. One caveat regarding localization of this lesion site is that lesions of the parahippocampus typically occur in concert with lesions of the medial lingual gyrus, the area described earlier as consistently involved in landmark agnosia. Can we be certain that landmark agnosia and anterograde disorientation actually result from lesions to two differentiable cortical areas? The report by Takahashi and Kawamura (in press), who studied the performance of four patients with TD, is helpful in this regard. They observed that the patient with damage restricted to the parahippocampus was impaired in the acquisition of novel topographical information (they tested scene learning), while the other patients with lesions that included the medial lingual gyrus displayed difficulty recognizing previously familiar scenes and buildings, in addition to an anterograde impairment.

Despite the case literature that argues for the primacy of the parahippocampus within the medial temporal lobe for way-finding, other lines of evidence continue to raise intriguing questions regarding the role of the hippocampus proper. Maguire and colleagues (2000) recently reported that London taxicab drivers, who are required to assimilate an enormous quantity of topographical information, have larger posterior hippocampi than control subjects. Moreover, the size of the posterior hippocampus across drivers was correlated with the number of years they had spent on the job! The neuroimaging literature reviewed in the next section has also found neural activity within hippocampal areas in the setting of topographically relevant tasks.

Functional Neuroimaging Studies

Functional neuroimaging studies of topographical representation fall into two broad categories: (1) those that have sought the neural substrates of the entire cognitive process of topographical representation and (2) those that have examined subcomponents of environmental knowledge.

In the first category, one of the earliest studies was that by Aguirre, Detre, Alsop, & D'Esposito (1996). The subjects were studied with functional MRI (fMRI) while they attempted to learn their way through a "virtual reality" maze. When the signal obtained during these periods was compared with that obtained while the subjects repetitively traversed a simple corridor, greater activity was observed within the parahippocampus bilaterally, the posterior parietal cortex, the retrosplenial cortex, and the medial occipital cortex. This study did not attempt to isolate the different cognitive elements that are presumed to make up the complex behavior of way-finding. Thus, the most we can conclude from this study (and studies of its kind) is that the regions identified are activated by some aspect of way-finding.

Since then, Maguire and colleagues have published a number of neuroimaging studies that present clever refinements of this basic approach: presenting subjects with virtual reality environments in which they perform tasks (Maguire, Frackowiak, & Frith, 1996b, 1997; Maguire, Frith, Burgess, Donnett, & O'Keefe, 1998a; Maguire et al., 1998b). A consistent finding in their work has been the presence of activity within the hippocampus proper, particularly in association with successful navigation in more complex and realistic virtual reality environments. Parahippocampal activity has also been a component of the activated areas, although Maguire has argued that this is driven more by the presence of landmarks within the testing environment than the act of navigation itself. The interested reader is referred to Maguire, Burgess, & O'Keefe (1999) for a cogent review.

Clearly, something interesting is happening in the hippocampus proper in association with navigation tasks. What is intriguing, however, is the absence of clinical or even neuropsychological findings of topographical impairments in association with lesions of this structure. The existence of this seeming conflict points to the inferential limitations of functional neuroimaging studies. The behaviors under study are enormously complicated, making any attempt to isolate them by cognitive subtraction (a standard technique of neuroimaging inference) questionable.

It will always be possible that activity in the hippocampus (or any other area) is the result of confounding and uncontrolled behaviors that differ between the two conditions. Even if we could be certain that we have isolated the cognitive process of navigation, it would still be possible to observe neural activity in cortical regions that are not necessary for this function (Aguirre, Zarahn, & D'Esposito, 1998b). Regardless, the individual contributions of areas of the medial temporal lobes to navigational abilities in humans remains an area of active investigation.

The second class of neuroimaging study has sought the neural correlates of particular subcomponents of environmental representation. At the most basic level of division, Aguirre and D'Esposito (1997) sought to demonstrate a dorsal-ventral dissociation of cortical responsiveness for manipulation of judgments about landmark identity and direction in environmental spaces. Their subjects became familiar with a complex virtual reality town over a period of a few days. During scanning, the subjects were presented with scenes from the environment and asked to either identify their current location or, if given the name of the place, to judge the compass direction of a different location. Consistent with the division of topographical representation outlined earlier, medial lingual areas responded during location identification, while posterior cingulate and posterior parietal areas responded during judgments about heading.

Further studies have refined this gross division. Aguirre and colleagues (1998a) tested the hypothesis that the causative lesion in landmark agnosia damages a substrate specialized for the perception of buildings and large-scale environmental landmarks. Using functional MRI, they identified a cortical area that has a greater neural response to buildings than to other stimuli, including faces, cars, general objects, and phase-randomized buildings. Across subjects, the voxels that evidenced "building" responses were located straddling the anterior end of the right lingual sulcus, which is in good agreement with the lesion sites reported for landmark agnosia. The finding of a "building-sensitive" cortex within the anterior, right lingual gyrus has been replicated by other groups (Ishai, Ungerlieder, Martin, & Schouten, 1999).

Epstein and his colleagues have studied the conditions under which parahippocampal activity is elicited. Their initial finding (Epstein & Kanwisher, 1998) was that perception of spatially extended scenes (either indoor or outdoors) elicited robust activation of the parahippocampus. These responses were equivalent whether the pictured rooms contained objects or were simply bare walls! In a series of follow-up studies (Epstein, Harris, Stanley, & Kanwisher, 1999), Epstein has found that activity in the parahippocampus is particularly sensitive to the encoding of new perceptual information regarding the appearance and layout of spatially extended scenes. These findings dovetail nicely with the pattern of anterograde deficits that have been reported in patients with parahippocampal damage.

Conclusions and Future Directions

The past decade has seen the development of several key insights into the nature of TD. Driven by the success of the cognitive neuroscience program, it is now possible to attribute varieties of topographical disorientation to particular impairments in cognitive function. When presented with a patient with TD, a series of simple questions and tests should be sufficient to place the patient within one of the four categories of disorientation described. Is the patient grossly disoriented within egocentric space? Can he find his way about places known to him prior to his injury? Does he make

now use of a different set of environmental cues, in place of large-scale features like buildings? Can he recognize landmarks but is uncertain of which direction to travel next? When the cognitive categorization is consonant with the lesion observed, the clinician can be fairly confident of the type of TD experienced by the patient.

In many cases, the degree of impairment improves over the months following the lesion, particularly in the case of egocentric and anterograde disorientation (Barrash, 1998). For those patients with landmark agnosia, encouragement in the use of environmental features other than large-scale landmarks may be helpful in returning the patient to a normal way-finding function.

The clinical syndrome of topographical disorientation remains an area of active investigation for several groups. More generally, the tools and models of cognitive neuroscience are now being applied to the problems of normative way-finding. Unresolved issues concern the relative contributions of areas of the medial temporal lobes, explicit demonstration of the representation of heading in the posterior cingulate gyrus and a better understanding of the development and representational properties of the lingual gyrus.

References

Acredolo, L. P. (1977). Developmental changes in the ability to coordinate perspectives of a large-scale space. *Developmental Psychology, 13,* 1–8.

Aguirre, G. K., & D'Esposito, M. (1997). Environmental knowledge is subserved by separable dorsal/ventral neural areas. *Journal of Neuroscience, 17,* 2512–2518.

Aguirre, G. K., & D'Esposito, M. (1999). Topographical disorientation: A synthesis and taxonomy. *Brain, 122,* 1613–1628.

Aguirre, G. K., Detre, J. A., Alsop, D. C., & D'Esposito, M. (1996). The parahippocampus subserves topographical learning in man. *Cerebral Cortex, 6,* 823–829.

Aguirre, G. K., Zarahn, E., & D'Esposito, M. (1998a). An area within human ventral cortex sensitive to "building" stimuli: Evidence and implications. *Neuron, 21,* 373–383.

Aguirre, G. K., Zarahn, E., & D'Esposito, M. (1998b). Neural components of topographical representation. *Proceedings of the National Academy of Sciences, U.S.A., 95,* 839–846.

Allen, G. L., Kirasic, K. C., Siegel, A. W., & Herman, J. F. (1979). Developmental issues in cognitive mapping: The selection and utilization of environmental landmarks. *Child Development, 50,* 1062–1070.

Anderson, R. A., Snyder, L. H., Li, C.-S., & Stricanne, B. (1993). Coordinate transformations in the representation of spatial information. *Current Opinion in Neurobiology, 3,* 171–176.

Appleyard, D. (1969). Why buildings are known. *Environment and Behavior, 1,* 131–156.

Barrash, J. (1998). A historical review of topographical disorientation and its neuroanatomical correlates. *Journal of Clinical and Experimental Neuropsychology, 20,* 807–827.

Barrash, J., Damasio, H., Adolphs, R., & Tranel, D. (2000). The neuroanatomical correlates of route learning impairment. *Neuropsychologia, 38,* 820–836.

Bisiach, E., Brouchon, M., Poncet, M., & Rusconi, M. (1993). Unilateral neglect and route description. *Neuropsychologia, 31,* 1255–1262.

Bohbot, V. D., Kalina, M., Stepankova, K., Spackova, N., Petrides, M., & Nadel, L. (1998). Spatial memory deficits in patients with lesions to the right hippocampus and to the right parahippocampal cortex. *Neuropsychologia, 36,* 1217–1238.

Byrne, R. W. (1982). Geographical knowledge and orientation. In A. W. Ellis (Ed.), *Normality and pathology in cognitive functions.* London: Academic Press.

Cammalleri, R., Gangitano, M., D'Amelio, M., Raieli, V., Raimondo, D., & Camarda, R. (1996). Transient topographical amnesia and cingulate cortex damage: A case report. *Neuropsychologia, 34,* 321–326.

Chen, L. L., Lin, L. H., Green, E. J., Barnes, C. A., & McNaughton, B. L. (1994). Head-direction cells in the rat posterior cortex. I. Anatomical distribution and behavioral modulation. *Experimental Brain Research, 101,* 8–23.

Cohen, N. J., & Eichenbaum, H. (1993). *Memory, amnesia and the hippocampal system.* Cambridge MA: MIT Press.

Cole, M., & Perez-Cruet, J. (1964). Prosopagnosia. *Neuropsychologia, 2,* 237–346.

DeRenzi, E. (1982). *Disorders of space exploration and cognition.* Chichester: Wiley.

DeRenzi, E., & Faglioni, P. (1962). Il disorientamento spaziale da lesione cerebrale. *Sistema Nervoso, 14,* 409–436.

Epstein, R., DeYoe, E. A., Press, D. Z., Rosen, A. C., & Kanwisher, N. (2001). Neuopsychological evidence for a topographical learning mechanism in parahippocampal cortex. *Cognitive Neuropsychology, 18,* 481–508.

Epstein, R., Harris, A., Stanley, D., & Kanwisher, N. (1999). The parahippocampal place area: Recognition, navigation, or encoding? *Neuron, 23,* 115–125.

Epstein, R., & Kanwisher, N. (1998). A cortical representation of the local visual environment. *Nature, 392*(6676), 598–601.

Farah, M. J. (1990). *Visual agnosia: Disorders of object recognition and what they tell us about normal vision.* Cambridge, MA: MIT Press.

Farrell, M. J. (1996). Topographical disorientation. *Neurocase, 2,* 509–520.

Funakawa, I., Mukai, K., Terao, A., Kawashima, S., & Mori, T. (1994). (A case of MELAS associated with prosopagnosia, topographical disorientation and PLED) *Rinsho Shinkeigaku (Clinical Neurology), 34,* 1052–1054.

Habib, M., & Sirigu, A. (1987). Pure topographical disorientation: A definition and anatomical basis. *Cortex, 23,* 73–85.

Hanley, J. R., & Davies, A. D. (1995). Lost in your own house. In R. Campbell & M. A. Conway (Eds.), *Broken memories* (pp. 195–208). Oxford: Blackwell.

Hécaen, H., Tzortzis, C., & Rondot, P. (1980). Loss of topographic memory with learning deficits. *Cortex, 16,* 525–542.

Holmes, G., & Horax, G. (1919). Disturbances of spatial orientation and visual attention with loss of stereoscopic vision. *Archives of Neurology and Psychiatry, 1,* 385–407.

Ishai, A., Ungerleider, L. G., Martin, A., Schouten, J. L., & Haxby, J. V. (1999). Distributed representation of objects in the human ventral visual pathway. *Proceedings of the National Academy of Sciences U.S.A., 96,* 9379–9384.

Jarrard, L. E. (1993). On the role of the hippocampus in learning and memory in the rat. *Behavioral and Neural Biology, 60,* 9–26.

Kase, C. S., Troncoso, J. F., Court, J. E., Tapia, J. F., & Mohr, J. P. (1977). Global spatial disorientation. Clinico-pathologic correlations. *Journal of the Neurological Sciences, 34,* 267–278.

Landis, T., Cummings, J. L., Benson, D. F., & Palmer, E. P. (1986). Loss of topographic familiarity. *Archives of Neurology, 43*, 132–136.

Levine, D. N., Warach, J., & Farah, M. J. (1985). Two visual systems in mental imagery: Dissociation of "what" and "where" in imagery disorders due to bilateral posterior cerebral lesions. *Neurology, 35*, 1010–1018.

Luzzi, S., Pucci, E., Di Bella, P., & Piccirilli, M. (2000). Topographical disorientation consequent to amnesia of spatial location in a patient with right parahippocampal damage. *Cortex, 36*, 427–434.

Maguire, E. A., Burgess, N., Donnett, J. G., Frackowiak, R. S., Frith, C. D., & O'Keefe, J. (1998b). Knowing where and getting there: A human navigation network. *Science, 280*, 921–924.

Maguire, E. A., Burgess, N., & O'Keefe, J. (1999). Human spatial navigation: Cognitive maps, sexual dimorphism, and neural substrates. *Current Opinion in Neurobiology, 9*, 171–177.

Maguire, E. A., Burke, T., Phillips, J., & Staunton, H. (1996a). Topographical disorientation following unilateral temporal lobe lesions in humans. *Neuropsychologia, 34*, 993–1001.

Maguire, E. A., Frackowiak, R. S. J., & Frith, C. D. (1996b). Learning to find your way: A role for the human hippocampal formation. *Proceedings of the Royal Society of London, Ser. B, 263*, 1745–1750.

Maguire, E. A., Frackowiak, R. S. J., & Frith, C. D. (1997). Recalling routes around London: Activation of the right hippocampus in taxi drivers. *Journal of Neuroscience, 17*, 7103–7110.

Maguire, E. A., Frith, C. D., Burgess, N., Donnett, J. G., & O'Keefe, J. (1998a). Knowing where things are: Parahippocampal involvement in encoding object locations in virtual large-scale space. *10*, 61–76.

Maguire, E. A., Gadian, D. G., Johnsrude, I. S., Good, C. D., Ashburner, J., Frackowiak, R. S., & Frith, C. D. (2000). Navigation-related structural change in the hippocampi of taxi drivers. *Proceedings of the National Academy of Sciences U.S.A., 97*, 4398–4403.

McCarthy, R. A., Evans, J. J., & Hodges, J. R. (1996). Topographical amnesia: Spatial memory disorder, perceptual dysfunction, or category-specific semantic memory impairment? *Journal of Neurology, Neurosurgery and Psychiatry, 60*, 318–325.

McNaughton, B. L., Mizumori, S. J., Barnes, C. A., Leonard, B. J., Marquis, M., & Green, E. J. (1994). Cortical representation of motion during unrestrained spatial navigation in the rat. *Cerebral Cortex, 4*, 27–39.

Meyer, O. (1900). Ein- und doppelseitige homonyme hemianopsie mit orientierungsstörungen. *Monatschrift für Psychiatrie und Neurologic, 8*, 440–456.

Milner, B. (1965). Visually-guided maze learning in man: Effects of bilateral hippocampal, bilateral frontal, and unilateral cerebral lesions. *Neuropsychologia, 3*, 317–338.

Milner, B., Corkin, S., & Teuber, H.-L. (1968). Further analysis of the hippocampal amnesic syndrome: 14-year follow-up study of HM. *Neuropsychologia, 6*, 215–234.

Morris, R. G., Garrud, P., Rawlins, J. N., & O'Keefe, J. (1982). Place navigation impaired in rats with hippocampal lesions. *Nature, 297*, 681–683.

Morris, R. G., Schenk, F., Tweedie, F., & Jarrard, L. F. (1990). Ibotenate lesions of the hippocampus and/or subiculum: Dissociating components of allocentric spatial learning. *European Journal of Neuroscience, 2*, 1016–1028.

Newcombe, F., & Ritchie, R. W. (1969). Dissociated visual perception and spatial deficits in focal lesions of the right hemisphere. *Journal of Neurology, 32*, 73–81.

O'Keefe, J., & Nadel, L. (1978). *The hippocampus as a cognitive map*. Oxford: Oxford University Press.

Pai, M. C. (1997). Topographic disorientation: Two cases. *Journal of the Formosan Medical Association, 96*, 660–663.

Pallis, C. A. (1955). Impaired identification of locus and places with agnosia for colours. *Journal of Neurology, Neurosurgery and Psychiatry, 18*, 218–224.

Passini, R., Rainville, C., & Habib, M. (2000). Spatiocognitive deficits in right parietal lesion and its impact on wayfinding: A case study. *Neurocase, 6*, 245–257.

Piaget, J., Inhelder, B., & Szeminska, A. (1960). *The child's conception of geometry*. New York: Basic Books.

Pick, H. L. (1993). Organization of spatial knowledge in children. In N. Eilan, R. McCarthy, & B. Brewer (Eds.), *Spatial representation* (pp. 31–42). Oxford: Blackwell.

Polk, T. A., & Farah, M. J. (1995). Brain localization for arbitrary stimulus categories: A simple account based on Hebbian learning. *Proceedings of the National Academy of Sciences U.S.A., 92*, 12370–12373.

Presson, C. C. (1987). The development of landmarks in spatial memory: The role of differential experience. *Journal of Clinical and Experimental Neuropsychology, 20*, 807–827.

Rempel-Clower, N. L., Zola, S. M., Squire, L. R., & Amaral, D. G. (1996). Three cases of enduring memory impairment after bilateral damage limited to the hippocampal formation. *Journal of Neuroscience, 16,* 5233–5255.

Rocchetta, A. I., Cipolotti, L., & Warrington, E. K. (1996). Topographical disorientation: Selective impairment of locomotor space? *Cortex, 32,* 727–735.

Ross, E. D. (1980). Sensory-specific and fractional disorders of recent memory in man: I. Isolated loss of visual recent memory. *Archives of Neurology, 37,* 193–200.

Scoville, W. B., & Milner, B. (1957). Loss of recent memory after bilateral hippocampal lesions. *Journal of Neurology, Neurosurgery and Psychiatry, 20,* 11–21.

Siegel, A. W., Kirasic, K. C., & Kail, R. V. (1978). Stalking the elusive cognitive map: The development of children's representations of geographic space. In J. F. Wohlwill & I. Altman (Eds.), *Human behavior and environment: Children and the environment* (Vol. 3). New York: Plenum.

Siegel, A. W., & White, S. H. (1975). The development of spatial representation of large-scale environments. In H. W. Reese (Ed.), *Advances in child development and behavior.* New York: Academic Press.

Stark, M., Coslett, B., & Saffran, E. M. (1996). Impairment of an egocentric map of locations: Implications for perception and action. *Cognitive Neuropsychology, 13,* 481–523.

Suzuki, K., Yamadori, A., Hayakawa, Y., & Fujii, T. (1998). Pure topographical disorientation related to dysfunction of the viewpoint-dependent visual system. *Cortex, 34,* 589–599.

Suzuki, K., Yamadori, A., Takase, S., Nagamine, Y., & Itoyama, Y. (1996). (Transient prosopagnosia and lasting topographical disorientation after the total removal of a right occipital arteriovenous malformation) *Rinsho Shinkeigaku (Clinical Neurology), 36,* 1114–1117.

Takahashi, N., & Kawamura, M. (in press). Pure topographical disorientation—The anatomical basis of topographical agnosia. *Cortex.*

Takahashi, N., Kawamura, M., Hirayama, K., & Tagawa, K. (1989). (Non-verbal facial and topographic visual object agnosia—a problem of familiarity in prosopagnosia and topographic disorientation) *No to Shinkei (Brain & Nerve), 41*(7), 703–710.

Takahashi, N., Kawamura, M., Shiota, J., Kasahata, N., & Hirayama, K. (1997). Pure topographic disorientation due to right retrosplenial lesion. *Neurology, 49,* 464–469.

Taube, J. S., Goodridge, J. P., Golob, E. J., Dudchenko, P. A., & Stackman, R. W. (1996). Processing the head direction cell signal: A review and commentary. *Brain Research Bulletin, 40,* 477–486.

Taylor, H., & Tversky, B. (1992). Spatial mental models derived from survey and route descriptions. *Journal of Memory & Language, 31,* 261–282.

Teng, E., & Squire, L. R. (1999). Memory for places learned long ago is intact after hippocampal damage. *Science, 400,* 675–677.

Thorndyke, P. (1981). Spatial cognition and reasoning. In J. Harvey (Ed.), *Cognition, social behavior, and the environment.* Hillsdale, NJ: Lawrence Erlbaum Associates.

Thorndyke, P. W., & Hayes, R. B. (1982). Differences in spatial knowledge acquired from maps and navigation. *Cognitive Psychology, 14,* 560–589.

Tohgi, H., Watanabe, K., Takahashi, H., Yonezawa, H., Hatano, K., & Sasaki, T. (1994). Prosopagnosia without topographagnosia and object agnosia associated with a lesion confined to the right occipitotemporal region. *Journal of Neurology, 241,* 470–474.

Vargha-Khadem, F., Gadian, D. G., Watkins, K. E., Connolly, A., Van Paesschen, W., & Mishkin, M. (1997). Differential effects of early hippocampal pathology on episodic and semantic memory. *Science, 277,* 376–380.

Whiteley, A. M., & Warrington, E. K. (1978). Selective impairment of topographical memory: A single case study. *Journal of Neurology, Neurosurgery and Psychiatry, 41,* 575–578.

Zola-Morgan, S., Squire, L. R., & Amaral, D. G. (1986). Human amnesia and the medial temporal region: Enduring memory impairment following a bilateral lesion limited to field CA1 of the hippocampus. *Journal of Neuroscience, 6,* 2950–2967.

6 Acquired Dyslexia: A Disorder of Reading

H. Branch Coslett

Case Report

Family members of the patient (W.T.), a 30-year-old right-handed woman, noted that she suddenly began to speak gibberish and lost the ability to understand speech. Neurological examination revealed only Wernicke's aphasia. Further examination revealed fluent speech, with frequent phonemic and semantic paraphasias. Naming was relatively preserved. Repetition of single words and phonemes was impaired. She repeated words of high imageability (e.g., desk) more accurately than words of low imageability (e.g., fate). Occasional semantic errors were noted in repetition; for example, when asked to repeat "shirt," she said "tie." Her writing of single words was similar to her repetition in that she produced occasional semantic errors and wrote words of high imageability significantly better than words of low imageability. A computed axial tomography (CAT) scan performed 6 months after the onset of her symptoms revealed a small cortical infarct involving a portion of the left posterior superior temporal gyrus.

W.T.'s reading comprehension was impaired; she performed well on comprehension tests involving high-imageability words, but was unable to reliably derive meaning from low-imageability words that she correctly read aloud. Of greatest interest was that her oral reading of single words was relatively preserved. She read approximately 95% of single words accurately and correctly read aloud five of the commands from the Boston Diagnostic Aphasia Examination (Goodglass & Kaplan, 1972). It is interesting that the variables that influenced her reading did not affect her writing and speech. For example, her reading was not altered by the part of speech (e.g., noun, verb, adjective) of the target word; she read nouns, modifiers, verbs, and even functors (e.g., words such as that, which, because, you) with equal facility. Nor was her reading affected by the imageability of the target word; she read words of low imageability (e.g., destiny) as well as words of high imageability (e.g., chair). W.T. also read words with irregular print-to-sound correspondences (e.g., yacht, tomb) as well as words with regular correspondence.

W.T. exhibited one striking impairment in her reading, an inability to read pronounceable nonword letter strings. For example, when shown the letter string "flig," W.T. could reliably indicate that the letter string was not a word.

Asked to indicate how such a letter string would be pronounced or "sounded out," however, she performed quite poorly, producing a correct response on only approximately 20% of trials. She typically responded by producing a visually similar real word (e.g., flag) while indicating that her response was not correct.

In summary, W.T. exhibited Wernicke's aphasia and alexia characterized by relatively preserved oral reading of real words, but impaired reading comprehension and poor reading of nonwords. Her pattern of reading deficit was consistent with the syndrome of phonological dyslexia. Her performance is of interest in this context because it speaks to contemporary accounts of the mechanisms mediating reading. As will be discussed later, a number of models of reading (e.g., Seidenberg & McClelland, 1989) invoke two mechanisms as mediating the pronunciation of letter strings; one is assumed to involve semantic mediation whereas the other is postulated to involve the translation of print into sound without accessing word-specific stored information—that is, without "looking up" a word in a mental dictionary. W.T.'s performance is of interest precisely because it challenges such accounts.

W.T.'s impaired performance on reading comprehension and other tasks involving semantics suggests that she is not reading aloud by means of a semantically based procedure. Similarly, her inability to read nonwords suggests that she is unable to reliably employ print-to-sound translation procedures. Her performance, therefore, argues for an additional reading mechanism by which word-specific stored information contacts speech production mechanisms directly.

Historical Overview of Acquired Dyslexia

Dejerine provided the first systematic descriptions of disorders of reading resulting from brain lesions in two seminal manuscripts in the late nineteenth century (1891, 1892). Although they were not the first descriptions of patients with reading disorders (e.g., Freund, 1889), his elegant descriptions of very different disorders provided the general theoretical framework that animated discussions of acquired dyslexia through the latter part of the twentieth century.

Dejerine's first patient (1891) manifested impaired reading and writing in the context of a mild aphasia after an infarction involving the left parietal lobe. Dejerine called this disorder "alexia with agraphia" and argued that the deficit was attributable to a disruption of the "optical image for words," which he thought to be supported by the left angular gyrus. This stored information was assumed to provide the template by which familiar words were recognized; the loss of the "optical images," therefore, would be expected to produce an inability to read familiar words. Although multiple distinct patterns of acquired dyslexia have been identified in subsequent investigations, Dejerine's account of alexia with agraphia represented the first well-studied investigation of the "central dyslexias" to which we will return.

Dejerine's second patient (1892) was quite different. This patient exhibited a right homonymous hemianopia and was unable to read aloud or for comprehension, but could write and speak well. This disorder, designated "alexia without agraphia" (also known as agnosic alexia and pure alexia), was attributed by Dejerine to a disconnection between visual information presented to the right hemisphere and the left angular gyrus, which he assumed to be critical for the recognition of words.

During the decades after the contributions of Dejerine, the study of acquired dyslexia languished. The relatively few investigations that were reported focused primarily on the anatomical underpinnings of the disorders. Although a number of interesting observations were reported, they were often either ignored or their significance was not appreciated. For example, Akelaitis (1944) reported a left hemialexia—an inability to read aloud words presented in the left visual field—in patients whose corpus callosum had been severed. This observation pro-vided powerful support for Dejerine's interpretation of alexia without agraphia as a disconnection syndrome.

In 1977, Benson sought to distinguish a third alexia associated with frontal lobe lesions. This disorder was said to be associated with a Broca aphasia as well as agraphia. These patients were said to comprehend "meaningful content words" better than words playing a "relational or syntactic" role and to exhibit greater problems with reading aloud than reading for comprehension. Finally, these patients were said to exhibit a "literal alexia" or an impairment in the identification of letters within words (Benson, 1977).

The study of acquired dyslexia was revitalized by the elegant and detailed investigations of Marshall and Newcombe (1966, 1973). On the basis of careful analyses of the words their subjects read successfully as well as a detailed inspection of their reading errors, these investigators identified distinctly different and reproducible types of reading deficits. The conceptual framework developed by Marshall and Newcombe (1973) has motivated many subsequent studies of acquired dyslexia (see Coltheart, Patterson, & Marshall, 1980; Patterson, Marshall, & Coltheart, 1985), and "information-processing" models of reading have been based to a considerable degree on their insights.

Experimental Research on Acquired Dyslexia

Reading is a complicated process that involves many different procedures and cognitive faculties. Before discussing the specific syndromes of acquired dyslexia, the processes mediating word recognition and pronunciation are briefly reviewed. The visual system efficiently processes a complicated stimulus that, at least for alphabet-based languages, is composed of smaller meaningful units, letters. In part because the number of letters is small in relation to the number of words, there is often a considerable visual similarity between words (e.g., same versus sane). In addition, the position of letters within the letter string is also critical to word identification (consider *mast* versus *mats*). In light of these factors, it is perhaps not surprising that reading places a substantial burden on the visual system and that disorders of visual processing or visual attention may substantially disrupt reading.

The fact that normal readers are so adept at word recognition has led some investigators to suggest that words are not processed as a series of distinct letters but rather as a single entity in a process akin to the recognition of objects. At least for normal readers under standard conditions, this does not appear to be the case. Rather, normal reading appears to require the identification of letters as alphabetic symbols. Support for this claim comes from demonstrations that presenting words in an unfamiliar form—for example, by alternating the case of the letters (e.g., wOrD) or introducing spaces between words (e.g., food)—does not substantially influence reading speed or accuracy (e.g., McClelland & Rumelhart, 1981). These data argue for a stage of letter identification in which the graphic form (whether printed or written) is transformed into a string of alphabetic characters (W-O-R-D), sometimes called "abstract letter identities."

As previously noted, word identification requires not only that the constituent letters be identified but also that the letter sequence be processed. The mechanism by which the position of letters within the stimulus is determined and maintained is not clear, but a number of accounts have been proposed. One possibility is that each letter is linked to a position in a word "frame" or envelope. Finally, it should be noted that under normal circumstances letters are not processed in a strictly serial fashion, but may be analyzed by the visual system in parallel (provided the words are not too long). Disorders of reading resulting from an impairment in the processing of the visual stimulus or the failure of this visual information to access stored knowledge appropriate to a letter string are designated "peripheral dyslexias" and are discussed later.

In "dual-route" models of reading, the identity of a letter string may be determined by a number of distinct procedures. The first is a "lexical" procedure in which the letter string is identified by matching it with an entry in a stored catalog of familiar words, or a visual word form system. As indicated in figure 6.1 and discussed later, this procedure, which in some respects is similar to looking up a word in a dictionary, provides access to the meaning and phonological form of the word and at least some of its syntactic properties. Dual-route models of reading also assume that the letter string can be converted directly to a phonological form by the application of a set of learned correspondences between orthography and phonology. In this account, meaning may then be accessed from the phonological form of the word.

Support for dual-route models of reading comes from a variety of sources. For present purposes, perhaps the most relevant evidence was provided by Marshall and Newcombe's (1973) ground-breaking description of "deep" and "surface" dyslexia. These investigators described a patient (G.R.) who read approximately 50% of concrete nouns (e.g., table, doughnut), but was severely impaired in the reading of abstract nouns (e.g., destiny, truth) and all other parts of speech. The most striking aspect of G.R.'s performance, however, was his tendency to produce errors that appeared to be semantically related to the target word (e.g., *speak* read as *talk*). Marshall and Newcombe designated this disorder "deep dyslexia."

These investigators also described two patients whose primary deficit appeared to be an inability to reliably apply grapheme-phoneme correspondences. Thus, J.C., for example, rarely applied the "rule of e" (which lengthens the preceding vowel in words such as "like") and experienced great difficulties in deriving the appropriate phonology for consonant clusters and vowel digraphs. The disorder characterized by impaired application of print-to-sound correspondences was called "surface dyslexia."

On the basis of these observations, Marshall and Newcombe (1973) argued that the meaning of written words could be accessed by two distinct procedures. The first was a direct procedure by which familiar words activated the appropriate stored representation (or visual word form), which in turn

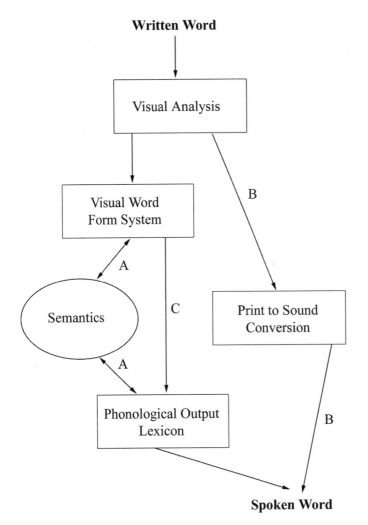

Figure 6.1
An information-processing model of reading illustrating the putative reading mechanisms.

activated meaning directly; reading in deep dyslexia, which was characterized by semantically based errors (of which the patient was often unaware), was assumed to involve this procedure. The second procedure was assumed to be a phonologically based process in which grapheme-to-phoneme or print-to-sound correspondences were employed to derive the appropriate phonology (or "sound out" the word); the reading of surface dyslexics was assumed to be mediated by this nonlexical procedure. Although a number of Marshall and Newcombe's specific hypotheses have subsequently been criticized, their argument that reading may be mediated by two distinct procedures has received considerable empirical support.

The information-processing model of reading depicted in figure 6.1 provides three distinct procedures for oral reading. Two of these procedures correspond to those described by Marshall and Newcombe. The first (labeled "A" in figure 6.1) involves the activation of a stored entry in the visual word form system and the subsequent access to semantic information and ultimately activation of the stored sound of the word at the level of the phonological output lexicon. The second ("B" in figure 6.1) involves the nonlexical grapheme-to-phoneme or print-to-sound translation process; this procedure does not entail access to any stored information about words, but rather is assumed to be mediated by access to a catalog of correspondences stipulating the pronunciation of phonemes.

Many information-processing accounts of the language mechanisms subserving reading incorporate a third procedure. This mechanism ("C" in figure 6.1) is lexically based in that it is assumed to involve the activation of the visual word form system and the phonological output lexicon. The procedure differs from the lexical procedure described earlier, however, in that there is no intervening activation of semantic information. This procedure has been called the "direct" reading mechanism or route. Support for the direct lexical mechanism comes from a number of sources, including observations that some subjects read aloud words that they do not appear to comprehend

(Schwartz, Saffran, & Marin, 1979; Noble, Glosser, & Grossman, 2000; Lambon Ralph, Ellis, & Franklin, 1995).

As noted previously, the performance of W.T. is also relevant. Recall that W.T. was able to read aloud words that she did not understand, suggesting that her oral reading was not semantically based. Furthermore, she could not read nonwords, suggesting that she was unable to employ a sounding-out strategy. Finally, the fact that she was unable to write or repeat words of low imageability (e.g., affection) that she could read aloud is important because it suggests that her oral reading was not mediated by an interaction of impaired semantic and phonological systems (cf. Hills & Caramazza, 1995). Thus, data from W.T. provide support for the direct lexical mechanism.

Peripheral Dyslexias

A useful starting point in the discussion of acquired dyslexia is provided by the distinction made by Shallice and Warrington (1980) between "peripheral" and "central" dyslexias. The former are conditions characterized by a deficit in the processing of visual aspects of the stimulus, which prevents the patient from achieving a representation of the word that preserves letter identity and sequence. In contrast, central dyslexias reflect impairment to the "deeper" or "higher" reading functions by which visual word forms mediate access to meaning or speech production mechanisms. In this section we discuss the major types of peripheral dyslexia.

Alexia without Letter-by-Letter Agraphia (Pure Alexia; Letter-by-Letter Reading)

This disorder is among the most common of the peripheral reading disturbances. It is associated with a left hemisphere lesion that affects the left occipital cortex (which is responsible for the analysis of visual stimuli on the right side of space) and/or the structures (i.e., left lateral geniculate nucleus of the thalamus and white matter, including callosal fibers from the intact right visual cortex) that provide input to this region of the brain. It is likely that the lesion either blocks direct visual input to the mechanisms that process printed words in the left hemisphere or disrupts the visual word form system itself (Geschwind & Fusillo, 1966; Warrington & Shallice, 1980; Cohen et al., 2000). Some of these patients seem to be unable to read at all, while others do so slowly and laboriously by a process that involves serial letter identification (often called "letter-by-letter" reading). Letter-by-letter readers often pronounce the letter names aloud; in some cases, they misidentify letters, usually on the basis of visual similarity, as in the case of N → M (see Patterson & Kay, 1982). Their reading is also abnormally slow and is often directly proportional to word length. Performance is not typically influenced by variables such as imageability, part of speech, and regularity of print-to-sound correspondences.

It was long thought that patients with pure alexia were unable to read, except letter by letter (Dejerine, 1892; Geschwind & Fusillo, 1966). There is now evidence that some of them do retain the ability to recognize letter strings, although this does not guarantee that they will be able to read aloud. Several different paradigms have demonstrated the preservation of word recognition. Some patients demonstrate a word superiority effect in that a letter is more likely to be recognized when it is part of a word (e.g., the R in WORD) than when it occurs in a string of unrelated letters (e.g., WKRD) (Bowers, Bub, & Arguin, 1996; Bub, Black, & Howell, 1989; Friedman & Hadley, 1992; Reuter-Lorenz & Brunn, 1990).

Second, some of them have been able to perform lexical decision tasks (determining whether a letter string constitutes a real word) and semantic categorization tasks (indicating whether a word belongs to a category, such as foods or animals) at above chance levels when words are presented too rapidly to support letter-by-letter reading (Shallice & Saffran, 1986; Coslett & Saffran, 1989a). Brevity of presentation is critical, in that longer exposure to the letter string seems to engage the letter-by-letter strategy, which appears to interfere with the ability to perform the covert reading task (Coslett, Saffran,

Greenbaum, & Schwartz, 1993). In fact, the patient may show better performance on lexical decisions in shorter (e.g., 250 ms) than in longer presentations (e.g., 2 seconds) that engage the letter-by-letter strategy, but do not allow it to proceed to completion (Coslett & Saffran, 1989a).

A compelling example comes from a previously reported patient who was given 2 seconds to scan the card containing the stimulus (Shallice & Saffran, 1986). The patient did not take advantage of the full inspection time when he was performing lexical decision and categorization tasks; instead, he glanced at the card briefly and looked away, perhaps to avoid letter-by-letter reading. The capacity for covert reading has also been demonstrated in two pure alexics who were unable to employ the letter-by-letter reading strategy (Coslett & Saffran, 1989b, 1992). These patients appeared to recognize words, but were rarely able to report them, although they sometimes generated descriptions that were related to the word's meaning (for example, cookies → "candy, a cake"). In some cases, patients have shown some recovery of oral reading over time, although this capacity appears to be limited to concrete words (Coslett & Saffran, 1989a; Buxbaum & Coslett, 1996).

The mechanisms that underlie "implicit" or "covert" reading remain controversial. Dejerine (1892), who provided the first description of pure alexia, suggested that the analysis of visual input in these patients is performed by the right hemisphere, as a result of the damage to the visual cortex on the left. (It should be noted, however, that not all lesions to the left visual cortex give rise to alexia. A critical feature that supports continued left hemisphere processing is the preservation of callosal input from the unimpaired visual cortex on the right.)

One possible explanation is that covert reading reflects recognition of printed words by the right hemisphere, which is unable to either articulate the word or (in most cases) to adequately communicate its identity to the language area of the left hemisphere (Coslett & Saffran, 1998; Saffran & Coslett, 1998). In this account, letter-by-letter reading is carried out by the left hemisphere using letter information transferred serially and inefficiently from the right hemisphere. Furthermore, the account assumes that when the letter-by-letter strategy is implemented, it may be difficult for the patient to attend to the products of word processing in the right hemisphere. Consequently, the patient's performance in lexical decision and categorization tasks declines (Coslett & Saffran, 1989a; Coslett et al., 1993). Additional evidence supporting the right hemisphere account of reading in pure alexia is presented later.

Alternative accounts of pure alexia have also been proposed (see Coltheart, 1998, for a special issue devoted to the topic). Behrmann and colleagues (Behrmann, Plaut, & Nelson, 1998; Behrmann & Shallice, 1995), for example, have proposed that the disorder is attributable to impaired activation of orthographic representations. In this account, reading is assumed to reflect the "residual functioning of the same interactive system that supported normal reading premorbidly" (Behrmann et al., 1998, p. 7).

Other investigators have attributed pure dyslexia to a visual impairment that precludes activation of orthographic representations (Farah & Wallace, 1991). Chialant & Caramazza (1998), for example, reported a patient, M.J., who processed single, visually presented letters normally and performed well on a variety of tasks assessing the orthographic lexicon with auditorily presented stimuli. In contrast, M.J. exhibited significant impairments in the processing of letter strings. The investigators suggest that M.J. was unable to transfer information specifying multiple letter identities in parallel from the intact visual processing system in the right hemisphere to the intact language-processing mechanisms of the left hemisphere.

Neglect Dyslexia

Parietal lobe lesions can result in a deficit that involves neglect of stimuli on the side of space that is contralateral to the lesion, a disorder referred to as *hemispatial neglect* (see chapter 1). In most cases, this disturbance arises with damage to the right parietal lobe; therefore attention to the left side

of space is most often affected. The severity of neglect is generally greater when there are stimuli on the right as well as on the left; attention is drawn to the right-sided stimuli at the expense of those on the left, a phenomenon known as *extinction*. Typical clinical manifestations include bumping into objects on the left, failure to dress the left side of the body, drawing objects that are incomplete on the left, and reading problems that involve neglect of the left portions of words, i.e., "neglect dyslexia."

With respect to neglect dyslexia, it has been found that such patients are more likely to ignore letters in nonwords (e.g., the first two letters in bruggle) than letters in real words (such as snuggle). This suggests that the problem does not reflect a total failure to process letter information but rather an attentional impairment that affects conscious recognition of the letters (e.g., Sieroff, Pollatsek, & Posner, 1988; Behrmann, Moscovitch, & Moser, 1990a; see also Caramazza & Hills, 1990b). Performance often improves when words are presented vertically or spelled aloud. In addition, there is evidence that semantic information can be processed in neglect dyslexia, and that the ability to read words aloud improves when oral reading follows a semantic task (Ladavas, Shallice, & Zanella, 1997).

Neglect dyslexia has also been reported in patients with left hemisphere lesions (Caramazza & Hills, 1990b; Greenwald & Berndt, 1999). In these patients the deficiency involves the right side of words. Here, visual neglect is usually confined to words and is not ameliorated by presenting words vertically or spelling them aloud. This disorder has therefore been termed a "positional dyslexia," whereas the right hemisphere deficit has been termed a "spatial neglect dyslexia" (Ellis, Young, & Flude, 1993).

Attentional Dyslexia

Attentional dyslexia is a disorder characterized by relatively preserved reading of single words, but impaired reading of words in the context of other words or letters. This infrequently described disorder was first described by Shallice and Warrington

(1977), who reported two patients with brain tumors involving (at least) the left parietal lobe. Both patients exhibited relatively good performance with single letters or words, but were significantly impaired in the recognition of the same stimuli when they were presented as part of an array. Similarly, both patients correctly read more than 90% of single words, but only approximately 80% of the words when they were presented in the context of three additional words. These investigators attributed the disorder to a failure of transmission of information from a nonsemantic perceptual stage to a semantic processing stage (Shallice & Warrington, 1977).

Warrington, Cipolotti, and McNeil (1993) reported a second patient, B.A.L., who was able to read single words, but exhibited a substantial impairment in the reading of letters and words in an array. B.A.L. exhibited no evidence of visual disorientation and was able to identify a target letter in an array of "X"s or "O"s. He was impaired, however, in the naming of letters or words when these stimuli were flanked by other members of the same stimulus category. This patient's attentional dyslexia was attributed to an impairment arising after words and letters had been processed as units.

More recently Saffran and Coslett (1996) reported a patient, N.Y., who exhibited attentional dyslexia. The patient had biopsy-proven Alzheimer's disease that appeared to selectively involve posterior cortical regions. N.Y. scored within the normal range on verbal subtests of the Wechsler Adult Intelligence Scale-Revised (WAIS-R), but was unable to carry out any of the performance subtests. He performed normally on the Boston Naming Test. N.Y. performed quite poorly in a variety of experimental tasks assessing visuospatial processing and visual attention. Despite his visuoperceptual deficits, however, N.Y.'s reading of single words was essentially normal. He read 96% of 200 words presented for 100 ms (unmasked). Like previously reported patients with this disorder, N.Y. exhibited a substantial decline in performance when asked to read two words presented simultaneously.

Of greatest interest, however, was the fact that N.Y. produced a substantial number of "blend" errors in which letters from the two words were combined to generate a response that was not present in the display. For example, when shown "flip shot," N.Y. responded "ship." Like the blend errors produced by normal subjects with brief stimulus presentation (Shallice & McGill, 1977), N.Y.'s blend errors were characterized by the preservation of letter position information; thus, in the preceding example, the letters in the blend response ("ship") retained the same serial position in the incorrect response. A subsequent experiment demonstrated that for N.Y., but not controls, blend errors were encountered significantly less often when the target words differed in case (desk, FEAR).

Like Shallice (1988; see also Mozer, 1991), Saffran and Coslett (1996) considered the central deficit in attentional dyslexia to be impaired control of a filtering mechanism that normally suppresses input from unattended words or letters in the display. More specifically, they suggested that as a consequence of the patient's inability to effectively deploy the "spotlight" of attention to a particular region of interest (e.g., a single word or a single letter), multiple stimuli fall within the attentional spotlight. Since visual attention may serve to integrate visual feature information, impaired modulation of the spotlight of attention would be expected to generate word blends and other errors reflecting the incorrect concatenation of letters.

Saffran and Coslett (1996) also argued that loss of location information contributed to N.Y.'s reading deficit. Several lines of evidence support such a conclusion. First, N.Y. was impaired relative to controls, both with respect to accuracy and response time in a task in which he was required to indicate if a line was inside or outside a circle. Second, N.Y. exhibited a clear tendency to omit one member of a double-letter pair (e.g., reed > "red"). This phenomenon, which has been demonstrated in normal subjects, has been attributed to the loss of location information that normally helps to differentiate two occurrences of the same object.

Finally, it should be noted that the well-documented observation that the blend errors of normal subjects as well as those of attentional dyslexics preserve letter position is not inconsistent with the claim that impaired location information contributes to attentional dyslexia. Migration or blend errors reflect a failure to link words or letters to a location in space, whereas the letter position constraint reflects the properties of the word-processing system. The latter, which is assumed to be at least relatively intact in patients with attentional dyslexia, specifies letter location with respect to the word form rather than to space.

Other Peripheral Dyslexias

Peripheral dyslexias may be observed in a variety of conditions involving visuoperceptual or attentional deficits. Patients with simultanagnosia, a disorder characterized by an inability to "see" more than one object in an array, are often able to read single words, but are incapable of reading text (see chapter 2). Other patients with simultanagnosia exhibit substantial problems in reading even single words.

Patients with degenerative conditions involving the posterior cortical regions may also exhibit profound deficits in reading as part of their more general impairment in visuospatial processing (e.g., Coslett, Stark, Rajaram, & Saffran, 1995). Several patterns of impairment may be observed in these patients. Some patients exhibit attentional dyslexia, with letter migration and blend errors, whereas other patients exhibiting deficits that are in certain respects rather similar do not produce migration or blend errors in reading or illusory conjunctions in visual search tasks. We have suggested that at least some patients with these disorders suffer from a progressive restriction in the domain to which they can allocate visual attention. As a consequence of this impairment, these patients may exhibit an effect of stimulus size so that they are able to read words in small print, but when shown the same word in large print see only a single letter.

Central Dyslexias

Deep Dyslexia

Deep dyslexia, initially described by Marshall and Newcombe in 1973, is the most extensively investigated of the central dyslexias (see Coltheart et al., 1980) and in many respects the most dramatic. The hallmark of this disorder is semantic error. Shown the word "castle," a deep dyslexic may respond "knight"; shown the word "bird," the patient may respond "canary." At least for some deep dyslexics, it is clear that these errors are not circumlocutions. Semantic errors may represent the most frequent error type in some deep dyslexics whereas in other patients they comprise a small proportion of reading errors. Deep dyslexics make a number of other types of errors on single-word reading tasks as well. "Visual" errors in which the response bears a strong visual similarity to the target word (e.g., book read as "boot") are common. In addition, "morphological" errors in which a prefix or suffix is added, deleted, or substituted (e.g., scolded read as "scolds"; governor read as "government") are typically observed.

Another defining feature of the disorder is a profound impairment in the translation of print into sound. Deep dyslexics are typically unable to provide the sound appropriate to individual letters and exhibit a substantial impairment in the reading of nonwords. When confronted with letter strings such as flig or churt, for example, deep dyslexics are typically unable to employ print-to-sound correspondences to derive phonology; nonwords frequently elicit "lexicalization" errors (e.g., flig read as "flag"), perhaps reflecting a reliance on lexical reading in the absence of access to reliable print-to-sound correspondences. Additional features of the syndrome include a greater success in reading words of high compared with low imageability. Thus, words such as table, chair, ceiling, and buttercup, the referent of which is concrete or imageable, are read more successfully than words such as fate, destiny, wish, and universal, which denote abstract concepts.

Another characteristic feature of deep dyslexia is a part-of-speech effect in which nouns are typically read more reliably than modifiers (adjectives and adverbs), which in turn are read more accurately than verbs. Deep dyslexics manifest particular difficulty in the reading of functors (a class of words that includes pronouns, prepositions, conjunctions, and interrogatives including that, which, they, because, and under). The striking nature of the part-of-speech effect may be illustrated by the patient who correctly read the word "chrysanthemum" but was unable to read the word "the" (Saffran & Marin, 1977)! Most errors in functors involve the substitution of a different functor (that read as "which") rather than the production of words of a different class, such as nouns or verbs. Since functors are in general less imageable than nouns, some investigators have claimed that the apparent effect of part of speech is in reality a manifestation of the pervasive imageability effect. There is no consensus on this point because other investigators have suggested that the part-of-speech effect is observed even if stimuli are matched for imageability (Coslett, 1991).

Finally, it should be noted that the accuracy of oral reading may be determined by context. This is illustrated by the fact that a patient was able to read aloud the word "car" when it was a noun, but not when the same letter string was a conjunction. Thus, when presented with the sentence, "Le car ralentit car le moteur chauffe" (The car slows down because the motor overheats), the patient correctly pronounced only the first instance of "car" (Andreewsky, Deloche, & Kossanyi, 1980).

How can deep dyslexia be accommodated by the information-processing model of reading illustrated in figure 6.1? Several alternative explanations have been proposed. Some investigators have argued that the reading of deep dyslexics is mediated by a damaged form of the left hemisphere-based system employed in normal reading (Morton & Patterson, 1980; Shallice, 1988; Glosser & Friedman, 1990). In such an account, multiple processing deficits must be hypothesized to accommodate the full range of symptoms characteristic of deep dyslexia.

First, the strikingly impaired performance in reading nonwords and other tasks assessing phonological function suggests that the print-to-sound conversion procedure is disrupted. Second, the presence of semantic errors and the effects of imageability (a variable thought to influence processing at the level of semantics) suggest that these patients also suffer from a semantic impairment (but see Caramazza & Hills, 1990a). Finally, the production of visual errors suggests that these patients suffer from impairment in the visual word form system or in the processes mediating access to the visual word form system.

Other investigators (Coltheart, 1980, 2000; Saffran, Bogyo, Schwartz, & Marin, 1980) have argued that reading by deep dyslexics is mediated by a system not normally used in reading—that is, the right hemisphere. We will return to the issue of reading with the right hemisphere later. Finally, citing evidence from functional imaging studies demonstrating that deep dyslexic subjects exhibit increased activation in both the right hemisphere and nonperisylvian areas of the left hemisphere, other investigators have suggested that deep dyslexia reflects the recruitment of both right and left hemisphere processes.

Phonological Dyslexia: Reading without Print-to-Sound Correspondences

First described in 1979 by Derouesne and Beauvois, phonological dyslexia is perhaps the "purest" of the central dyslexias in that, at least in some accounts, the syndrome is attributable to a selective deficit in the procedure mediating the translation from print into sound. Single-word reading in this disorder is often only mildly impaired; some patients, for example, correctly read 85–95% of real words (Funnell, 1983; Bub, Black, Howell, & Kartesz, 1987). Some phonological dyslexics read all different types of words with equal facility (Bub et al., 1987), whereas other patients are relatively impaired in the reading of functors (Glosser & Friedman, 1990).

Unlike the patients with surface dyslexia described later, the regularity of print-to-sound correspondences is not relevant to their performance; thus, phonological dyslexics are as likely to correctly pronounce orthographically irregular words such as colonel as words with standard print-to-sound correspondences such as administer. Most errors in response to real words bear a visual similarity to the target word (e.g., topple read as "table"). The reader is referred to a special issue of *Cognitive Neuropsychology* for a discussion of this disorder (Coltheart, 1996).

The striking and theoretically relevant aspect of the performance of phonological dyslexics is a substantial impairment in the oral reading of nonword letter strings. We have examined patients with this disorder, for example, who read more than 90% of real words of all types yet correctly pronounced only approximately 10% of nonwords. Most errors in nonwords involve the substitution of a visually similar real word (e.g., phope read as "phone") or the incorrect application of print-to-sound correspondences (e.g., stime read as "stim" to rhyme with "him").

Within the context of the reading model depicted in figure 6.1, the account for this disorder is relatively straightforward. Good performance with real words suggests that the processes involved in normal "lexical" reading—that is, visual analysis, the visual word form system, semantics, and the phonological output lexicon—are at least relatively preserved. The impairment in reading nonwords suggests that the print-to-sound translation procedure is disrupted.

Recent explorations of the processes involved in reading nonwords have identified a number of distinct procedures involved in this task (see Coltheart, 1996). If these distinct procedures may be selectively impaired by brain injury, one might expect to observe different subtypes of phonological dyslexia. Although the details are beyond the scope of this chapter, Coltheart (1996) has recently reviewed evidence suggesting that different subtypes of phonological dyslexia may be observed.

Finally, it should be noted that several investigators have suggested that phonological dyslexia is not attributable to a disruption of a reading-specific

component of the cognitive architecture, but rather to a more general phonological deficit. Support for this assertion comes from the observation that the vast majority of phonological dyslexics are impaired on a wide variety of nonreading tasks that assess phonology.

Phonological dyslexia is, in certain respects, similar to deep dyslexia, the critical difference being that semantic errors are not observed in phonological dyslexia. Citing the similarity of reading performance and the fact that deep dyslexics may evolve into phonological dyslexics as they improve, it has been argued that deep and phonological dyslexia are on a continuum of severity (Glosser & Friedman, 1990).

Surface Dyslexia: Reading without Lexical Access

Surface dyslexia, first described by Marshall and Newcombe (1973), is a disorder characterized by the relatively preserved ability to read words with regular or predictable grapheme-to-phoneme correspondences, but substantially impaired reading of words with "irregular" or exceptional print-to-sound correspondences. Thus, patients with surface dyslexia typically are able to read words such as state, hand, mosquito, and abdominal quite well, whereas they exhibit substantial problems reading words such as colonel, yacht, island, and borough, the pronunciation of which cannot be derived by sounding-out strategies. Errors in irregular words usually consist of "regularizations"; for example, surface dyslexics may read colonel as "kollonel." These patients read nonwords (e.g., blape) quite well. Finally, it should be noted that all surface dyslexics that have been reported to date read at least some irregular words correctly. Patients will often read high-frequency irregular words (e.g., have, some), but some surface dyslexics have been reported to read such low-frequency and highly irregular words as sieve and isle.

As noted earlier, some accounts of normal reading postulate that familiar words are read aloud by matching a letter string to a stored representation of the word and retrieving the pronunciation by a mechanism linked to semantics or by a direct route. Since this process is assumed to involve the activation of the sound of the whole word, performance would not be expected to be influenced by the regularity of print-to-sound correspondences. The fact that this variable significantly influences performance in surface dyslexia suggests that the deficit in this syndrome is in the mechanisms mediating lexical reading, that is, in the semantically mediated and direct reading mechanisms. Similarly, the preserved ability to read words and nonwords demonstrates that the procedures by which words are sounded out are at least relatively preserved.

In the context of the information-processing model discussed previously, how would one account for surface dyslexia? Scrutiny of the model depicted in figure 6.1 suggests that at least three different deficits may result in surface dyslexia. First, this disorder may arise from a deficit at the level of the visual word form system that disrupts the processing of words as units. As a consequence of this deficit, subjects may identify "sublexical" units (e.g., graphemes or clusters of graphemes) and identify words on the basis of print-to-sound correspondences. Note that in this account, semantics and output processes would be expected to be preserved. The patient J.C. described by Marshall and Newcombe (1973) exhibited at least some of the features of this type of surface dyslexia. For example, in response to the word listen, JC said "Liston" (a former heavyweight champion boxer) and added "that's the boxer," demonstrating that he was able to derive phonology from print and subsequently access meaning.

In the model depicted in figure 6.1, one might also expect to encounter surface dyslexia with deficits at the level of the output lexicon (see Ellis, Lambon Ralph, Morris, & Hunter, 2000). Support for such an account comes from patients who comprehend irregular words yet regularize these words when asked to read them aloud. For example, M.K. read the word "steak" as "steek" (as in seek) before adding, "nice beef" (Howard & Franklin, 1987). In this instance, the demonstration that M.K. was able to provide appropriate semantic information indi-

cates that he was able to access meaning directly from the written word and suggests that the visual word form system and semantics were at least relatively preserved.

One might also expect to observe surface dyslexia in patients exhibiting semantic loss. Indeed, most patients with surface dyslexia (often in association with surface dysgraphia) exhibit a significant semantic deficit (Shallice, Warrington, & McCarthy, 1983; Hodges, Patterson, Oxbury, & Funnell, 1992). Surface dyslexia is most frequently observed in the context of semantic dementia, a progressive degenerative condition characterized by a gradual loss of knowledge in the absence of deficits in motor, perceptual, and, in some instances, executive function (see chapter 4).

Note, however, that the information-processing account of reading depicted in figure 6.1 also incorporates a lexical but nonsemantic reading mechanism by which patients with semantic loss would be expected to be able to read even irregular words not accommodated by the grapheme-to-phoneme procedure. In this account, then, surface dyslexia is assumed to reflect impairment in both the semantic and lexical, but not nonsemantic mechanisms. It should be noted in this context that the "triangle" model of reading developed by Seidenberg and McClelland (1989; also see Plaut, McClelland, Seidenberg, & Patterson, 1996) provides an alternative account of surface dyslexia. In this account, to which we briefly return later, surface dyslexia is assumed to reflect the disruption of semantically mediated reading.

Reading and the Right Hemisphere

One controversial issue regarding reading concerns the putative reading capacity of the right hemisphere. For many years investigators argued that the right hemisphere was "word-blind" (Dejerine, 1892; Geschwind, 1965). In recent years, however, several lines of evidence have suggested that the right hemisphere may possess the capacity to read (Coltheart, 2000; Bartolomeo, Bachoud-Levi, Degos, & Boller, 1998). Indeed, as previously noted, a number of investigators have argued that the reading of deep dyslexics is mediated at least in part by the right hemisphere.

One seemingly incontrovertible finding demonstrating that at least some right hemispheres possess the capacity to read comes from the performance of a patient who underwent a left hemispherectomy at age 15 for treatment of seizures caused by Rasmussen's encephalitis (Patterson, Varga-Khadem, & Polkey, 1989a). After the hemispherectomy, the patient was able to read approximately 30% of single words and exhibited an effect of part of speech; she was unable to use a grapheme-to-phoneme conversion process. Thus, as noted by the authors, this patient's performance was similar in many respects to that of patients with deep dyslexia, a pattern of reading impairment that has been hypothesized to reflect the performance of the right hemisphere.

The performance of some split-brain patients is also consistent with the claim that the right hemisphere is literate. These patients may, for example, be able to match printed words presented to the right hemisphere with an appropriate object (Zaidel, 1978; Zaidel & Peters, 1983). It is interesting that the patients are apparently unable to derive sound from the words presented to the right hemisphere; thus they are unable to determine if a word presented to the right hemisphere rhymes with a spoken word.

Another line of evidence supporting the claim that the right hemisphere is literate comes from an evaluation of the reading of patients with pure alexia and optic aphasia. We reported data, for example, from four patients with pure alexia who performed well above chance in a number of lexical decision and semantic categorization tasks with briefly presented words that they could not explicitly identify. Three of the patients who regained the ability to explicitly identify rapidly presented words exhibited a pattern of performance consistent with the right hemisphere reading hypothesis. These patients read nouns better than functors and words of high imageability (e.g., chair) better than words of low imageability (e.g., destiny). In addition, both

patients for whom data are available demonstrated a deficit in the reading of suffixed (e.g., flowed) compared with pseudo-suffixed (e.g., flower) words. These data are consistent with a version of the right hemisphere reading hypothesis, which postulates that the right hemisphere lexical-semantic system primarily represents high imageability nouns. In this account, functors, affixed words, and low-imageability words are not adequately represented in the right hemisphere.

An important additional finding is that magnetic stimulation applied to the skull, which disrupts electrical activity in the brain below, interfered with the reading performance of a partially recovered pure alexic when it affected the parieto-occipital area of the right hemisphere (Coslett & Monsul, 1994). The same stimulation had no effect when it was applied to the homologous area on the left. Additional data supporting the right hemisphere hypothesis come from the demonstration that the limited whole-word reading of a pure alexic was lost after a right occipito-temporal stroke (Bartolomeo et al., 1998).

Although a consensus has not yet been achieved, there is mounting evidence that at least for some people, the right hemisphere is not word-blind, but may support the reading of some types of words. The full extent of this reading capacity and whether it is relevant to normal reading, however, remain unclear.

Functional Neuromaging Studies of Acquired Dyslexia

A variety of experimental techniques including position emission tomography (PET), functional magnetic resonance imaging (fMRI), and evoked potentials have been employed to investigate the anatomical basis of reading in normal subjects. As in other domains of inquiry, differences in experimental technique (e.g., stimulus duration) (Price, Moore, & Frackowiak, 1996) and design have led to some variability in the localization of putative components of reading systems. Attempts to precisely localize components of the cognitive architecture of reading are also complicated by the interactive nature of language processes. Thus, since word recognition may lead to automatic activation of meaning and phonology, tasks such as written-word lexical decisions, which in theory may require only access to a visual word form system, may also activate semantic and phonological processes (see Demonet, Wise, & Frackowiak, 1993). Despite these potential problems, there appears to be at least relative agreement regarding the anatomical basis of several components of the reading system (see Fiez & Petersen, 1998; Price, 1998).

A number of studies suggest that early visual analysis of orthographic stimuli activates Brodmann areas 18 and 19 bilaterally (Petersen, Fox, Snyder, & Raichle, 1990; Price et al., 1996; Bookheimer, Zeffiro, Blaxton, Gaillard, & Theodore, 1995; Indefrey et al., 1997; Hagoort et al., 1999). For example, Petersen et al. (1990) reported extrastriate activation with words, nonwords, and even false fonts.

As previously noted, most accounts of reading postulate that after initial visual processing, familiar words are recognized by comparison with a catalog of stored representations that is often termed the "visual word-form system." A variety of recent investigations involving fMRI (Cohen et al., 2000, Puce, Allison, Asgari, Gore, & McCarthy, 1996), PET (e.g., Beauregard et al., 1997), and direct recording of cortical electrical activity (Nobre, Allison, & McCarthy, 1994) suggest that the visual word-form system is supported by the inferior occipital or inferior temporo-occipital cortex; the precise localization of the visual word form system in cortex, however, varies somewhat from study to study.

Recent strong support for this localization comes from an investigation by Cohen et al. (2000) of five normal subjects and two patients with posterior callosal lesions. These investigators presented words and nonwords for lexical decision or oral reading to either the right or left visual fields. They found initial unilateral activation in what was thought to be area V4 in the hemisphere to which

the stimulus was projected. More important, however, in normal subjects, activation was observed in the left fusiform gyrus (Talairach coordinates −42, −57, −6), which was independent of the hemisphere to which the stimulus was presented. The two patients with posterior callosal lesions were more impaired in the processing of letter strings presented to the right than to the left hemisphere; fMRI in these subjects demonstrated that the region of the fusiform gyrus described earlier was activated in the callosal patients only by stimuli presental to the left hemisphere. As noted by the investigators, these findings are consistent with the hypothesis that the hemialexia demonstrated by the callosal patients is attributable to a failure to access the visual word-form system in the left fusiform gyrus.

It should be noted, however, that alternative localizations of the visual word-form system have been proposed. Petersen et al. (1990) and Bookheimer et al. (1995), for example, have suggested the medial extrastriate cortex as the relevant site for the visual word-form system. In addition, Howard et al. (1992), Price et al. (1994), and Vandenberghe, Price, Wise, Josephs, & Frackowiak (1996) have localized the visual word-form system to the left posterior temporal lobe. Evidence against this localization has been presented by Cohen et al. (2000).

Several studies have suggested that retrieval of phonology for visually presented words may activate the posterior superior temporal lobe or the left supramarginal gyrus. For example, Vandenberghe et al. (1996), Bookheimer et al. (1995), and Menard, Kosslyn, Thompson, Alpert, & Rauch (1996) reported that reading words activated Brodmann area 40 to a greater degree than naming pictures, raising the possibility that this region is involved in retrieving phonology for written words.

The left inferior frontal cortex has also been implicated in phonological processing with written words. Zatorre, Meyer, Gjedde, & Evans (1996) reported activation of this region in tasks involving discrimination of final consonants or phoneme monitoring. In addition, the contrast between reading of pseudo-words and regular words has been reported to activate the left frontal operculum (Price et al., 1996), and this region was activated by a lexical decision test with written stimuli (Rumsey et al., 1997).

Deriving meaning from visually presented words requires access to stored knowledge or semantics. While the architecture and anatomical bases of semantic knowledge remain controversial and are beyond the scope of this chapter, a variety of lines of evidence reviewed by Price (1998) suggests that semantics are supported by the left inferior temporal and posterior inferior parietal cortices. The role of the dorsolateral frontal cortex in semantic processing is not clear; Thompson-Schill, D'Esposito, Aguirre, & Farah (1997) and other investigators (Gabrieli, 1998) have suggested that this activation is attributable to "executive" processing, including response selection rather than semantic processing.

Conclusions and Future Directions

Our discussion to this point has focused on a "box-and-arrow" information-processing account of reading disorders. This account has not only proven useful in terms of explaining data from normal and brain-injured subjects but has also predicted syndromes of acquired dyslexia. One weakness of these models, however, is the fact that the accounts are largely descriptive and underspecified.

In recent years, a number of investigators have developed models of reading in which the architecture and procedures are fully specified and implemented in a fashion that permits an empirical assessment of their performance. One computational account of reading has been developed by Coltheart and colleagues (Coltheart & Rastle, 1994; Rastle & Coltheart, 1999). Their "dual-route cascaded" model is a computational version of the dual-route theory similar to that presented in figure 6.1. This account incorporates a "lexical" route (similar to "C" in figure 6.1) as well as a "nonlexical" route by which the pronunciation of graphemes is computed on the basis of position-specific correspondence rules. This model accommodates a wide range of findings from the literature on normal reading.

A fundamentally different type of reading model was developed by Seidenberg and McClelland and subsequently elaborated by Plaut, Seidenberg, and colleagues (Seidenberg & McClelland, 1989; Plaut, Seidenberg, & McClelland, Patterson 1996). This account belongs to the general class of parallel distributed processing or connectionist models. Sometimes called the "triangle" model, this approach differs from information-processing accounts in that it does not incorporate word-specific representations (e.g., visual word forms, output phonological representations). In this account, the subjects are assumed to learn how written words map onto spoken words through repeated exposure to familiar and unfamiliar words. Word pronunciations are learned by the development of a mapping between letters and sounds generated on the basis of experience with many different letter strings. The probabilistic mapping between letters and sounds is assumed to provide the means by which both familiar and unfamiliar words are pronounced.

This model not only accommodates an impressive array of the classic findings in the literature on normal reading but also has been "lesioned" in an attempt to reproduce the reading patterns characteristic of dyslexia. For example, Patterson et al. (1989b) have attempted to accommodate surface dyslexia by disrupting semantically mediated reading, and Plaut and Shallice (1993) generated a performance pattern similar to that of deep dyslexia by lesioning a somewhat different connectionist model.

A full discussion of the relative merits of these models as well as approaches to understanding reading and acquired dyslexia is beyond the scope of this chapter. It would appear likely, however, that investigations of acquired dyslexia will help us to choose between competing accounts of reading and that these models will continue to offer critical insights into the interpretation of data from brain-injured subjects.

Acknowledgments

This work was supported by National Institutes of Health grant RO1 DC02754.

References

Akelaitis, A. J. (1944). A study of gnosis, praxis and language following section of the the corpus callosum and anterior commissure. *Journal of Neurosurgery*, *1*, 94–102.

Andreewsky, E., Deloche, G., & Kossanyi, P. (1980). Analogy between speed reading and deep dyslexia: towards a procedural understanding of reading. In M. Coltheart, K. Patterson, & J. C. Marshall (Eds.), *Deep dyslexia*. London: Routledge and Kegan Paul.

Bartolomeo, P., Bachoud-Levi, A-C., Degos, J-D., & Boller, F. (1998). Disruption of residual reading capacity in a pure alexic patient after a mirror-image right-hemispheric lesion. *Neurology*, *50*, 286–288.

Beauregard, M., Chertkow, H., Bub, D., Murtha, S., Dixon, R., & Evans, A. (1997). The neural substrate for concrete, abstract and emotional word lexica: A positron emission computed tomography study. *Journal of Cognitive Neuroscience*, *9*, 441–461.

Behrmann, M., Moscovitch, M., & Mozer, M. C. (1990a). Directing attention to words and non-words in normal subjects and in a computational model: Implications for neglect dyslexia. *Cognitive Neuropsychology*, *8*, 213–248.

Behrmann, M., Moscovitch, M., Black, S. E., & Mozer, M. (1990b). Perceptual and conceptual mechanisms in neglect dyslexia. *Brain*, *113*, 1163–1183.

Behrmann, M., & Shallice, T. (1995). Pure alexia: a non-spatial visual disorder affecting letter activation. *Cognitive Neuropsychology*, *12*, 409–454.

Behrmann, M., Plaut, D. C., & Nelson, J. (1998). A literature review and new data supporting an interactive account of letter-by-letter reading. *Cognitive Neuropsychology*, *15*, 7–52.

Benson, D. F. (1977). The third alexia. *Archives of Neurology*, *34*, 327–331.

Bookheimer, S. Y., Zeffiro, T. A., Blaxton, T., Gaillard, W., & Theodore, W. (1995). Regional cerebral blood flow during object naming and word reading. *Human Brain Mapping*, *3*, 93–106.

Bowers, J. S., Bub, D. N., & Arguin, M. (1996). A characterization of the word superiority effect in a case of letter-by-letter surface alexia. *Cognitive Neuropsychology*, *13*, 415–442.

Bub, D., Black, S. E., Howell, J., & Kertesz, A. (1987). Speech output processes and reading. In M. Coltheart, G. Sartori, & R. Job (Eds.), *Cognitive Neuropsychology of Language*. Hillsdale, NJ: Lawrence Erlbaum Associates.

Bub, D. N., Black, S., & Howell, J. (1989). Word recognition and orthographic context effects in a letter-by-letter reader. *Brain and Language*, *36*, 357–376.

Buxbaum, L. J., & Coslett, H. B. (1996). Deep dyslexic phenomenon in pure alexia. *Brain and Language*, *54*, 136–167.

Caramazza, A., & Hills, A. E. (1990a). Where do semantic errors come from? *Cortex*, *26*, 95–122.

Caramazza, A., & Hills, A. E. (1990b). Levels of representation, coordinate frames and unilateral neglect. *Cognitive Neuropsychology*, *7*, 391–455.

Chialant, D., & Caramazza, A. (1998). Perceptual and lexical factors in a case of letter-by-letter reading. *Cognitive Neuropsychology*, *15*, 167–202.

Cohen, L., Dehaene, S., Naccache L., Lehericy, S., Dehaene-Lambertz, G., Henaff, M.-A., & Michel, F. (2000). The visual word form area. *Brain*, *123*, 291–307.

Coltheart, M. (1980). Deep dyslexia: A right hemisphere hypothesis. In M. Coltheart, K. Patterson, & J. C. Marshall (Eds.), *Deep dyslexia*. London: Routledge and Kegan Paul.

Coltheart, M. (1996). Phonological dyslexia: past and future issues. *Cognitive Neuropsychology*, *13*, 749–762.

Coltheart, M. (1998). Letter-by-letter reading. *Cognitive Neuropsychology*, *15*(3) (Special issue).

Coltheart, M. (2000). Deep dyslexia is right-hemisphere reading. *Brain and Language*, *71*, 299–309.

Coltheart, M., Patterson, K., & Marshall, J. C. (Eds.) (1980). *Deep dyslexia*. London: Routledge and Kegan Paul.

Coltheart, M., & Rastle, K. (1994). Serial processing in reading aloud: Evidence for dual-route models of reading. *Journal of Experimental Psychology: Human Perception and Performance*, *20*, 1197–1211.

Coslett, H. B. (1991). Read but not write "idea": Evidence for a third reading mechanism. *Brain and Language*, *40*, 425–443.

Coslett, H. B., & Monsul, N. (1994). Reading with the right hemisphere: Evidence from transcranial magnetic stimulation. *Brain and Language*, *46*, 198–211.

Coslett, H. B., & Saffran, E. M. (1989a). Evidence for preserved reading in "pure alexia." *Brain*, *112*, 327–359.

Coslett, H. B., & Saffran, E. M. (1989b). Preserved object identification and reading comprehension in optic aphasia. *Brain*, *112*, 1091–1110.

Coslett, H. B., & Saffran, E. M. (1992). Optic aphasia and the right hemisphere: A replication and extension. *Brain and Language*, *43*, 148–161.

Coslett, H. B., & Saffran, E. M. (1998). Reading and the right hemisphere: Evidence from acquired dyslexia. In M. Beeman & C. Chiarello (Eds.), *Right hemisphere language comprehension* (pp. 105–132). Mahwah, NJ: Lawrence Erlbaum Associate.

Coslett, H. B., Saffran, E. M., Greenbaum, S., & Schwartz, H. (1993). Preserved reading in pure alexia: The effect of strategy. *Brain*, *116*, 21–37.

Coslett, H. B., Stark, M., Rajaram, S., & Saffran, E. M. (1995). Narrowing the spotlight: A visual attentional disorder in Alzheimer's disease. *Neurocase*, *1*, 305–318.

Déjerine, J. (1891). Sur un cas de cécité verbale avec agraphie suivi d'autopsie. *Compte Rendu des Séances de la Societé de Biologie*, *3*, 197–201.

Déjerine, J. (1892). Contribution à l'étude anatomopathologique et clinique des différentes variétés de cécité verbale. *Compte Bendu des Séances de la Société de Biologie*, *4*, 61–90.

Demonet, J. F., Wise, R., & Frackowiak, R. S. J. (1993). Language functions explored in normal subjects by positron emission tomography: A critical review. *Human Brain Mapping*, *1*, 39–47.

Derouesne, J., & Beauvois, M-F. (1979). Phonological processing in reading: Data from dyslexia. *Journal of Neurology, Neurosurgery and Psychiatry*, *42*, 1125–1132.

Ellis, A. W., Young, A. W., & Flude, B. M. (1993). Neglect and visual language. In I. H. Robinson & J. C. Marshall (Eds.), *Unilateral neglect: Clinical and experimental studies*. Mahwah, NW: Lawrence Erlbaum Associates.

Ellis, A. W., Lambon Ralph, M. A., Morris, J., & Hunter, A. (2000). Surface dyslexia: Description, treatment and interpretation. In E. Funnell (Ed.), *Case studies in the neuropsychology of reading*. Hove, East Sussex, UK: Psychology Press.

Farah, M. J., & Wallace, M. A. (1991). Pure alexia as a visual impairment: A reconsideration. *Cognitive Neuropsychology*, *8*, 313–334.

Fiez, J. A., & Petersen, S. E. (1998). Neuroimaging studies of word reading. *Proceedings of The National Academy of Sciences U.S.A.*, *95*, 914–921.

Freund, D. C. (1889). Über optische aphasia und seelenblindheit. *Archiv Psychiatrie und Nervenkrankheiten*, *20*, 276–297.

Friedman, R. B., & Hadley, J. A. (1992). Letter-by-letter surface alexia. *Cognitive Neuropsychology*, *9*, 185–208.

Funnell, E. (1983). Phonological processes in reading: New evidence from acquired dyslexia. *British Journal of Psychology*, *74*, 159–180.

Gabrieli, J. D. (1998). The role of the left prefrontal cortex in language and memory. *Proceedings of the National Academy of Science U.S.A.*, *95*, 906–913.

Geschwind, N. (1965). Disconnection syndromes in animals and man. *Brain*, *88*, 237–294, 585–644.

Geschwind, N., & Fusillo, M. (1966). Color-naming defects in association with alexia. *Archives of Neurology*, *15*, 137–146.

Glosser, G., & Friedman, R. B. (1990). The continuum of deep/phonological dyslexia. *Cortex*, *26*, 343–359.

Goodglass, H., & Kaplan, E. (1972). *Boston Diagnostic Aphasia Examination*. Philadelphia: Lea and Febiger.

Greenwald, M. L., & Berndt, R. S. (1999). Impaired encoding of abstract letter code order: Severe alexia in a mildly aphasic patient. *Cognitive Neuropsychology*, *16*, 513–556.

Hagoort, P., Indefrey, P., Brown, P., Herzog, H., Steinmetx, H., & Seitz, R. J. (1999). The neural circuitry involved in the reading of German words and pseudowords: A PET study. *Journal of Cognitive Neuroscience*, *11*, 383–398.

Hills, A. E., & Caramazza, A. (1995). Converging evidence for the interaction of semantic and sublexical phonological information in accessing lexical representations for spoken output. *Cognitive Neuropsychology*, *12*, 187–227.

Hodges, J. R., Patterson, K., Oxbury, S., & Funnell, E. (1992). Semantic dementia: Progressive fluent aphasia with temporal lobe atrophy. *Brain*, *115*, 1783–806.

Howard, D., & Franklin, S. (1987). Three ways for understanding written words, and their use in two contrasting cases of surface dyslexia (together with an odd routine for making "orthographic" errors in oral word production). In

A. Allport, D. Mackay, W. Prinz, & E. Scheerer (Eds.), *Language perception and production*. New York: Academic Press.

Howard, D., Patterson, K., Wise, R., Brown, W. D., Friston, K., Weiller, C., & Frackowiak, R. (1992). The cortical localization of the lexicons. *Brain, 115,* 1769–1782.

Indefrey, P. I., Kleinschmidt, A., Merboldt, K.-D., Kruger, G., Brown, C., Hagoort, P., & Frahm, J. (1997). Equivalent responses to lexical and nonlexical visual stimuli in occipital cortex: A functional magnetic resonance imaging study. *Neuroimage, 5,* 78–81.

Ladavas, E., Shallice, T., & Zanella, M. T. (1997). Preserved semantic access in neglect dyslexia. *Neuropsychologia, 35,* 257–270.

Lambon Ralph, M. A., Ellis, A. W., & Franklin, S. (1995). Semantic loss without surface dyslexia. *Neurocase, 1,* 363–369.

Marshall, J. C., & Newcombe, F. (1966). Syntactic and semantic errors in paralexia. *Neuropsychologia, 4,* 169–176.

Marshall, J. C., & Newcombe, F. (1973). Patterns of paralexia: A psycholinguistic approach. *Journal of Psycholinguistic Research, 2,* 175–199.

McClelland, J. L., & Rumelhart, D. E. (1981). An interactive activation model of context effects in letter perception: Part I. An account of basic findings. *Psychology Review, 88,* 375–407.

Menard, M. T., Kosslyn, S. M., Thompson, W. L., Alpert, N. M., & Rauch, S. L. (1996). Encoding words and pictures: A positron emission computed tomography study. *Neuropsychologia, 34,* 185–194.

Morton, J., & Patterson, K. E. (1980). A new attempt at an interpretation, or, an attempt at a new interpretation. In M. Coltheart, K. Patterson, & J. C. Marshall (Eds.), *Deep dyslexia* (pp. 91–118). London: Routledge and Kegan Paul.

Mozer, M. C. (1991). *The perception of multiple objects.* Cambridge, MA: MIT Press.

Noble, K., Glosser, G., & Grossman, M. (2000). Oral reading in dementia. *Brain and Language, 74,* 48–69.

Nobre, A. C., Allison, T., & McCarthy, G. (1994). Word recognition in the human inferior temporal lobe. *Nature, 372,* 260–263.

Patterson, K., & Kay, J. (1982). Letter-by-letter reading: Psychological descriptions of a neurological syndrome. *Quarterly Journal of Experimental Psychology, 34A,* 411–441.

Patterson, K. E., Marshall, J. C., & Coltheart, M. (Eds.) (1985). *Surface dyslexia.* London: Routledge and Kegan Paul.

Patterson, K. E., Vargha-Khadem, F., & Polkey, C. F. (1989a). Reading with one hemisphere. *Brain, 112,* 39–63.

Patterson, K. E., Seidenberg, M. S., & McClelland, J. L. (1989b). Connections and disconnections: Acquired dyslexia in a computational model of reading processes. In R. G. M. Morris (Ed.), *Parallel distributed processing: Implications for psychology and neurobiology.* Oxford: Oxford University Press.

Petersen, S. E., Fox, P. T., Snyder, A. Z., & Raichle, M. E. (1990). Activation of extrastriate and frontal cortical areas by words and word-like stimuli. *Science, 249,* 1041–1044.

Plaut, D. C., & Shallice, T. (1993). Deep dyslexia: A case study in connectionist neuropsychology. *Cognitive Neuropsychology, 10,* 377–500.

Plaut, D. C., McClelland, J. L., Seidenberg, M. S., & Patterson, K. (1996). Understanding normal and impaired word reading: Computational principles in quasi-regular domains. *Psychological Review, 103,* 56–115.

Price, C. J. (1998). The functional anatomy of word comprehension and production. *Trends in Cognitive Sciences, 2,* 281–288.

Price, C. J., Moore, C. J., & Frackowiak, R. S. J. (1996). The effect of varying stimulus rate and duration on brain activity during reading. *Neuroimage, 3,* 40–52.

Price, C. J., Wise, R. J. S., Watson, J. D. G., Patterson, K., Howard, D., & Frackowiak, R. S. J. (1994). Brain activity during reading: The effects of exposure duration and task. *Brain, 117,* 1255–1269.

Puce, A., Allison, T., Asgari, M., Gore, J. C., & McCarthy, G. (1996). Differential sensitivity of human visual cortex to faces, letter strings and textures: A functional resonance imaging study. *Journal of Neuroscience, 16,* 5205–5215.

Rastle, K., & Coltheart, M. (1999). Serial and Strategic Effects in Reading Aloud. *Journal of Experimental Psychology: Human Perception and Performance, 25,* 482–503.

Reuter-Lorenz, P. A., & Brunn, J. L. (1990). A prelexical basis for letter-by-letter reading: A case study. *Cognitive Neuropsychology, 7,* 1–20.

Rumsey, J. M., Horwitz, B., Donohue, B. C., Nace, K., Maisog, J. M., & Andreason, P. (1997). Phonological and orthographic components of word recognition. A PET-rCBF study. *Brain, 120,* 739–759.

Saffran, E. M., Bogyo, L. C., Schwartz, M. F., & Marin, O. S. M. (1980). Does deep dyslexia reflect right-hemisphere reading? In M. Coltheart, K. Patterson, & J. C. Marshall (Eds.), *Deep dyslexia* (pp. 381–406). London: Routledge and Kegan Paul.

Saffran, E. M., & Coslett, H. B. (1996). "Attentional dyslexia" in Alzheimer's disease: A case study. *Cognitive Neuropsychology, 13,* 205–228.

Saffran, E. M., & Coslett, H. B. (1998). Implicit vs. letter-by-letter reading in pure alexia: A tale of two systems. *Cognitive Neuropsychology, 15,* 141–166.

Saffran, E. M., & Marin, O. S. M. (1977). Reading without phonology: Evidence from aphasia. *Quarterly Journal of Experimental Psychology, 29,* 515–525.

Schwartz, M. F., Saffran, E. M., & Marin, O. S. M. (1979). Dissociation of language function in dementia: A case study. *Brain and Language, 7,* 277–306.

Seidenberg, M. S., & McClelland, J. L. (1989). A distributed, developmental model of word recognition and naming. *Psychological Review, 96,* 523–568.

Sieroff, E., Pollatsek, A., & Posner, M. (1988). Recognition of visual letter strings following injury to the posterior visual spatial attention system. *Cognitive Neuropsychology, 5,* 427–449.

Shallice, T. (1988). *From neuropsychology to mental structure.* Cambridge: Cambridge University Press.

Shallice, T., & Saffran, E. M. (1986). Lexical processing in the absence of explicit word identification: Evidence from a letter-by-letter reader. *Cognitive Neuropsychology, 3,* 429–458.

Shallice, T., & McGill, J. (1977). The origins of mixed errors. In J. Reguin (Ed.), *Attention and Performance* (Vol. VII, pp. 193–208). Hillsdale, NJ: Lawrence Erlbaum Associates.

Shallice, T., & Warrington E. K. (1977). The possible role of selective attention in acquired dyslexia. *Neuropsychologia, 15,* 31–41.

Shallice, T., & Warrington, E. K. (1980). Single and multiple component central dyslexic syndromes. In M. Coltheart, K. Patterson, & J. C. Marshall (Eds.), *Deep dyslexia.* London: Routledge and Kegan Paul.

Shallice, T., Warrington, E. K., & McCarthy, R. (1983). Reading without semantics. *Quarterly Journal of Experimental Psychology, 35A,* 111–138.

Sieroff, E., Pollatsek, A., & Posner, M. I. (1988). Recognition of visual letter strings following injury to the posterior visual spatial attention system. *Cognitive Neuropsychology, 5,* 427–449.

Thompson-Schill, S. L., D'Esposito, M., Aguirre, G. K., & Farah, M. J. (1997). Role of the left inferior prefrontal cortex in retrieval of semantic knowledge: A reevaluation. *Proceedings of the National Academy of Sciences U.S.A., 94,* 14792–14797.

Vandenberghe, R., Price, C., Wise, R., Josephs, O., & Frackowiak, R. S. (1996). Functional anatomy of a common semantic system for words and pictures. *Nature, 383,* 254–256.

Warrington, E., & Shallice, T. (1980). Word-form dyslexia. *Brain, 103,* 99–112.

Warrington, E. K., Cipolotti, L., & McNeil, J. (1993). Attentional dyslexia: A single case study. *Neuropsychologia, 31,* 871–886.

Zaidel, E. (1978). Lexical organization in the right hemisphere. In P. Buser & A. Rougeul-Buser (Eds.), *Cerebral correlates of conscious experience.* Amsterdam; Elsevier.

Zaidel, E., & Peters, A. M. (1983). Phonological encoding and ideographic reading by the disconnected right hemisphere: Two case studies. *Brain and Language, 14,* 205–234.

Zatorre, R. J., Meyer, E., Gjedde, A., & Evans, A. C. (1996). PET studies of phonetic processing of speech: Review, replication and reanalysis. *Cerebral Cortex, 6,* 21–30.

7 Acalculia: A Disorder of Numerical Cognition

Darren R. Gitelman

Arithmetic is being able to count up to twenty without taking off your shoes.
—Mickey Mouse

Although descriptions of calculation deficits date from the early part of this century, comprehensive neuropsychological and neuroanatomical models of this function have been slow to develop. This lag may reflect several factors, including an initial absence of nomenclature accurately describing calculation deficits, difficulty separating calculation disorders from disruptions in other domains, and, more fundamentally, the multidimensional nature of numerical cognition, which draws upon perceptual, linguistic, and visuospatial skills during both childhood development and adult performance. The goal of this chapter is to review the cognitive neuroscience and behavioral neuroanatomy underlying these aspects of numerical processing, and the lesion-deficit correlations that result in acalculia. Recommended tests at the bedside are outlined at the end of the chapter since the theoretical motivations for those tests will have been discussed by that point.

Case Report

C.L., a 55-year-old right-handed woman, sought an evaluation for problems with writing and calculations. These symptoms had been present for approximately 1 year and had led her to resign from her position as a second-grade teacher. In addition to writing and calculation deficits, both spelling and reading had declined. Lapses of memory occurred occasionally. Despite these deficits, daily living activities remained intact.

Examination revealed an alert, cooperative, and pleasant woman who was appropriately concerned about her predicament. She was fully oriented, but had only a vague knowledge of current events. She could not recite the months in normal order and her verbal fluency was reduced for lexical items (five words). After ten trials she was able to repeat four words from immediate memory,

and could then recall all four words after 10 minutes. This performance suggested that she did not have a primary memory disorder. There was mild hesitancy to her spontaneous speech, but no true word-finding pauses. She did well on confrontation naming, showing only mild hesitation on naming parts of objects. Only a single phonemic paraphasia was noted. Her comprehension was preserved, and reading was slow but accurate, including reading numbers. Writing was very poor. She had severe spelling difficulties, even for simple words, including regular and irregular forms. Calculations were severely impaired. For example, she said that 8 + 4 was 11 and could not calculate 4 × 12. Mild deficits were noted for finger naming and left-right orientation. Thus she manifested all four components of Gerstmann's syndrome (acalculia, agraphia, right-left confusion, and finger agnosia). Difficulties in target scanning and mild simultanagnosia were present. Clock drawing showed minimal misplacement of numbers, but she could not copy a cube. Lines were bisected correctly. Her general physical examination and elementary sensorimotor neurological examination showed no focal deficits.

Because of her relatively young age and unusual presentation, an extensive workup was performed. A variety of laboratory tests were unremarkable. A brain magnetic resonance imaging (MRI) scan showed moderate atrophic changes. Single-photon emission computed tomography showed greater left than right parietal perfusion deficits (figure 7.1).

The patient in this case report clearly had difficulty with calculations. The most significant other cognitive deficits were in writing and certain restricted aspects of naming (e.g., finger naming). The description of this case reports a simple, classic neurological approach to the evaluation of her calculation deficit. However, it will soon be shown that the examination barely touched upon the rich cognitive neurology and neuropsychology underlying human numerical cognition. The case also illustrates two important points regarding calculations that will be expanded upon later: (1) Calculation deficits do not necessarily represent general disturbances in intellectual abilities; for example, in this patient, language functions (outside of writing) and memory

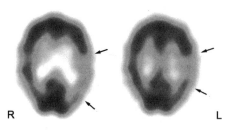

Figure 7.1
Two representative slices from the single-photon emission computed tomography scan for C.L. The areas of predominant left frontoparietal hypoperfusion are indicated by arrows. Perfusion was also reduced in similar areas on the right compared with normal subjects, but the extent was much less dramatic than the abnormalities on the left.

R   L

were generally preserved. (2) The cerebral perfusion deficits, particularly in the left parietal cortex, and the patient's anarithmetia are consistent with the prominent role of this region in several aspects of calculations.

Historical Perspective and Early Theories of Calculation

The development of numerical cognitive neuroscience has paralleled that of many other cognitive disorders. Early on in the history of this field, lesion-deficit correlations suggested the presence of discrete centers for calculation. Subsequently, views based on equipotentiality prevailed, and calculation deficits were thought to reflect generalized disruptions of brain function (Spiers, 1987). Current views preserve the concepts of regional specialization and multiregional integration through the theoretical formulation that complex cognitive functions, such as calculations, are supported by large-scale neural networks.[1]

The phrenologist Franz Josef Gall was probably the first to designate a cerebral source for numbers, in the early 1800s, which he attributed to the inferior frontal regions bilaterally (Kahn & Whitaker, 1991). No patient-related information, however,

was provided for this conjecture. The first patient-based description of an acquired calculation disorder was provided in 1908 by Lewandowsky and Stadelman. Their patient developed calculation deficits following removal of a left occipital hematoma. The resulting calculation disturbance clearly exceeded problems in language or deficits in other aspects of cognition. Thus, these authors were the first to report that calculation disturbances could be distinct from other language deficits.

Subsequently, several cases were reported in which calculation disturbances appeared to follow left retrorolandic lesions or bilateral occipital damage (Poppelreuter, 1917; Sittig, 1917; Peritz, 1918, summarized by Boller & Grafman, 1983). Peritz also specifically cited the left angular gyrus as a center for calculations (Boller & Grafman, 1983).

Henschen first used the term *acalculia* to refer to an inability to perform basic arithmetical operations (Henschen, 1920; Boller & Grafman, 1983; Kahn & Whitaker, 1991). He also postulated that calculations involved several cortical centers, including the inferior frontal gyrus for number pronunciation, both the angular gyrus and intraparietal sulcus for number reading, and the angular gyrus alone for writing numbers. Significantly, he also recognized that calculation and language functions are associated but independent (Boller & Grafman, 1983; Kahn & Whitaker, 1991).

Several subsequent analyses have documented the distinctions between acalculia and aphasia, and have demonstrated that calculation deficits are unlikely to be related to a single brain center (i.e., they are not simply localized to the angular gyrus). Berger, for example, documented three cases of acalculia that had lesions in the left temporal and occipital cortices but not in the angular gyrus (Berger, 1926; Boller & Grafman, 1983; Kahn & Whitaker, 1991). Berger also suggested that the various brain areas underlying calculation worked together to produce these abilities, thus heralding large-scale network theories of brain organization (Mesulam, 1981; Selemon & Goldman-Rakic, 1988; Alexander, Crutcher, & Delong, 1990;

Dehaene & Cohen, 1995). Another important distinction noted by Berger was the difference between secondary acalculia (i.e., those disturbances due to cognitive deficits in attention, memory language, etc.), and primary acalculia, which appeared to be independent of other cerebral disorders (Boller & Grafman, 1983).

Other early authors postulated a variety of additional deficits that could interfere with calculations, such as altered spatial cognition (Singer & Low, 1933; Krapf, 1937; Critchley, 1953), disturbed sensorimotor transformations (possibly having to do with the physical manipulation of quantities) (Krapf, 1937), altered numerical mental representations and calculation automaticity (Leonhard, 1939; Critchley, 1953), and abnormal numerical and symbolic semantics (Cohn, 1961; Boller & Grafman, 1983; Kahn & Whitaker, 1991). Consistent with this plethora of potential cognitive deficits, an increasing number of cognitive processes (e.g., ideational, verbal, spatial, and constructional) were hypothesized to support numerical functions, and correspondences were developed between cortical areas and the cognitive functions they were thought to serve (Boller & Grafman, 1983; Kahn & Whitaker, 1991).

The parietal lobes have long been considered to be a fundamental cortical region for calculation processes. From 1924 to 1930, Josef Gerstmann published a series of articles describing a syndrome that now bears his name. He described the association of lesions in the left parietal cortex with deficits in writing, finger naming, right-left orientation and calculations (Gerstmann, 1924, 1927, 1930). Gerstmann attributed this disorder to a disturbance of "body schema," which he thought was coordinated through the parietal lobes. The existence and cohesiveness of this syndrome has been both praised (Strub & Geschwind, 1974) and challenged (Benton, 1961; Poeck & Orgass, 1966; Benton, 1992).

It has also been unclear how disturbances in body schema would explain acalculia except at a superficial level (e.g., children learn calculations by counting on their fingers; therefore a disturbance in finger

naming may lead to a disturbance in calculations). More recently, it has been suggested that the Gerstmann syndrome may represent a disconnection between linguistic and visual-spatial systems (Levine, Mani, & Calvanio, 1988). This explanation may be particularly important for understanding how neural networks supporting language or symbolic manipulation and those supporting spatial cognition interact with each other and contribute to calculations. This particular point is discussed further in the section on network models of calculations.

Aside from the parietal contributions to number processing, other authors, focusing on the visual aspects of numerical manipulation, have considered the occipital lobes to be particularly important (Krapf, 1937; Goldstein, 1948). Another debate has concentrated on the hemispheric localization of arithmetical functions. Although calculation deficits occur more commonly with lesions to the left hemisphere, they can also be seen with right hemisphere injury (Henschen, 1919; Critchley, 1953; Hécaen, 1962). Others, such as Goldstein (1948), doubted the right hemisphere's involvement in this function.

More recently, Collignon et al. and Grafman et al. documented calculation performance in series of patients with right or left hemisphere damage (Collingnon, Leclercq & Mahy, 1977; Grafman, Passafiume, Faglioni, & Boller, 1982). In both reports, disturbances of calculation followed injury to either hemisphere; however, acalculia occurred more often in patients with left hemisphere lesions. Grafman et al. (1982) also demonstrated that left retrorolandic lesions impaired calculations more than left anterior or right-sided lesions.

In 1961, Hècaen et al. published a report on a large series of patients (183) with posterior cortical lesions and calculation disorders (Hécaen, Angelergues, & Hovillier, 1961). Three main types of calculation deficits were noted: (1) One group had alexia and agraphia for digits with or without alexia and agraphia for letters. In this group, calculations appeared to be impaired secondary to disturbances in visual aspects of numerical input and output. (2) A second group showed problems with the spatial organization of numbers and tended to write numbers in the wrong order or invert them. (3) The third group had difficulty performing arithmetical operations, but their deficits were not simply attributable to problems with the comprehension or production of numbers. This group was defined as having anarithmetia.

The importance of this report was severalfold: It confirmed the distinctions between aphasia and acalculia; it demonstrated the importance of the parietal cortex to calculations (among other retrorolandic regions); it demonstrated the separability of comprehension, production, and computational operations in the calculation process; and it suggested that both hemispheres contribute to this function (Boller & Grafman, 1983). This report was also the first to attempt a comprehensive cognitive description of calculation disorders, rather than considering them as disconnected and unrelated syndromes.

Grewel (1952, 1969) stressed the symbolic nature of calculation and that abnormalities in the semantics and syntax of number organization could also define a series of dyscalculias. He noted that the essential aspects of our number system are based on the principles underlying the Hindu system: (1) ten symbols (0–9) are all that is necessary to define any number; (2) a digit's value in a number is based on its position (place value); and (3) zero indicates the absence of power (Grewel 1952, 1969; Boller & Grafman, 1983). Therefore calculation disorders might reflect abnormalities of digit selection or digit placement. These features are particularly important in modern concepts of numerical comprehension and production (McCloskey, Caramazza, & Basili, 1985).

Grewel also suggested several additional types of primary acalculia. For example, asymbolic acalculia referred to problems in comprehending or manipulating mathematical symbols, while asyntactic acalculia described problems in comprehending and producing numbers (Grewel, 1952, 1969). Although many of the anatomical associations he reported are not in use today, they illuminated the

multiple cortical areas associated with this function (Grewel, 1952, 1969).

Comprehensive Neuropsychological Theories of Calculation

By the early 1970s, a variety of case reports and group lesion studies had suggested a number of basic facts about arithmetical functions: (1) It was likely that calculation abilities represented a collection of cognitive functions separate from but interdependent with other intellectual abilities such as language, memory, and visual-spatial functions. Therefore, significant calculation deficits could occur, with less prominent disturbances across several other cognitive domains. (2) A number of brain regions appeared to be important for calculations, including the parietal, posterior temporal, and occipital cortices, and possibly the frontal cortex.[2] Additional lesion sites are discussed further later. (3) Both hemispheres were thought to contribute to calculation performance, but lesions of the left hemisphere more often produced deficits in calculations and resulted in greater impairments in performance. (4) There were likely to be several different types of deficits that resulted in acalculia, for example, the asymbolic and asyntactic acalculias of Grewel (Grewel, 1952, 1969).

Despite these theoretical advances, there was still debate about the distinctness and localizability of calculations as a function (Collingnon et al., 1977; Spiers, 1987). More problematic had been the lack of a coherent theoretical framework to explain either the operational principles or the functional–anatomical correlations underlying calculation abilities. Further understanding of the neuropsychology and functional anatomy of calculations benefited from the development of theoretically constrained case studies (Spiers, 1987) and the use of mental chronometry to specify the underlying neuropsychological processes (Posner, 1986). In recent years, a variety of brain mapping methods have also contributed to our understanding of the brain regions subserving this function.

Current psychological approaches to numerical cognition have attempted to incorporate many of these aspects of numerical processing into a comprehensive theoretical framework. This forumulation includes how numbers are perceived (visually, verbally, etc.), the nature of numerical representations in the brain, the variety of numerical operations (number comparison, counting, approximation, and arithmetical computations), and how these perceptual, representational, and operational functions relate to one another.

McCloskey formulated one of the first comprehensive calculation theories by outlining number processing and computational mechanisms (McCloskey et al., 1985). However, Dehaene has argued that approximation and quantification processes constitute an important aspect of the calculation system and were not explicitly modeled in McCloskey's formulations (McCloskey et al., 1985; Dehaene & Cohen, 1995, 1997; Dehaene, Dehaene-Lambertz, & Cohen, 1998).

A general schematic representing a synthesis of various models for calculations is shown in figure 7.2. Most current calculation theories include each of the systems in figure 7.2, although the nature of the interrelationships among these processes has been debated considerably. Recent theories, such as the popular triple-code model of Dehaene, attempt to integrate neuropsychological theories of calculation with network theories of the associated brain anatomy (Dehaene & Cohen, 1995). Details of these neurocognitive systems and the nature of deficits following their injury are reviewed later.

Number Processing

As illustrated in figure 7.2, a number-processing system is central to our ability to comprehend and produce a variety of numerical formats.[3] Numbers can be written as numerals or words (e.g., 47 versus forty-seven) or they can be spoken. There are also lexical and syntactic aspects of number processing

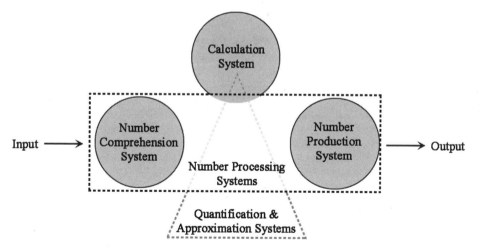

Figure 7.2
Schematic of systems supporting calculations and number processing. The functions concerned with quantification and approximation were not explicitly included in the original model outlined by McCloskey Caramazzza, Basili (1985), but have been added because of their demonstrated importance to numerical cognition (Dehaene & Cohen, 1995). The positions of quantification and approximation operations in the model represent both a foundation supporting the development of numerical cognition and an important numerical resource used by adults in number processing and calculations.

(McCloskey et al., 1985). Lexical processing involves the identification of individual numerals within a number. For example, lexical processing of the number 447 establishes that there are two 4s and one 7. An example of a lexical error would be to interpret this number as 457. This demonstrates maintenance of the overall number quantity (as opposed to saying "forty-five"), but an individual digit has been misidentified.

Syntactic processing defines the order and relationship of the numerical elements to each other and is closely associated with the concept of place value. An example of a syntactic error would be writing the number four-hundred forty seven as 40047. Although this answer contains the elements 400 and 47, combining them in this manner violates the syntactic relationships in the original number (McCloskey et al., 1985).

As part of the set of lexical functions, mechanisms have also been posited for the phonological processing of numbers (i.e., processing spoken words for numbers), and the graphemic processing of numbers (i.e., processing written number forms). However, phonological and graphemic mechanisms have not been attributed to syntactic functions since spoken and written verbal number forms appear to require similar syntactic processing (i.e., the syntactic relationships among the elements of forty-four and 44 are identical). Phonological and graphemic mechanisms have also not been distinguished for Arabic numerals, which occur only in written form (McCloskey et al., 1985). An outline of possible cognitive subcomponents for number processing is shown in figure 7.3.

General support for the functions delineated in this schema has been neuropsychologically demonstrated by finding patients who show dissociations in their number-processing abilities following various brain lesions (traumatic, vascular, etc.). Unfortunately, in the acalculia literature, precise localization of lesions for most patients is lacking. Over the past several years, however, data from functional neuroimaging studies have started to provide more precise information on brain–behavior relationships in this area.

In order to illustrate these deficits in number processing, specific aspects of patients' case histories are provided here. However, room does not permit a complete elaboration of each report, and the interested reader is encouraged to review the source material for this detail. Patients are identified as they were in the original publication. Some patients

NUMBER PROCESSING MECHANISMS

Number Comprehension   **Number Production**

Arabic mechanisms   *Arabic mechanisms*

    Lexical   Lexical
    Syntactic   Syntactic

Verbal mechanisms   *Verbal mechanisms*

    Lexical   Lexical

      Phonologic   Phonologic
      Graphemic   Graphemic

    Syntactic   Syntactic

Figure 7.3
Outline of proposed neuropsychological mechanisms subserving number processing. (Adapted from McCloskey, Caramazza, & Basili, 1985.)

are included several times because they illustrate several types of number and/or calculation deficits.

Comprehension versus Production Dissociations

Both Benson and Denckla (1969) and Singer and Low (1933) have described patients with relatively preserved number comprehension, but impaired production. Case 1 of Benson and Denckla (1969), for example, could identify a verbally specified number (i.e., when asked to find the number eighty, the patient could point to 80), but could not write down the Arabic numerals for a verbally presented number (i.e., the patient could not write 80). This patient could also select the correct answers to calculations when allowed to choose from several responses, but could not generate the correct answer in either spoken or written form.

The patient's ability to identify numerals and to correctly select answers to calculations implied that the mechanisms for comprehending and adding numbers were intact. In addition, although number production was impaired, her responses were usually of the proper magnitude, suggesting that she made lexical rather than syntactic errors. Thus when given the problem of adding 4 + 5, case 1 verbally responded "eight," wrote "5," and chose "9" from a list. The only anatomical localization described is that the lesion was initially associated with a mild right hemiparesis, a fluent aphasia, altered cortical sensory function (agraphesthesia), and a right homonymous hemianopia, suggesting a lesion affecting the left posterior temporal and inferior parietal cortices.

The other example of preserved comprehension but impaired production is given by Singer and Low's (1933) report. Their patient developed acalculia following accidental carbon monoxide poisoning, so there was no focal lesion. This patient demonstrated intact number comprehension by correctly indicating the larger of two numerals and by identifying verbally specified numbers. Although he was able to write one and two-digit numerals to dictation, he made syntactic errors for numerals with three or more digits (e.g., for two-hundred forty-two he wrote 20042).

Patients with preserved number production but deficits in comprehension are more difficult to differentiate since it may be unclear if the numbers produced are correct. For example, if the number 47 is misunderstood and then written as 43, it would be difficult to know whether comprehension or production was impaired. However, some understanding of the true deficit may be gained through testing performance on quantification operations (i.e., counting, subitizing, and estimating). Thus a patient may be able to produce the correct answer when asked to count a set of objects, or to estimate whether a calculation is correct. Furthermore, patients with intact production and differential preservation of either Arabic numeral or verbal comprehension also allow demonstration of a production-comprehension dissociation (see the reports on patients H.Y. and K. below; McCloskey et al., 1985).

Notational Dissociations (Arabic Numerals and Verbal Descriptions)

Double dissociations in processing Arabic numerals and verbal numbers were seen in patients H.Y. and K. described by McCloskey et al. (1985), and two patients described by Berger (1926). Patient H.Y., for example, was able to indicate which of two Arabic numerals was larger (i.e., he could correctly choose when shown 4 and 3), but he performed at chance level when judging visually presented verbal numbers (i.e., he could not choose correctly when shown four and three). This pattern shows a comprehension deficit for verbal numbers. Patient K. showed the opposite notational deficit. K. could judge visually presented verbal numbers, but not Arabic numerals (McCloskey et al., 1985).

Berger's patients showed notational dissociations for production rather than comprehension (Berger, 1926). Thus one patient of Berger's provided correct spoken responses, but incorrect written responses to simple calculations. The second patient showed correct written, but incorrect spoken responses. Unfortunately no anatomical information is available for H.Y., K., or Berger's cases.

Lexical versus Syntactic Dissociations

Dissociations in lexical versus syntactic processing have been described in several patients. A lexical but not syntactic production deficit was described by Benson and Denckla in case 1 noted earlier (Benson and Denckla, 1969), and R.R. of McCloskey et al. (1985). For example, R.R. responded "fifty-five thousand" when shown the number 37,000 (McCloskey et al., 1985). This answer is considered syntactically correct because it is of the same general magnitude as the correct response. If R.R. had instead responded "thirty-seven hundred" when shown 37,000, this would have been classified as a syntactic error because the numerals are correct, but the number is of the wrong magnitude. R.R. also performed number comparisons without error, confirming a deficit in production but not comprehension.

Syntactic but not lexical production errors were reported for Singer and Low's patient and for patient V.O. of McCloskey et al. (Singer and Low, 1933; McCloskey et al., 1985). V.O., for example, produced numbers such as 40037000 when asked to write four hundred thirty-seven thousand.

When lexical disturbances are present, errors can show the influence of lexical class. There appear to be three primary lexical classes for numbers in common use: ones (i.e., 1–9), teens (i.e., 10–19), and tens (i.e., 20–90). Patients such as R.R. tend to stay within a lexical class when producing the incorrect response (e.g., saying "seven" but not "fourteen" or "fifty-two" in response to the number three, or saying "sixteen" but not "five" or "thirty-seven" in response to the number thirteen). However, there is no tendency to select from the same tens class. Thus, patients are equally likely to choose numbers in the twenties, forties, or sixties when shown the number 23. Similarly, number proximity does not appear to influence lexical accuracy in these patients, and they are as likely to choose 4, 6, or 8 in response to the number 7. These findings suggest a categorical specificity to lexical class that is not influenced by the "semantic" value of the number itself. Although McCloskey et al. (1985) have sug-

gested this implies separate lexical systems underlying each number class, category specificity could also arise as a consequence of the frequency and pattern of usage for a number class rather than from the magnitude values of that class (Ashcraft, 1987).

Phonological versus Graphemic Dissociations

Independent disruptions in the processing of spoken versus written numbers suggest dissociations in phonological versus graphemic mechanisms. McCloskey et al. (1985) provide an example of this dissociation through their patient H.Y., who was unable to compare two written-out numbers (e.g., indicating whether six or five is larger), but could perform the task when the numbers were spoken. This performance suggests a deficit in comprehending written numbers or graphemes, but not spoken numbers or phonemes (McCloskey et al., 1985). Although the lesion leading to H.Y.'s disturbed graphemic comprehension was not reported, the deficit bears a similarity to the findings in pure alexia, suggesting a possible anatomical localization.

Patients with pure alexia are unable to read words, but have no difficulty writing or understanding language presented by the auditory route (see Chapter 6). Anatomically, most cases of pure alexia have damage to the left medial occipital cortex and the splenium of the corpus callosum. The left occipital damage results in a right homonymous hemianopia and eliminates input from the left hemisphere visual system to language networks on the left. Information from the intact right occipital cortex also cannot reach the language system because the concomitant involvement of the splenium of the corpus callosum disconnects visual information from the right hemisphere to the left hemisphere language system. Patients with pure alexia are not aphasic, because their auditory language performance is intact. Similarly, patient H.Y. did not have an underlying deficit in number comprehension because performance following auditory presentation was correct, but there seemed to be a disconnection between visual number input and the numerical comprehension system, suggesting a possible left occipital location to his lesion.

In fact, alexia for numerals is often, but not always, associated with alexia for words and has a similar anatomical localization in the left occipito-temporal cortex (McNeil & Warrington, 1994; Cohen & Dehaene, 1995). However, some patients have shown dissociable deficits in reading numerals and words, suggesting nonoverlapping but proximate brain regions for these functions. (Hécaen & Angelergues, 1961; Hécaen et al., 1961; Hécaen, 1962).

Patients with alexia for numerals may also reveal different capabilities of the left and right hemispheres for numerical processing. As discussed later, the left hemisphere is generally necessary for exact calculations, but both hemispheres appear to contain the neural machinery for quantification and approximation. Evidence for this organization was provided by Cohen and Dehaene (1995) in their description of patients G.O.D. and S.M.A. Both patients suffered infarctions in the medial left occipitotemporal cortex, resulting in a right homonymous hemianopia and pure alexia for words and numerals. Both patients showed increasing error rates for reading multidigit numerals compared with single digits. They also both had difficulty adding visually presented numbers, but performed very well when numbers were presented by the auditory route. Despite these deficits, the patients were able to compare visually presented numerals with a very high accuracy. This performance is consistent with a disconnection of visual information from the left hemisphere networks necessary for exact calculations. However, visual information was able to reach right hemisphere regions that are capable of number comparison (Cohen & Dehaene, 1995).

Similar dissociations between comparison and computation have been seen in split-brain patients (i.e., patients with division of the corpus callosum due to either surgery or an ischemic lesion) (Gazzaniga & Smylie, 1984; Dehaene & Cohen, 1995). In these reports, split-brain patients were able to compare digits when the stimuli were flashed to either hemifield. However, they were able to read numerals or perform simple arithmetical operations only when the numerals were flashed to the right hemifield. Taken together, the findings in patients with alexia for numerals and in split-brain patients suggest that both hemispheres contain the neural machinery for numeral recognition and comparison, but that only the left hemisphere is generally capable of performing calculations or naming numerals.

Anatomical Relationships and Functional Imaging

While lesion and neuropsychological data have generally not provided sufficient information to decide on the location of many numerical processing functions, the results from brain mapping techniques such as position emission tomography (PET), functional magnetic resonance imaging (fMRI), and event-related potentials (ERP) have helped to illuminate some of the functional–anatomical relationships for number processing.

Allison et al. used intracranial ERP recordings to identify areas in the fusiform and inferior temporal gyri that were responsive to numerals (Allison, McCarthy, Nobre, Puce, & Belger, 1994). These regions only partially overlapped with areas responsive to letter strings, a result that is consistent with previous observations of dissociations between letter and numeral reading in patients with pure alexia (Hécaen et al., 1961). Polk and Farah (1998) using fMRI and a surface coil over the left hemisphere found a left-sided occipitotemporal area in six subjects that responded more to letters than to numerals, but did not find any areas more responsive to numerals than to letters. However, these authors noted the reduced sensitivity of this technique and that it would have specifically missed activations in the right hemisphere.

Pinel, Le Clec'h, van de Moortele, Naccache, LcBihan, & Dehaene (1999) used event-related fMRI to examine various aspects of number processing, including visual identification (Arabic numerals versus spelled out numbers) and comparison of magnitude (numerical distance). The task produced a large number of activations (forty-seven) overlying frontal (precentral and prefrontal), parietal, occipital, fusiform, and cingulate cortices and the thalamus. Notational effects were seen in the right fusiform gyrus (greater activation for Arabic numerals than spelled-out numbers) and the left superior, precentral gyrus (slight prolongation of the hemodynamic response for spelled-out numbers than for Arabic numerals) (Pinel et al., 1999).

Although lesion information and brain mapping data for numerical processing are limited, the available information suggests that the fusiform gyrus and nearby regions of bilateral visual association cortex are closely associated with support of numerical notation and numerical lexical access. It is also tempting to speculate that the syntactic aspects of number processing are served by left posterior frontal regions, perhaps in the superior precentral gyrus (by analogy with syntactic processing areas for language), but this has not been shown conclusively.

Calculation Operations

Aside from mechanisms for processing numbers, a separate set of functions has been posited for performing arithmetical operations. Deficits in this area were formerly described as anarithmetia or primary acalculia (Boller & Grafman, 1985). The major neuropsychological abnormalities of this subsystem have been hypothesized to consist of deficits in (1) processing operational symbols or words, (2) retrieving memorized mathematical facts, (3) performing simple rule-based operations, and (4) executing multistep calculation procedures (McCloskey et al., 1985). Patients showing dissociated abilities for each of these operations have provided support for this organizational scheme.

Numerical Symbol Processing

Grewel was one of the first authors to codify deficits in comprehending the operational symbols of calculation. A disorder that he called "asymbolia,"

which had been documented in patients as early as 1908, was characterized by difficulty recognizing operational symbols, but no deficits in understanding the operations themselves (Lewandowsky & Stadelmann, 1908; Eliasberg & Feuchtwanger, 1922; Grewel, 1952, 1969). A separate deficit also noted by Grewel in the patients of Sittig and Berger was a loss of conceptual understanding of mathematical operations (i.e., an inability to describe the meaning of an operation) (Sittig, 1921; Berger, 1926; Grewel, 1952).

Ferro and Bothelho described a patient who developed a deficit corresponding to Grewel's asymbolia following a left occipitotemporal lesion (Ferro & Botelho, 1980). Although the patient had an anomic aphasia, reading and writing of words were preserved. The patient could also read and write single and multidigit numerals, and had no difficulty performing verbally presented calculations. This performance demonstrated intact conceptual knowledge of basic arithmetical operations. Although the patient frequently misnamed operational symbols in visually presented operations, she could then perform the misnamed operation correctly. Thus, when presented with 3×5, she said "three plus five," and responded "eight."

Retrieval of Mathematical Facts

Remarkably, patients can show deficits in retrievals of arithmetical facts (impaired recall of "rote" values for multiplication on division tables) despite an intact knowledge of calculation procedures. Warrington (1982) first described a patient (D.R.C.) with this dissociation. Following a left parieto-occipital hemorrhage, patient D.R.C. had difficulty performing even simple calculations despite preservation of other numerical abilities, such as accurately reading and writing numbers, comparing numbers, estimating quantities, and properly defining arithmetical operations that he could not perform correctly. D.R.C.'s primary deficit therefore appeared to be in the recall of memorized computational facts. Patients with similar deficits had been alluded to in earlier reports by Grewel

(1952, 1969) and Cohn (1961), but their analyses did not exclude possible disturbances in number processing.

Patient M.W. reported by McCloskey et al. (1985) also showed deficits in the retrieval of facts from memorized tables. This patient's performance was particularly striking because he retrieved incorrect values for operations using single digits even though multistep calculations were performed flawlessly (e.g., carrying operations and rule-based procedures were correct despite difficulties in performing single-digit operations). He further demonstrated intact knowledge for arithmetical procedures by using table information that he could remember, to derive other answers. For example, he could not spontaneously recall the answer to 7×7. However, he could recall the answers to 7×3 and 7×10, and was able to use these results to calculate the solution to 7×7. Comprehension of both numerals and simple procedural rules was shown by his nearly flawless performance on problems such as $1 \times N$ despite numerous errors for other computations (e.g., $9 \times N$).

One interesting aspect of M.W.'s performance on multiplication problems, and also the performance of similar patients, is that errors tend to be both "within table" and related to the problem being calculated. "Within table" refers to responses coming from the set of possible answers to commonly memorized single-digit multiplication problems. For example, a related, within-table error for 6×8 is 56 (i.e., the answer to 7×8). Errors that are not within table (e.g., 59 or 47), or not related to the problem (e.g., 55 or 45), are much less likely to occur. Another important issue in the pattern of common deficits is that the errors vary across the range of table facts. Thus the patient may have great difficulty retrieving 8×8 or 8×7, while having no difficulty retrieving 8×6 or 9×7. The variability of deficits following brain injury (e.g., impairment of $8 \times 9 = 72$ but not $7 \times 9 = 63$) may somehow reflect the independent mental representations of these facts (Dehaene, 1992; McCloskey, 1992).

One model for the storage of arithmetical facts, which attempts to account for these types of deficits,

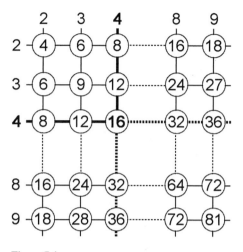

Figure 7.4
Schematic of a tabular representation for storing multiplication facts. Activation of a particular answer occurs by searching the corresponding rows and columns of the table to their point of intersection, as indicated by the bold numbers and lines. (Adapted from McCloskey, Aliminosa, & Sokol, 1991.)

is that of a tabular lexicon (figure 7.4). The figure shows that during recall, activation is hypothesized to spread among related facts (the bold lines in figure 7.4). This mechanism may account for both the within-table and the relatedness errors noted earlier (Stazyk, Ashcraft, & Hamann, 1982). Two other behaviors are also consistent with a "tabular" organization of numerical facts: (1) repetition priming, or responding more quickly to an identical previously seen problem and (2) error priming, which describes the increased probability of responding incorrectly after seeing a problem that is related but not identical to one shown previously (Dehaene, 1992).

Other calculation error types are noted in table 7.1. The nomenclature used in the table is derived from the classification scheme suggested by Sokol et al., although the taxonomy has not been universally accepted (Sokol, McCloskey, Cohen, & Aliminosa, 1991). Two general categories of errors

Table 7.1
Types of calculation errors

Error type	Description	Example
Commission		
Operand	The correct answer to the problem shares an operand with the original equation.	$5 \times 8 = 48$. The answer is correct for 6×8, which shares the operand 8 with the original equation.
Operation	The answer is correct for a different mathematical operation on the operands.	$3 \times 5 = 8$. The answer is correct for addition.
Indeterminate	The answer could be classified as either an operand or an operational error.	$4 \times 4 = 8$. The answer is true for 2×4 or $4 + 4$.
Table	The answer comes from the range of possible results for a particular operation, but is not related to the problem.	$4 \times 8 = 30$. The answer comes from the "table" of single-digit multiplication answers.
Nontable	The answer does not come from the range of results for that operation.	$5 \times 6 = 23$. There are no single-digit multiplication problems whose answer is 23.
Omission	The answer is not given.	$3 \times 7 =$

are errors of omission (i.e., failing to respond) and errors of commission (i.e., responding with the incorrect answer). As shown in table 7.1, there are several types of commission errors, some of which seem to predominate in different groups. Operand errors are the most common error type seen in normal subjects (Miller, Perlmutter, & Keating, 1984; Campbell & Graham, 1985). Patients can show a variety of dissociated error types. For example, Sokol et al. (1991) described patient P.S., who primarily made operand errors, while patient G.E. made operation errors. Although the occurrences of these errors were generally linked to left hemisphere lesions, there has been no comprehensive framework linking error type to particular lesion locations.

Rules and Procedures

An abnormality in the procedures of calculation is the third type of deficit leading to anarithmetia. Procedural deficits can take several forms, including errors in simple rules, in complex rules, or in complex multistep procedures. Examples of simple rules would include $0 \times N = 0$, $0 + N = N$, and $1 \times$ $N = N$ operations.[4] An example of a complex rule would be knowledge of the steps involved in multiplication by 0 in the context of executing a multidigit multiplication. Complex procedures would include the organization of intermediate products in multiplication or division problems, and multiple carrying or borrowing operations in multidigit addition and subtraction problems, respectively.

Several authors have shown that in normal subjects, rule-based problems are solved more quickly than nonrule-based types (Parkman & Groen, 1971; Groen & Parkman, 1972; Parkman, 1972; Miller et al., 1984), although occasional slower responses have been found (Parkman, 1972; Stazyk et al., 1982). Nevertheless, the available evidence suggests that rule-based and nonrule-based problems are solved differently, and can show dissociations in a subject's performance (Sokol et al., 1991; Ashcraft, 1992).

Patient P.S., who had a large left hemisphere hemorrhage, was reported by Sokol et al. (1991) as showing evidence for a deficit in simple rules, specifically multiplication by 0. This patient made patchy errors in the retrieval of table facts (0% errors for 9×8, to 52% errors for 4×4), but missed 100% of the $0 \times N$ problems. This performance suggested that the patient no longer had access to the rule for solving $0 \times N$ problems. Remarkably, during the last part of testing, the patient appeared to recover knowledge of this rule and began to perform $0 \times N$ operations flawlessly. During the same time period, performance on calculations of the $M \times N$ type showed only minimal improvement across blocks.

Patient G.E., reported by Sokol et al. (1991), suffered a left frontal contusion and demonstrated a dissociation in simple versus complex rule-based computations. This patient made errors when performing the simple rule computation of $0 \times N$ (always reporting the result as $0 \times N = N$), but he was able to multiply by 0 correctly within a multidigit calculation. In this setting he recalled the complex rule of using 0 as a placeholder in the partial products of multiplication problems.

More complex procedural deficits are illustrated in figure 7.5. Patient 1373, cited by McCloskey et al. (1985), showed good retrieval of table facts, but impaired performance of multiplication procedures. In one case, shown in figure 7.5A, he failed to shift the intermediate multiplication products one column to the left. Note that the individual arith-

metical operations in figure 7.5A are performed correctly, but the answer is nonetheless incorrect because of this procedural error.

Other deficits in calculation procedures have included incorrect performance of carrying and/or borrowing operations, as shown by patients V.O. and D.L. of McCloskey et al. (1985) (figure 7.5B), and confusing steps in one calculation procedure with those of another, as in patients W.W. and H.Y. of McCloskey et al. (1985) (figure 7.5C).

Arithmetical Dissociations

Individual arithmetical operations have also revealed dissociations among patients. For example, patients have been described with intact division, but impaired multiplication (patient 1373) (McCloskey et al., 1985) and intact multiplication and addition, but impaired subtraction and/or division (Berger, 1926), among other dissociations (Dehaene & Cohen, 1997). Several theories have tried to account for the apparent random dissociations among operations. One explanation is that separate processing streams underlie each arithmetical operation (Dagenbach & McCloskey, 1992). Another possibility is that each operation may be differentially linked to verbal, quantification (see later discussion), or other cognitive domains (e.g., working memory) (Dehaene & Cohen, 1995, 1997).

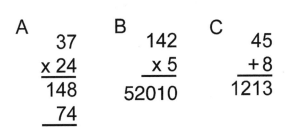

Figure 7.5
Examples of various calculation errors. (*A*) Multiplication: failure to shift the second intermediate product. (*B*) Multiplication: omission of the carrying operation and each partial product is written in full. (*C*) Addition: addend not properly carried, i.e., 8 is added to 5 and then incorrectly again added to 4. Each partial addend has then been placed on a single line. (Adapted from McCloskey, Caramazza, & Basili, 1985.)

Based on this concept, each arithmetical operation may require different operational strategies for a solution. These cognitive links may depend partly on previous experience (e.g., knowledge of multiplication tables) and partly on the strategies used to arrive at a solution. For example, multiplication and addition procedures are often retrieved through the recall of memorized facts. Simple addition operations can also be solved by counting strategies, an option not readily applicable to multiplication. Subtraction and division problems, on the other hand, are more frequently solved de novo, and therefore require access to several cognitive processes, such as verbal mechanisms (e.g., recalling multiplication facts to perform division), quantification operations (counting), and working memory. Differential injury to these cognitive domains may be manifest as a focal deficit for a particular arithmetical operation. The deficits in patient M.A.R. reported by Dehaene and Cohen (1997) support this cognitive organization.

This patient had a left inferior parietal lesion and could recall simple memorized facts for solving addition and multiplication problems, but did not perform as well when calculating subtractions. This performance suggested that M.A.R. had access to some memorized table facts, but that the inferior parietal lesion may have led to deficits in the calculation process itself. Patient B.O.O., also reported by Dehaene and Cohen (1997), had a lesion in the left basal ganglia and demonstrated greater deficits in multiplication than in either addition or subtraction. In this case, recall of rote-learned table facts was impaired, leading to multiplication deficits, but the patient was able to use other strategies for solving addition and subtraction problems.

Despite these examples, functional associations are not able to easily explain the dramatic dissociations reported in some patients, such as the one described by Lampl et al. Their patient had a left parietotemporal hemorrhage and had a near inability to perform addition, multiplication, or division, but provided 100% correct responses on subtraction problems (Lampl, Eshel, Gilad, & Sarova-Pinhas, 1994).

Anatomical Relationships and Functional Imaging

The most frequent cortical site of damage causing anarithmetia is the left inferior parietal cortex (Dehaene & Cohen, 1995). While several roles have been proposed for this region (access to numerical memories, quantification operations, semantic numerical relations) (Warrington, 1982; Dehaene & Cohen, 1995), one general way to conceive of this area is that it may provide a link between verbal processes and magnitude or spatial numerical relations.

Other lesion sites reported to cause anarithmetia include the left basal ganglia (Whitaker, Habinger, & Ivers, 1985; Corbett, McCusker, & Davidson, 1986; Hittmair-Delazer, Semenza, & Denes, 1994) and more rarely the left frontal cortex (Lucchelli & DeRenzi, 1992). The patient reported by Hittmair-Delazer and colleagues had a left basal ganglia lesion and particular difficulty mentally calculating multiplication and division problems (with increasing deficits for larger operands) despite 90% accuracy on mental addition and subtraction (Hittmair-Delazer et al., 1994). He was able to use complex strategies to solve multiplication problems in writing (e.g., solving $8 \times 6 = 48$ as $8 \times 10 = 80 \div 2 = 40 + 8 = 48$), demonstrating an intact conceptual knowledge of arithmetic and an ability to sequence several operations. However, automaticity for recall of multiplication and division facts was reduced and was the primary disturbance that interfered with overall calculation performance.

Similarly, patients with aphasia following left basal ganglia lesions may show deficits in the recall of highly automatized knowledge (Aglioti & Fabbro, 1993). Brown and Marsden (1998) have hypothesized that one role of the basal ganglia may be to enhance response automaticity through the linking of sensory inputs to "programmed" outputs (either thoughts or actions). Such automated or programmed recall may be necessary for the online manipulation of rote-learned arithmetical facts such as multiplication tables.

Deficits in working memory and sequencing behaviors have also been seen following basal ganglia lesions. The patient reported by Corbett et al. (1986), for example, had a left caudate infarction, and was able to perform single but not multidigit operations. The patient also had particular difficulty with calculations involving sequential processing and the use of working memory. The patient of Whitaker et al., who also had a left basal ganglia lesion, demonstrated deficits for both simple and multistep operations (Whitaker, Habiger, & Ivers, 1985). Thus basal ganglia lesions may interfere with calculations via several potentially dissociable mechanisms that include (1) deficits in automatic recall, (2) impairments in sequencing, and (3) disturbances in operations requiring working memory.

Calculation deficits following frontal lesions have been difficult to characterize precisely, possibly because these lesions often result in deficits in several interacting cognitive domains (e.g., deficits in language, working memory, attention, or executive functions). Grewel, in fact, insisted that "frontal acalculia must be regarded as a secondary acalculia" (Grewel, 1969, p. 189) precisely because of the concurrent intellectual impairments with these lesions. However, when relatively pure deficits have been seen following frontal lesions, they appear to involve more complex aspects of calculations, such as the execution of multistep procedures or understanding the concepts underlying particular operations such as the calculation of percentages (Lucchelli and DeRenzi, 1992). Studies by Fasotti and colleagues have suggested that patients with frontal lesions have difficulty translating arithmetical word problems into an internal representation, although they did not find significant differences in performance among patients with left, right, or bilateral frontal lesions (Fasotti, Eling, & Bremer, 1992). Functional imaging studies, detailed later, strongly support the involvement of various frontal sites in calculations, but these analyses have also not excluded frontal activations that are due to associated task requirements (e.g., working memory or eye movements).

In contrast to the significant calculation abnormalities seen with left hemisphere lesions, deficits in calculations are rare following right hemisphere injuries. However, when groups of patients with right and left hemisphere lesions were compared, there was evidence that comparisons of numerical magnitude are more affected by right hemisphere injuries (Dahmen, Hartje et al., 1982; Rosselli & Ardila, 1989). Patients with right hemisphere lesions may at times demonstrate "spatial acalculia." Hécaen defined this as difficulty in the spatial organization of digits (Hécaen et al., 1961). Nevertheless, the calculation deficits after right hemisphere lesions tend to be mild and the performance of patients with these lesions may not be distinguishable from that of normal persons (Jackson & Warrington, 1986).

Using an ^{133}Xe nontomographic scanner, Roland and Friberg in 1985 provided the first demonstration of functional brain activations for a calculation task (serial subtractions of 3 beginning at 50 compared with rest) (Roland & Friberg, 1985). All subjects had activations on the left, over the middle and superior prefrontal cortex, the posterior inferior frontal gyrus, and the angular gyrus. On the right, activations were seen over the inferior frontal gyrus, the rostral middle and superior frontal gyri, and the angular gyrus (figure 7.6) (lightest gray areas). Because the task and control conditions were not designed to isolate specific cognitive aspects of calculations (i.e., by subtractive, parametric, or factorial design), it is difficult to ascribe specific neurocognitive functions to each of the activated areas in this experiment. Nevertheless, the overall pattern of activations, which include parietal and frontal regions, anticipated the results in subsequent studies, and constituted the only functional imaging study to investigate calculations until 1996 (Grewel, 1952, 1969; Boller & Grafman, 1983; Roland & Friberg, 1985; Dehaene & Cohen, 1995).

The past 5 years have seen a large increase in the number of studies examining this cognitive domain. However, one difficulty in comparing the results has been that individual functional imaging calculation studies have tended to differ from one another along

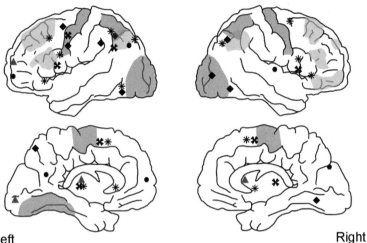

Left   Right

Figure 7.6
Cortical and subcortical regions activated by calculation tasks. Symbols are used to specify activations when the original publications either indicated the exact sites of activation on a figure, or provided precise coordinates. Broader areas of shading represent either activations in large regions of interest (Dehaene, Tzourio, Frak, Raynaud, Cohen, Mehler, & Mazoyer, 1996), or the low resolution of early imaging techniques (Roland & Friberg, 1985). Key: Light gray areas: serial 3 subtractions versus rest (Roland & Friberg, 1985). Triangle: calculations (addition or subtraction) versus reading of equations (Sakurai, Momose, Iwata, Sasaki, & Kanazeu, 1996). Dark gray areas: multiplication versus rest (Dehaene, Tzourio, Frak, Raynaud, Cohen, Mehler, Mazoyer, 1996). Circle: exact versus approximate calculations (addition) (Dehaene, Spelke, Pinel, Stanescu, & Tsivikin, 1999). Diamond: multiplication of two single digits versus reading numbers composed of 0 and 1 (Zago, Pesenti, Mellet, Crevello, Mazoyer, & Tzourio-Mazoyer, 2000). Asterisk: verification of addition and subtraction problems versus identifying numbers containing a 0 (Menon, Rivera, White, Glover, & Reiss, 2000). Cross: addition, subtraction, or division of two numbers (one to two digits) versus number repetition (Cowell, Egan, Code, Harasty, 2000). More complete task descriptions are listed in tables 7.2 and 7.3. The brain outline for figures 7.6 and 7.8 was adapted from Dehaene, Tzourio, Frak, Raynaud, Cohen, Mehler, & Mazoyer, 1996. Activations are plotted bilaterally if they are within ±3 mm of the midline or are cited as bilateral in the original text. The studies generally reported coordinates in Montreal Neurological Institute space. Only Cowell, Egan, Code, Harasty, Watso (2000), and Sathian, Simon, Peterson, Patel, Hoffman, & Grafton (1999) for figure 7.8, reported locations in Talairach coordinates (Talairach & Tournoux, 1988). Talairach coordinates were converted to MNI space using the algorithms defined by Matthew Brett (http://www.mrc-cbu.cam.ac.uk/Imaging/mnispace.html) (Duncan, Seitz, Kolodny, Bor, Herzog, Ahmed, Newell, & Emsile, 2000). Note that the symbol sizes do not reflect the activation sizes. Thus hemispheric asymmetries, particularly those based on activation size, are not demonstrated in this figure or in figure 7.8.

multiple methodological dimensions: imaging modality (PET versus fMRI), acquisition technique (block versus event-related fMRI), arithmetical operation (addition, subtraction, multiplication, etc.), mode and type of response (oral versus button press, generating an answer versus verifying a result), etc. These differences have at least partly contributed to the seemingly disparate functional–anatomical correlations among studies (figure 7.7). However, rather than focusing on the disparities in these reports and trying to relate activation differences post hoc to methodological variations, a more informative approach may be to look for areas of commonality (Démonet, Fiez Paulesu, Petersen, Zatorre, 1996; Poeppel, 1996).

As indicated in figures 7.6 and 7.7, the set of regions showing the most frequent activations across studies included the bilateral dorsal lateral prefrontal cortex, the premotor cortex (precentral gyrus and sulcus), the supplementary motor cortex, the inferior parietal lobule, the intraparietal sulcus, and the posterior occipital cortex-fusiform gyrus (Roland & Friberg, 1985; Dehaene et al., 1996; Sakurai, Momose, Iwata, Sasaki, & Kanazawa, 1996; Pinel et al., 1999; Cowell, Egan, Code, Harasty, & Watson, 2000; Menon, Rivera, White, Glouer, & Reiss, 2000; Zago et al., 2000). When examined regionally, six out of eight studies demonstrated dorsal lateral prefrontal or premotor activations, and seven of eight had activations in the posterior parietal cortex. In addition, ten out of sixteen areas were more frequently activated on the left across studies, which is consistent with lesion-deficit correlations indicating the importance of the left hemisphere for performing exact calculations.

Other evidence regarding the left hemisphere's importance to calculations comes from a study by Dehaene and colleagues (Dehaene, Spelke Pinel, Stanesczu, & Tsivikin, 1999). In their initial psychophysics task, bilingual subjects were taught exact or approximate sums involving two, two-digit numbers in one of their languages (native or non-native language training was randomized). They were then tested again in the language used for initial training or in the "untrained" language on a subset of the learned problems and on a new set of problems. The subjects showed a reaction time cost (i.e., a slower reaction time) when answering previously learned problems in the untrained language regardless of whether this was the subject's native or non-native language.

There was also a reaction time cost for solving novel problems. The presence of a reaction time cost when performing learned calculations in a language different from training or when solving novel problems is consistent with the hypothesis that exact arithmetical knowledge is accessed in a language-specific manner, and thus is most likely related to left-hemisphere linguistic or symbolic abilities.

In contrast, when they were performing approximate calculations, subjects showed neither a language-based nor a novel problem-related effect on reaction times. This result suggests that approximate calculations may take place via a language-independent route and thus may be more bilaterally distributed.

The fMRI activation results from Dehaene et al. (1999) were consistent with these behavioral results in that exact calculations activated a left-hemisphere predominant network of regions (figures 7.6–7.7), while approximate calculations (figures 7.8–7.9) showed a more bilateral distribution of activations. An additional ERP experiment in this study confirmed this pattern of hemispheric asymmetry, with exact calculations showing an earlier (216–248 ms) left frontal negativity, while approximate calculations produced a slightly later (256–280 ms) bilateral parietal negativity (Dehaene et al., 1999).

In a calculation study using PET imaging, which compared multiplying two, two-digit numbers with reading numbers composed of 1 or 0 or recalling memorized multiplication facts, Zago et al. (2000) made the specific point that perisylvian language regions, including Broca's and Wernicke's areas, were actually deactivated as calculation-related task requirements increased. This finding was felt to be consistent with other studies showing relative independence between language and calculation deficits

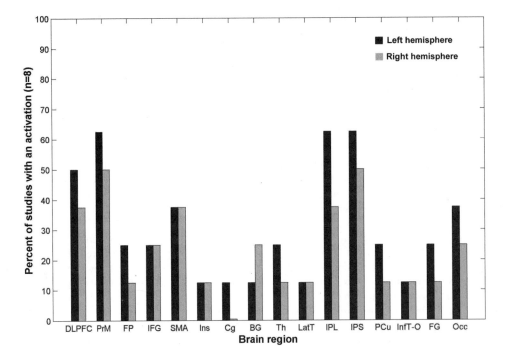

Figure 7.7
Number of studies showing activations for exact calculations organized by region and by hemisphere. Ten out of sixteen areas have a greater number of studies showing activation in the left hemisphere as opposed to the right. The graph also indicates that the frontal, posterior parietal, and, to a lesser extent, occipital cortices are most commonly activated in exact computational tasks. The small bar near 0 for the right cingulate gyrus region is for display purposes. The value was actually 0. Key: DLPFC, dorsal lateral prefrontal cortex; PrM, premotor cortex (precentral gyrus and precentral sulcus); FP, prefrontal cortex near frontal pole; IFG, posterior inferior frontal gyrus overlapping Broca's region on the left and the homologous area on the right; SMA, supplementary motor cortex; Ins, insula; Cg, cingulate gyrus; BG, basal ganglia, including caudate nucleus and/or putamen; Th, thalamus; LatT, lateral temporal cortex; IPL, inferior parietal lobule; IPS, intraparietal sulcus; PCu, precuneus; InfT-O, posterior lateral inferior temporal gyrus near occipital junction; FG, fusiform or lingual gyrus region; Occ, occipital cortex.

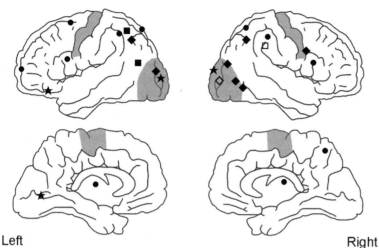

Figure 7.8
Cortical and subcortical activations for tasks of quantification, estimation, or number comparison. See figure 7.6 for details of figure design. Key: Dark gray areas: number comparison versus rest (Dehaene, Tzourio, Frak, Raynaud, Cohen, Mehler, & Mazoyer, 1996). Squares: number comparison with specific inferences for distance effects; closed squares are for numbers closer to the target, open squares are for numbers farther from the target (Pinel Le Clec'h, van der Moortele, Naccache, Le Bihan, & Dehaene, 1999). Open diamond: subitizing versus single-target identification (Sathian, Simon, Peterson, Patel, Hoffman, Graftor, 1999). Closed diamond: counting multiple targets versus subitizing (Sathian, Simon, Peterson, Patel, Hoffman, Grafton, 1999). Closed article: approximate versus exact calculations (addition) (Dehaene, Spelke, Pinel, Starescu, Tsivikin, 1999). Star: estimating numerosity versus estimating shape (Fink, Marshall, Gurd, Weiss, Zafiris, Shah, Zilles, 2000).

in some patients (Warrington, 1982; Whetstone, 1998).

Zago et al. (2000) also noted that the left precentral gyrus, intraparietal sulcus, bilateral cerebellar cortex, and right superior occipital cortex were activated in several contrasts and that similar activations had been reported in previous calculation studies (Dehaene et al., 1996, Dehaene et al., 1999; Pinel et al., 1999; Pesenti et al., 2000). Because of these results, Zago and colleagues (2000) suggested that given the motor or spatial functions of several of these areas, they could represent a developmental trace of a learning strategy based on counting fingers. As support for this argument, the authors noted that certain types of acalculia, such as Gerstmann's syndrome, also produce finger identi-

fication deficits, dysgraphia, and right-left confusion, and that these deficits are consistent with the potential role of these regions in hand movements and acquisition of information in numerical magnitude.

However, these areas are also important for visual-somatic transformations, working memory, spatial attention, and eye movements, which were not controlled for in this experiment (Jonides et al., 1993; Paus, 1996; Nobre et al., 1997; Courtney, Petit, Maisog, Ungerleider, & Haxby, 1998; Gitelman et al., 1999; LaBar, Gitelman, Parrish, & Mesulam, 1999; Gitelman, Parrish, LaBar, & Mesulam, 2000; Zago et al., 2000). Also, because covert finger movements and eye movements were not monitored, it is difficult to confidently ascribe

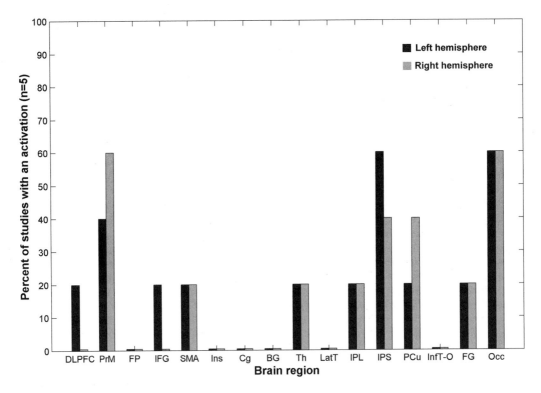

Figure 7.9
Number of studies showing activations for quantification and approximation operations organized by region and by hemisphere. Activations are more bilaterally distributed, by study, than for exact calculations (figure 7.7). In addition, the posterior parietal and occipital cortices now show the predominant activations, with lesser activations frontally. The small bars near 0 for several of the regions were added for display purposes. The values were actually 0. See figure 7.7 for abbreviations.

activations in these regions solely to the representation of finger movements.

One region not displayed in figure 7.6 is the cerebellum. Activation of the cerebellum was seen in only two studies reviewed here. Menon et al. (2000) saw bilateral midcerebellar activations when their subjects performed the most difficult computational task (table 7.2). Zago et al. (2000) saw right cerebellar activation for the combined contrasts (conjunction) of retrieving multiplication facts and de novo computations versus reading the digits 1 or 0. Thus cerebellar activations are most likely to be

seen when relatively complex or novel computations are compared with simpler numerical perception tasks. Cerebellar activation may therefore represent a difficulty effect.

Quantification and Approximation

Quantification is the assessment of a measurable numerical quantity (numerosity) of a set of items. It is among the most basic of arithmetical operations and may play a role in both the childhood development of calculation abilities and the numerical

Table 7.2
Description of functional imaging tasks for exact calculations

Study	Modality	Paradigm	Response
Roland, Fribery 1985	^{133}Xe	Serial three subtractions from 50 versus rest	Silent
Rueckert et al., 1996	fMRI Block design	Serial three subtractions from a 3-digit integer versus counting forward by ones	Silent
Sakurai et al., 1996	PET	Addition or subtraction of two numbers (2 digits and 1 digit) versus reading calculation problems	Oral
Dehaene et al., 1996	PET	Multiply two 1-digit numbers versus compare two numbers	Silent
Dehaene et al., 1999	fMRI Block design	Subjects pretrained on sums of two 2-digit numbers During the task, subjects selected correct answer (two choices). For exact calculations, one answer was correct and the tens digit was off by one in the other. For approximate calculations, the correct answer was rounded to the nearest multiple of ten. The incorrect answer was 30 units off.	Silent: two-choice button press
Cowell et al., 2000	PET	Addition or subtraction or division of two numbers (1–2 digits) versus number repetition	Oral
Menon et al., 2000	PET	Verify addition and subtraction of problems with three operands versus identify numbers containing the numeral 0	Silent: single-choice button press
Zago et al., 2000	PET	Multiply two 2-digit numbers versus reading numbers consisting of just zeros and ones	Oral

processes of adults (Spiers, 1987). Despite the basic nature of quantification operations, they were not included in some early models of calculations (McCloskey et al., 1985). Three quantification processes have been described: counting, subitizing, and estimation (Dehaene, 1992). Counting is the assignment of an ordered representation of quantity to any arbitrary collection of objects (Gelman & Gallistel, 1978; Dehaene, 1992). Subitizing is the rapid quantification of small sets of items (usually less than five); and estimation is the "less accurate" rapid quantification of larger sets (Dehaene, 1992).

Subitizing and Counting

Because subitizing and to an extent counting operations appear to be largely distinct from language abilities, these operations may be of considerable importance for understanding the calculation abilities of prelinguistic human infants and even (nonlinguistic) animals. Jokes about Clever Hans aside,[5] there is ample evidence that animals possess simple counting abilities (Dehaene, 1992; Gallistel & Gelman, 1992).

More important, young children possess counting abilities from an early age, and there is good evidence that even very young infants can subitize, suggesting that this ability may be closely associated with the operation of basic perceptual processes (Dehaene, 1992). Four-day-old infants, for example, can discriminate between one and two and two and three displayed objects (Bijeljac-Babic, Bertoncini, Mehler, 1993), and 6–8-month-old infants demonstrate detection of cross-modal (visual and auditory) numerical correspondence (Starkey, Spelke, & Gelman, 1983; Starkey, Spelke, & Gelman, 1990). Although quantification abilities may be bilaterally represented in the brain, the right hemisphere is thought to demonstrate some advantage for these operations (Dehaene & Cohen, 1995).

Estimation and Approximation

The use of estimation operations in simple calculations may have a role in performing these operations nonlinguistically or in allowing the rapid rejection of "obviously" incorrect answers. For example, if quantification can be conceived as encoding numbers on a mental "number line," then addition can be likened to mentally joining the number line segments and examining the total line length to arrive at the answer (Gallistel and Gelman, 1992). As with a physical line, the precision of the measurement is hypothesized to decline with increasing line length (Weber's law[6]) (Dehaene, 1992).

An example of the role of estimation in calculations is provided by examining subjects' performance in verification tasks. In these tasks, the subjects are asked to verify an answer to an arithmetic problem (e.g., $5 \times 7 = 36$?). The speed of classifying answers as incorrect increases (i.e., decreased reaction time) with increasing separation between the proposed and correct results ("split effect") (Ashcraft & Battaglia, 1978; Ashcraft & Stazyk, 1981). The response to glaringly incorrect answers (e.g., $4 \times 5 = 1000$?) can be so rapid as to suggest that estimation processes may be operating in parallel with exact "fact-based" calculations (Dehaene, Dehaene-Lambertz, & Cohen, 1998).

Further evidence that some magnitude operations can be approximated by a spatially extended mental number line comes from numerical comparison tasks. During these tasks, subjects judge whether two numbers are the same or different while reaction times are measured. Experiments show that the time to make this judgment varies inversely with the distance between the numbers. Longer reaction times are seen as numbers approach each other. In one experiment, Hinrichs et al. showed that it was quicker to compare 51 and 65 than to compare 59

and 65 (Hinrichs, Yurko, & Hu, 1981). If numbers were simply compared symbolically, there should have been no reaction time difference in this comparison since it should have been sufficient to compare the tens digits in both cases. This finding has been interpreted as showing that numbers can be compared as defined quantities and not just at a symbolic level (Dehaene, Dupoux, & Mehler, 1990).

Case studies of several patients have provided further support for the importance of quantification processes and the independence of these processes from exact calculations. Patient D.R.C. of Warrington suffered a left temporoparieto-occipital junction hemorrhage (~3 cm diameter) and subsequently had difficulty recalling arithmetical facts for addition, subtraction, and multiplication, yet he usually gave answers of reasonable magnitude when asked to solve problems. For example, he said "13 roughly" for the problem "5 + 7" (Warrington, 1982). A similar phenomenon occurred in the patient N.A.U. of Dehaene and Cohen (1991). This patient sustained head trauma, which produced a very large left temporoparieto-occipital hemorrhage (affecting most of the parietal, posterior temporal, and anterior occipital cortex). Although N.A.U. could not directly calculate 2 + 2, he could reject 9 but not 3 as a possible answer, which is consistent with access to an estimation process. N.A.U. could also compare numbers (possibly by using magnitude comparison), even ones he could not read explicitly, if they were separated by more than one digit. However, he performed at chance level when deciding if a number was odd or even. Although this dissociation may seem incongruous, one hypothesis is that parity decisions require exact and not approximate numerical knowledge, consistent with the inability of this patient to perform exact calculations.

Grafman et al. described a patient who suffered near total destruction of the left hemisphere from a gunshot wound, leaving only the occipital and parasagittal cortex remaining on the left (Grafman, Kampen, Rosenberg, & Salazar, 1989). Despite an inability to perform multidigit calculations, he could compare multidigit numerals with excellent accuracy, suggesting that intact right hemisphere mechanisms were sufficient for performing this comparison task. The opposite dissociation (increased deficits in approximation despite some preservation of rote-learned arithmetic) was seen in patient H.Ba. reported by Guttmann (1937). H.Ba. was able to perform simple calculations, but had difficulty with number comparisons and quantity estimation. Unfortunately, no anatomical information regarding H.Ba.'s lesions was provided since his deficits were developmental.

Overall, these studies strongly support the hypotheses that the cognitive processes underlying exact calculations and those related to estimating magnitude can be dissociated. In addition, left hemisphere regions seem clearly necessary for the performance of exact calculations, while estimation tasks may be more closely associated with the right hemisphere or possibly are bilaterally represented.

Anatomical Relationships and Functional Imaging

Figure 7.8 shows the combined activations from five studies of quantification or approximation operations, including subitizing, counting, number comparison, and approximate computations (Dehaene et al., 1996; Dehaene et al., 1999; Pinel et al., 1999; Sathian et al., 1999; Fink et al., 2000). The paradigms for these studies are summarized in table 7.3. In comparison with the data from studies of exact calculations (figures 7.6 and 7.7), approximation and magnitude operations (figures 7.8 and 7.9) show relatively more parietal and occipital and less

Table 7.3
Description of functional imaging tasks for approximation and quantification

Study	Modality	Paradigm	Response
Dehaene et al., 1996	PET	Multiply two 1-digit numbers versus compare two numbers	Silent
Dehaene et al., 1999	fMRI Block design	Subjects were pretrained on sums of two 2-digit numbers. During fMRI, subjects were shown a two-operand addition problem and a single answer. They pressed buttons to choose if the answer was correct or incorrect. For exact calculations, one answer was correct, while the tens digit was off by one in the other. For approximate calculations, the correct answer was was the actual result rounded to the nearest multiple of 10 (e.g., 25 + 28 = 53, so 50 was shown to subjects). The incorrect answer was 30 units off.	Silent: dual-choice button press
Pinel et al., 1999	fMRI Event related	Number comparison: Is a target number (shown as a word or a numeral) larger or smaller than 5?	Silent: single-choice button press
Sathian et al., 1999	PET	Subjects saw an array of 16 bars and reported the number of vertical bars. When 1–4 vertical bars were present, the subjects were assumed to identify magnitude by subitizing; when 5–8 vertical bars were present, they were assumed to be counting.	Oral
Fink et al., 2000	fMRI Block design	In the numerosity condition, subjects indicated if four dots were present. In the shape condition, subjects indicated if the dots formed a square.	Silent: dual-choice button press

frontal activity. In addition, the left-right asymmetry seen in figure 7.7 is no longer apparent.

Sathian et al. (1999) examined regions activated by tasks of counting and subitizing. Subitizing, which has been linked to preattentive and "pop-out" types of processes, resulted in activation of the right middle and inferior occipital gyrus (figure 7.8). The left hemisphere showed a homologous activation, which did not quite reach the threshold for significance, and is not shown in the figure. A small right cerebellar activation was also found just below threshold. Similar occipital predominant activations were also obtained by Fink et al. (2000) for a task that basically involved subitizing (deciding if four dots were present when shown three, four, or five dots) versus estimating shape.

Counting, in contrast to subitizing, according to Sathian et al. (1999), activated broad regions of the bilateral occipitotemporal, superior parietal, and right premotor cortices (figure 7.8). Based on these results, Sathian et al. suggested that counting processes may involve spatial shifts of attention (among the objects to be counted) and attention-mediated top-down modulation of the visual cortex.

Although the parietal cortex has been hypothesized to support numerical comparison operations (Dehaene and Cohen, 1995), this area was non-significantly activated ($p = 0.078$) in a PET study examining comparison operations (Dehaene et al., 1996). Instead, the contrast between number comparison and resting state conditions demonstrated significant activations in the bilateral occipital, premotor, and supplementary motor cortices (figure 7.8) (dark gray areas) (Dehaene et al., 1996). One possible explanation for the minimal parietal activation in this study is that the task involved repeated comparisons of two numerals between 1 and 9. In the case of small numerosities, it has been suggested that seeing a numeral may evoke quantity representations that are similar to seeing the same number of objects, and may engender automatic subitization. Hence, the task may have stressed operations related to number identification and covert subitizing processes more than the authors anticipated. Therefore the occipitotemporal cortex rather than the

parietal cortex may have been preferentially activated (Sathian et al., 1999; Fink et al., 2000).

A subsequent study of number comparison used event-related fMRI while the subjects decided whether a target numeral (between 1 and 9) was larger or smaller than the number 5 (Pinel et al., 1999). Distance effects (i.e., whether the numbers were closer to or farther from 5) were seen in the left intraparietal sulcus and the bilateral inferior, posterior parietal cortices, which is consistent with the hypothesized parietal involvement in magnitude processing (figure 7.8). The authors also noted that this study showed an apparent greater left hemisphere involvement for number comparison, while a previous study had suggested more involvement of the right hemisphere (Dehaene, 1996).

Numerical Representations

One issue of considerable debate has been the manner in which numerical relations are internally encoded. For example, are problems handled differently if they are presented as Arabic numerals ($2 + 6 = 8$), Roman numerals ($II + VI = 8$), or words (two plus six equals eight)? McCloskey and colleagues have maintained that the various number-processing and calculation mechanisms communicate via a single abstract representation of quantity (Sokol et al., 1991). Others have strongly disagreed with this approach and have suggested that internal representational codes may vary (encoding complex theory) according to input or output modality, task requirements, learning strategies, etc. (Campbell & Clark, 1988), or even according to the subject's experience (preferred entry code hypothesis) (Noël & Seron, 1993). Another approach, discussed later, is that there are specific representations (words, numerals, or magnitude) linked to particular calculation processes, and this suggestion is embodied by the triple-code model of Dehaene (Dehaene, 1992).

Considerable evidence exists attesting to the importance of an internal representation of magnitude. One example is the presence of the numerical distance effect. As previously noted, this effect is demonstrated by subjects taking longer to make comparison judgments for numbers that are closer in magnitude to one another. The effect has been demonstrated across a variety stimulus input types, including Arabic numerals (Moyer & Landauer, 1967; Sekuler, Rubin, & Armstrong, 1971), spelled-out numbers (Foltz, Poltrock, & Potts, 1984), dot patterns (Buckley & Gillman, 1974), and Japanese kana and kanji ideograms (Takahashi & Green, 1983). The occurrence of this effect regardless of the format of the stimulus has suggested that it is not mediated by different input codes for each format, but rather through a common representation of magnitude (Sokol et al., 1991).

Evidence for an opposing set of views, i.e., that numerical processing can take place via a variety of representational codes, has also been amassed. One prediction of "multicode" models is that input and/or response formats may influence the underlying calculations beyond effects attributable to simple sensory mechanisms. In the single-code model, since all calculations are based on an amodal representation of the number, it should not matter how the number is presented once this transcoding has taken place. A single-code model would suggest that differences in adding 5 + 6 and V + VI would be solely attributable to the transcoding operation.

In support of additional codes, Gonzalez and Kolers (1982, 1987) found that differences in reaction times to Arabic and Roman numerals showed an interaction with number size (i.e., there was a greater differential for IV + 5 = IX, than for II + 1 = III). This difference implied that the calculation process might have been affected by a combination of the input format and the numerical magnitude of the operands. A single-code model would predict that while calculations might be slower for a given input format, they should not be disproportionately slower for larger numbers in that format.

A second set of experiments addressed the possibility that the slower reaction time for Roman numerals was simply due to slowed numerical comprehension of this format. The subjects were trained in naming Roman numerals for several days, until they showed no more than a 10% difference in

naming times between Arabic and Roman numerals. Despite this additional training, differences in reaction time remained beyond the time differences attributable to numerical comprehension alone. This result again suggested that numerical codes may depend on the input format, and may influence calculations differentially. Countering these arguments, Sokol and colleagues (1991) have noted that naming numbers and comprehending them for use in calculations are different processes and may proceed via different initial mechanisms.

Synthesizing the various views for numerical representation, Dehaene (1992) has proposed that three codes can account for differences in input, output, and processing of numbers. These representations include a visual Arabic numeral, an auditory word frame, and an analog magnitude code. Each of these codes has its own input and output procedures and is interfaced with preferred aspects of calculations. The visual Arabic numeral can be conceived of as a string of digits, which can be held in a visual-spatial scratchpad. This code is necessary for multidigit operations and parity judgments. The auditory word frame consists of the syntactic and lexical elements that describe a number. This code is manipulated by language processing systems and is important for counting and the recall of memorized arithmetical facts. Finally, the analog magnitude code contains semantic information about the physical quantity of a number and can be conceived of as a spatially oriented number line. This code provides information, for example, that 20 is greater than 10 as a matter of quantity and is not just based on a symbolic relationship (Dehaene, 1992). The magnitude code is particularly important for estimation, comparison, approximate calculations, and subitizing operations (Dehaene, 1992).

Several lines of evidence make a compelling argument for this organization over that of a single-code model. (1) Multidigit operations appear to involve the manipulation of spatially oriented numbers (Dahmen et al., 1982; Dehaene, 1992), and experiments have suggested that parity judgments are strongly influenced by Arabic numeral formats

(Dehaene, 1992; Dehaene, Bossini, & Giraux, 1993). (2) The preference of bilingual subjects for performing calculations in their native language is consistent with the storage of (at least) addition and multiplication tables in some linguistic format (Gonzalez & Kolers, 1987; Dehaene, 1992; Noël & Seron, 1993). (3) The presence of distance effects on reaction time when comparing numbers and the presence of the "SNARC" effect both suggest that magnitude codes play a significant role in certain approximation processes (Buckley & Gillman, 1974; Dehaene et al., 1993). SNARC is an acronym for *spatial-numerical association of response codes* and refers to an interaction between number size and the hand used for response when making various numerical judgments. Responses to relatively small numbers are quicker with the left hand, while responses to relatively large numbers are quicker with the right hand. (Relative in this case refers to the set of given numbers for a particular judgment task, Fias, Brysbaert, Geypens, & d'Ydewalle, 1996).

This effect has been interpreted as evidence for a mental number line (spatially extended from left to right in left-to-right reading cultures). Thus small numbers are associated with the left end of a virtual number line and would be perceived by the right hemisphere, resulting in faster left-hand reaction times. The opposite would be true for large numbers. This effect has been confirmed by several authors, and argues for the existence of representation of magnitude at some level (Fias et al., 1996; Bächtold, Baumüller, & Brugger, 1998). Fias et al. (1996) have also found evidence for the SNARC effect when subjects transcode numbers from Arabic numerals to verbal formats. This effect, some might argue, demonstrates the existence of an obligatory magnitude representation in what should be an asemantic task (i.e., one would presume that the transcoding operation of eight → 8 should not require the representation of quantity for its success). However, Dehaene (1992) has suggested that even though one code may be necessary for the performance of a task (in this case the visual Arabic numeral form), other codes (such as the magnitude

representation) may be "incidentally" activated simply as a consequence of numerical processing, and then could influence performance (Deloche and Seron 1982a,b, 1987; McCloskey et al., 1985).

Network Models of Calculations

Despite the explanatory power of current models for some aspects of calculations, they all have tended to take a modular rather than a network approach to the organization of this higher cortical function. One description of the triple-code model, for example, was that it represented a "layered modular architecture" (Dehaene, 1992). Because they resort to modularity, current models ultimately fail at some level to provide a flexible architecture for understanding numerical cognition. The distinctions between modular and network models of cognition are subtle, however, and on first pass it may not be clear to the reader how or why this distinction is so important. An example will illustrate this point.

The triple-code model proposes that calculations are subserved by several functional-anatomical groups of cortical regions. One group centered in the parietal lobe serves quantification; a group centered around the perisylvian cortex serves linguistic functions; another group centered in the dorsolateral prefrontal cortex serves working memory; and so on. The discreteness of these functional groups potentially engenders a (false) sense of distinctness in how these regions are proposed to interact with numbers. Thus magnitude codes are proposed to be necessary for number comparisons while memorized linguistic codes are proposed to underlie multiplication. The result is a nearly endless debate about the right code for a particular job, with investigators proposing ever more clever tasks whose purpose is to finally identify the specific psychophysiological code (re: "center") underlying a particular task.

Similar distinctions have been proposed in other domains and found to be wanting. For example, in the realm of spatial attention, it had long been argued whether neglect was due to sensory-representational or motor-exploratory disturbances (Heilman and Valenstein, 1972; Bisiach, Luzzatti, & Perani, 1979). In fact, as suggested by large-scale network theories, the exploratory and representational deficits of neglect go hand in hand, since one's exploration of space actually takes place within the mind's representational schema (Droogleever-Fortuyn, 1979; Mesulam, 1981, 1999).

An alternative view of the codes underlying numerical operations is that they are innumerable and therefore, in a sense, unknowable (Campbell & Clark, 1988). This viewpoint is also not tenable because the brain must make decisions based on abstractions from basic, and fundamentally measurable, sensory and motor processes (Mesulam 1981, 1998).

Thus one important concept of a large-scale network theory is that while cortical regions may be specialized for a particular operation, they participate in higher cognitive functions, not as autonomously operating modules, but rather as interactive epicenters. Use of the term *epicenter*, in this case, implies that complex cortical functions arise as a consequence of brain regions being both specialized for various operations and integrated with other cortical and subcortical areas. There are several consequences for a cerebral organization based on these concepts (Mesulam 1981, 1990):

1. Cortical regions are unlikely to interact with only a single large-scale network. They are more likely to participate in several cognitive networks, so damage to any particular region may affect a number of intellectual functions. (Only the primary sensory and motor cortices appear to have a one-to-one mapping of structure to function, e.g., V1 and specific areas of the visual field.)

Thus areas of the parietal and frontal cortices participating in calculations are unlikely to serve only the computation of quantities or the recall of rote arithmetical answers, respectively. Instead, lesions of the left inferior parietal cortex, for example, are likely to disrupt calculation operations as well as other aspects of spatial and/or linguistic processing. Likewise, the apparently rare association of frontal injury with pure anarithmetia may occur because lesions of the frontal lobes so often interfere with a broad array of linguistic, working memory, and executive functions that they give the appearance that any calculation deficit is secondary.

2. Disruptions of any part of a large-scale network can lead to deficits that were not originally considered to be part of the lesioned area's repertoire of operations. For example, in the realm of language, although nonfluent aphasias are more likely to be associated with lesions in Broca's area, this type of aphasia can also follow from lesions in the posterior perisylvian cortex (Caplan, Hildebrandt, & Makris, 1996). Similarly, while calculation deficits most commonly follow left parietal cortex lesions, they can also be seen after left basal ganglia lesions (Whitaker et al., 1985; Hittmair-Delazer et al., 1994; Dehaene & Cohen, 1995). This result seems less mysterious when it is realized that the basal ganglia participate in large-scale networks that include frontal, temporal, and parietal cortices (Alexander et al., 1990).

3. The psychophysical codes or representations of a cognitive operation are all potentially activated during performance of a function. A corollary to this statement is that the activation of a particular cognitive code is dynamic and highly dependent on shifting task contingencies for a particular cognitive operation. Thus the codes underlying calculations are neither unbounded nor constrained to be activated individually. Rather, activation of specific representations is dependent on spatial, linguistic, and perceptual processes, among others, which interact to give rise to various cognitive functions. The activation of a specific representational code depends on the task requirements and a subject's computational strategy. Similar dependence of brain activations on varying contingencies has also been found in studies of facial processing (Wojciulik, Kanwisher, & Driver, 1998).

An attempt to organize the large-scale neural network for calculations could therefore proceed along the following lines: There are likely to be areas in the visual unimodal association cortex (around the fusiform and lingual gyri) whose function is specialized for discriminating various forms of numbers (numerals or words). Evidence suggests that areas for identifying numerals or verbal forms of numbers are likely to be closely allied, but are probably not completely overlapping. There are also data to suggest that their separation may arise as a natural consequence of various perceptual processes (Polk & Farah, 1998). These sensory object-form regions are then linked with higher-order areas supporting the linguistic or symbolic associations necessary for calculations, and also areas supporting concepts of numerical quantity (Dehaene & Cohen, 1995). The latter "magnitude" areas may be organized to reflect mechanisms associated with spatial and/or object processing and thereby provide a nonverbal sense of amount or quantity. Magnitude regions may be located within the posterior parietal cortex as part of areas that assess spatial extent and distributed quantities. Finally, the linguistic aspects of number processing are almost certainly linked at some level to language networks or areas involved with processing symbolic representations, such as the dorsolateral prefrontal cortex and/or the parietal cortex.

Links among the areas supporting the visual-verbal, linguistic, and magnitude aspects of numbers thereby form a large-scale neural network from which all other numerical processes are derived. The cortical epicenters of this network are likely to be located in the inferior parietal cortex (most likely intersecting with the intraparietal sulcus), the dorsolateral prefrontal cortex (probably close to the precentral gyrus), and the temporoparietal-occipital junction. Similar connections are likely to exist in both hemispheres, although the left hemisphere is proposed to coordinate calculations overall, particularly when the task requires some form of linguistic (verbal or numeral) response or requires symbolic manipulation. Additional connections of this network with different parts of the limbic system could provide episodic numerical memories or even emotional associations.

Other important connections would include those involving the frontal poles. This is an area that appears critical for organizing complex executive functions, particularly when the task involves branching contingencies, and may be necessary for complex calculations (Koechlin, Basso, Pietrini, Panzer, & Grafman, 1999). Subcortical connections would include the basal ganglia (particularly on the left) and thalamus. The critical difference between this proposed model and the triple-code model would be the a priori constraint of various "codes" based on specific brain-behavior relationships, and the distributed nature of the representations.

Bedside Testing

Based on the preceding discussion, testing for acalculia should focus on several areas of numerical cognition and should also document deficits in other cognitive domains. Clearly, deficits in attention, working memory, language, and visual-spatial skills should be sought. Testing for these functions is reviewed elsewhere in this volume. More specific testing for calculation deficits should cover the areas of numerical processing, quantification, and calculations proper. The test originally proposed by Boller and Faglioni (see Grafman et al., 1982; Boller & Grafman, 1985) represents a good starting point for the clinician. It contains problems testing numerical comparison and the four basic mathematical operations. Recommended tests for examining calculations are outlined below.

1. Numerical processing

a. Reading Arabic numerals and spelled-out numbers (words)

b. Writing Arabic numerals and spelled-out numbers to dictation

c. Transcoding from Arabic numerals to spelled-out numbers and vice versa

2. Quantification

a. Counting the number of several small (1–9) sets of dots or other objects

b. Estimating the quantity of larger collections of objects

3. Calculations

Testing should include both single-digit and multidigit problems. Multidigit operations should include carrying and borrowing procedures. Simple rules such as $0 \times N$, $0 + N$, and $1 \times N$ should be tested as well.

a. Addition

b. Multiplication

c. Subtraction

d. Division

Other tests, such as solving word problems (e.g., Jane had one dollar and bought two apples costing thirty cents each. How much money does she have left?), more abstract problems (e.g., $a \times (b + c) = (a \times b) + (a \times c)$), and higher mathematical concepts such as square root and logarithms can be tested, although the clinical associations are less clear.

Conclusions and Future Directions

Although this chapter began with a simple case report outlining some general aspects of acalculia and associated deficits, subsequent sections have illustrated the dissection of this function into a rich array of cognitive operations. Many questions about this cognitive function remain, however, including the nature of developmental deficits in calculations. For example, a patient reported by Romero et al. had developmental dyscalculia and dysgraphia and particular difficulty recalling multiplication facts despite normal intelligence and normal visual-spatial abilities (Romero, Granetz, Makale, Manly, & Grafman, 2000). Magnetic resonance spectroscopy demonstrated reduced N-acetyl-aspartate, creatine, and choline in the left inferior parietal lobule, suggesting some type of injury to this area although no structural lesion could be seen.

While parietal lesions can certainly disrupt learned calculations, current theories are not able to fully explain why this patient could not adopt an alternative means of learning the multiplication tables, such as remembering multiplication facts as individual items of verbal material. Based on this

case, it is clear that at some point in the learning process, multiplication facts are not just isolated verbal memories, as suggested by Dehaene and Cohen (1997), but must be learned within the context of other processes subserved by the left parietal lobe (possibly quantification). This hypothesis would also be consistent with a large-scale network approach to this function.

The functional–anatomical relationships underlying the most basic aspects of calculations and numerical processing are also far from being definitively settled, while those related to more abstract mathematical procedures have not yet been explored. Furthermore, to what extent eye movements, working memory, or even basic motor processes (i.e., counting fingers) could be contributing to calculations is also unclear. The range of processes participating in calculations suggests that this function has few equals among cognitive operations in terms of integration across a multiplicity of cognitive domains. By viewing the brain areas underlying these functions as part of intersecting large-scale neural networks, it is hoped that it will be possible to understand how their interactions support this complex cognitive function.

Acknowledgments

This work was supported by National Institute of Aging grant AG00940.

Notes

1. One overview of large-scale neural networks and their application to several cognitive domains can be found in Mesulam (1990).

2. In this case, critical refers to directly affecting calculations, as opposed to some other indirect relationship. For example, patients with frontal lesions can have profound deficits in attention and responsiveness. This will impair calculation performance in a secondary, but not necessarily in a primary, fashion (Grewel, 1969).

3. Deficits in production refer to writing the incorrect number, not to dysgraphia.

4. $0 \times N$ refers to multiplication of any number by 0. This notation also includes the commuted problem of $N \times 0$. The result is a rule because it is true for all numbers, N.

5. Clever Hans was a horse who supposedly could calculate and perform a variety of linguistic tasks. It was eventually shown that Clever Hans possessed no particular mathematical abilities, but primarily intuited his owner's nonconscious body language, which communicated the answers (Hediger, 1981).

6. In this context, Weber's law essentially says that objective numerical differences may seem subjectively smaller when they are contrasted with larger numbers (Dehaene, 1992).

References

Aglioti, S., & Fabbro, F. (1993). Paradoxical selective recovery in a bilingual aphasic following subcortical lesions. *NeuroReport, 4*, 1359–1362.

Alexander, G. E., Crutcher, M. D., & DeLong, M. R. (1990). Basal ganglia-thalamocortical circuits: Parallel substrates for motor, oculomotor, "prefrontal" and "limbic" functions. *Progress in Brain Research 85*, 119–146.

Allison, T., McCarthy, G., Nobre, A., Puce, A., & Belger, A. (1994). Human extrastriate visual cortex and the perception of faces, words, numbers, and colors. *Cerebral Cortex, 4*, 544–554.

Ashcraft, M. H. (1987). Children's knowledge of simple arithmetic: A developmental model and simulation. In J. Bisanz, C. J. Brainerd, & R. Kail (Eds.), *Formal methods in developmental psychology: Progress in cognitive developmental research* (pp. 302–338). New York: Springer-Verlag.

Ashcraft, M. H. (1992). Cognitive arithmetic: A review of data and theory. *Cognition, 44*, 75–106.

Ashcraft, M. H., & Battaglia, J. (1978). Cognitive arithmetic: Evidence for retrieval and decision processes in mental addition. *Journal of Experimental Psychology: Human Learning and Memory, 4*, 527–538.

Ashcraft, M. H., & Stazyk, E. H. (1981). Mental addition: A test of three verification models. *Memory and Cognition, 9*, 185–196.

Bächtold, D., Baumüller, M., & Brugger, P. (1998). Stimulus-response compatibility in representational space. *Neuropsychologia, 36*, 731–735.

Benson, D. F., & Denckla, M. B. (1969). Verbal paraphasia as a source of calculation disturbance. *Archives of Neurology, 21*, 96–102.

Benton, A. L. (1961). The fiction of the "Gerstmann syndrome". *Journal of Neurology, Neurosurgery and Psychiatry, 24*, 176–181.

Benton, A. L. (1992). Gerstmann's syndrome. *Archives of Neurology, 49*, 445–447.

Berger, H. (1926). Über rechenstörungen bei herderkrankungen des grosshirns. *Archiv für Psychiatrie und Nervenkrankheiten, 78*, 238–263.

Bijeljac-Babic, R., Bertoncini, J., & Mehler, J. (1993). How do 4-day-old infants categorize multisyllabic utterances? *Developmental Psychology, 29*, 711–721.

Bisiach, E., Luzzatti, C., & Perani, D. (1979). Unilateral neglect, representational schema and consciousness. *Brain, 102*, 609–618.

Boller, F., & Grafman, J. (1983). Acalculia: Historical development and current significance. *Brain and Cognition, 2*, 205–223.

Boller, F., & Grafman, J. (1985). Acalculia. In P. J. Vinker, G. W. Bruyn, H. L. Klawans, & J. A. M. Frederiks (Eds.), *Handbook of clinical neurology* (vol. 45, pp. 473–481). Amsterdam: Elsevier.

Brown, P., & Marsden, C. D. (1998). What do the basal ganglia do? *Lancet, 351*, 1801–1804.

Buckley, P. B., & Gillman, C. B. (1974). Comparisons of digits and dot patterns. *Journal of Experimental Psychology, 103*, 1131–1136.

Campbell, J. I. D., & Clark, J. M. (1988). An encoding-complex view of cognitive number processing: Comment on McCloskey, Sokol, and Goodman (1986). *Journal of Experimental Psychology: General, 117*, 204–214.

Campbell, J. I. D., & Graham, D. J. (1985). Mental multiplication skill: Structure, process, and acquisition. *Canadian Journal of Psychology, 39*, 338–366.

Caplan, D., Hildebrandt, N., & Makris, N. (1996). Location of lesions in stroke patients with deficits in syntactic processing in sentence comprehension. *Brain, 119*, 933–949.

Cohen, L., & Dehaene, S. (1995). Number processing in pure alexia: The effect of hemispheric asymmetries and task demands. *Neurocase: Case Studies in Neuropsychology, Neuropsychiatry & Behavioral Neurology, 1*, 121–137.

Cohn, R. (1961). Dyscalculia. *Archives of Neurology, 4*, 301–307.

Collingnon, R., Leclercq, C., & Mahy, J. (1977). Etude de la sémiologie des troubles de calcul observés aú cours des lésions corticales. *Acta Neurologica Belgica*, *77*, 257–275.

Corbett, A. J., McCusker, E. A., & Davidson, O. R. (1986). Acalculia following a dominant-hemisphere subcortical infarct. *Archives of Neurology*, *43*, 964–966.

Courtney, S. M., Petit, L., Maisog, J. M., Ungerleider, L. G., & Haxby, J. V. (1998). An area specialized for spatial working memory in human frontal cortex. *Science*, *279*, 1347–1351.

Cowell, S. F., Egan, G. F., Code, C., Harasty, J., & Watson, J. D. (2000). The functional neuroanatomy of simple calculation and number repetition: A parametric PET activation study. *NeuroImage*, *12*, 565–573.

Critchley, M. (1953). *The parietal lobes*. London: Edward Arnold.

Dagenbach, D., & McCloskey, M. (1992). The organization of arithmetic facts in memory: Evidence from a brain-damaged patient. *Brain and Cognition*, *20*, 345–366.

Dahmen, W., Hartje, W., Bussing, A., & Sturm, W. (1982). Disorders of calculation in aphasic patients—spatial and verbal components. *Neuropsychologia*, *20*, 145–153.

Dehaene, S. (1992). Varieties of numerical abilities. *Cognition*, *44*, 1–42.

Dehaene, S. (1996). The organization of brain activations in number comparison: Event-related potentials and the additive-factors method. *Journal of Cognitive Neuroscience*, *8*, 47–68.

Dehaene, S., Bossini, S., & Giraux, P. (1993). The mental representation of parity and number magnitude. *Journal of Experimental Psychology: General*, *122*, 371–396.

Dehaene, S., & Cohen, L. (1991). Two mental calculation systems: A case study of severe acalculia with preserved approximation. *Neuropsychologia*, *29*, 1045–1074.

Dehaene, S., & Cohen, L. (1995). Towards an anatomical and functional model of number processing. *Mathematical Cognition*, *1*, 83–120.

Dehaene, S., & Cohen, L. (1997). Cerebral pathways for calculation: Double dissociation between rote verbal and quantitative knowledge of arithmetic. *Cortex*, *33*, 219–250.

Dehaene, S., Dehaene-Lambertz, G., & Cohen, L. (1998). Abstract representations of numbers in the animal and human brain. *Trends in Neurosciences*, *21*, 355–361.

Dehaene, S., Dupoux, E., & Mehler, J. (1990). Is numerical comparison digital? Analogical and symbolic effects in two-digit number comparison. *Journal of Experimental Psychology: Human Perception and Performance*, *16*, 626–641.

Dehaene, S., Spelke, E., Pinel, P., Stanescu, R., & Tsivikin, S. (1999). Sources of mathematical thinking: Behavioral and brain-imaging evidence. *Science*, *284*, 970–974.

Dehaene, S., Tzourio, N., Frak, V., Raynaud, L., Cohen, L., Mehler, J., & Mazoyer, B. (1996). Cerebral activations during number multiplication and comparison: A PET study. *Neuropsychologia*, *34*, 1097–1106.

Deloche, G., & Seron, X. (1982a). From three to 3: A differential analysis of skills in transcoding quantities between patients with Broca's and Wernicke's aphasia. *Brain*, *105*, 719–733.

Deloche, G., & Seron, X. (1982b). From one to 1: An analysis of a transcoding process by means of neuropsychological data. *Cognition*, *12*, 119–149.

Deloche, G., & Seron, X. (1987). Numerical transcoding: A general production model. In G. Deloche & X. Seron (Eds.), *Mathematical disabilities: A cognitive neuropsychological perspective* (pp. 137–170). Hillsdalte, NJ: Lawrence Erlbaum Associates.

Démonet, J. F., Fiez, J. A., Paulesu, E., Petersen, S. E., & Zatorre, R. J. (1996). PET studies of phonological processing: A critical reply to Poeppel. *Brain and Language*, *55*, 352–379.

Droogleever-Fortuyn, J. (1979). On the neurology of perception. *Clinical Neurology and Neurosurgery*, *81*, 97–107.

Duncan, J., Seitz, R. J., Kolodny, J., Bor, D., Herzog, H., Ahmed, A., Newell, F. N., & Emslie, H. (2000). A neural basis for general intelligence. *Science*, *289*, 457–460.

Eliasberg, W., & Feuchtwanger, E. (1922). Zur psychologischen und psychopathologischen untersuchung und theorie des erworbenen schwachsinns. *Zeitschrift für die gesamte Neurologie und Psychiatrie*, *75*, 516.

Fasotti, L., Eling, P. A. T. M., & Bremer, J. J. (1992). The internal representation of arithmetical word problem sentences: Frontal and posterior-injured patients compared. *Brain and Cognition*, *20*, 245–263.

Ferro, J. M., & Botelho, M. A. S. (1980). Alexia for arithmetical signs. A cause of disturbed calculation. *Cortex*, *16*, 175–180.

Fias, W., Brysbaert, M., Geypens, F., & d'Ydewalle, G. (1996). The importance of magnitude information in numerical processing: Evidence from the SNARC effect. *Mathematical Cognition*, *2*, 95–110.

Fink, G. R., Marshall, J. C., Gurd, J., Weiss, P. H., Zafiris, O., Shah, N. J., & Zilles, K. (2000). Deriving numerosity and shape from identical visual displays. *NeuroImage*, *13*(1), 46–55.

Foltz, G. S., Poltrock, S. E., & Potts, G. R. (1984). Mental comparison of size and magnitude: Size congruity effects. *Journal of Experimental Psychology: Learning, Memory, and Cognition*, *10*, 442–453.

Gallistel, C. R., & Gelman, R. (1992). Preverbal and verbal counting and computation. *Cognition*, *44*, 43–74.

Gazzaniga, M. S., & Smylie, C. E. (1984). Dissociation of language and cognition: A psychological profile of two disconnected right hemispheres. *Brain*, *107*, 145–153.

Gelman, R., & Gallistel, C. R. (1978). *The child's understanding of number*. Cambridge, MA: Harvard University Press.

Gerstmann, J. (1924). Fingeragnosie: Eine umschriebene storung der orientierung am eigenen korper. *Wiener Klinische Wochenschrift*, *37*, 1010–1012.

Gerstmann, J. (1927). Fingeragnosie und isolierte agraphi-ein neues syndrom. *Zeitschrift für die gesamte Neurologie und Psychiatrie*, *108*, 152–177.

Gerstmann, J. (1930). Zur Symptomatologie der hirnlasionen im ubergangsgebiet der unteren parietal-und mittleren occipital windung. *Nervenarzt*, *3*, 691–695.

Geschwind, N. (1965). Disconnection syndromes in animals and man. *Brain*, *88*, 237–294.

Gitelman, D. R., Nobre, A. C., Parrish, T. B., Labar, K. S., Kim, Y. H., Meyer, J. R., & Mesulam, M. M. (1999). A large-scale distributed network for covert spatial attention: Further anatomical delineation based on stringent behavioral and cognitive controls. *Brain*, *122*, 1093–1106.

Gitelman, D. R., Parrish, T. B., LaBar, K. S., & Mesulam, M. M. (2000). Real-time monitoring of eye movements using infrared video-oculography during functional magnetic resonance imaging of the frontal eye fields. *NeuroImage*, *11*(1), 58–65.

Goldstein, K. (1948). *Language and language disturbances*. New York: Grune & Stratton.

Gonzalez, E. G., & Kolers, P. A. (1982). Mental manipulation of arithmetic symbols. *Journal of Experimental Psychology: Learning, Memory, and Cognition*, *8*, 308–319.

Gonzalez, E. G., & Kolers, P. A. (1987). Notational constraints on mental operations. In G. Deloche & X. Seron (Eds.), *Mathematical disabilities: A cognitive neuropsychological perspective* (pp. 27–42). Hillsdale, NJ: Lawrence Erlbaum Associates.

Grafman, J., Kampen, D., Rosenberg, J., & Salazar, A. (1989). Calculation abilities in a patient with a virtual left hemispherectomy. *Behavioral Neurology*, *2*, 183–194.

Grafman, J., Passafiume, D., Faglioni, P., & Boller, F. (1982). Calculation disturbances in adults with focal hemispheric damage. *Cortex*, *18*, 37–50.

Grewel, F. (1952). Acalculia. *Brain*, *75*, 397–407.

Grewel, F. (1969). The acalculias. In J. A. M. Frederiks (Ed.), *Handbook of clinical neurology* (Vol. 4, pp. 181–194), P. J. Vinken, G. W. Bruyn, & H. L. Klawans Elsevier, Amsterdam.

Groen, G. J., & Parkman, J. M. (1972). A chronometric analysis of simple addition. *Psychological Review*, *79*, 329–343.

Guttmann, E. (1937). Congenital arithmetic disability and acalculia (Henschen). *British Journal of Medical Psychology*, *16*, 16–35.

Hécaen, H. (1962). Clinical symptomatology in right and left hemispheric lesions. In V. B. Mountcastle (Ed.), *Interhemispheric relations and cerebral dominance* (pp. 215–243). Baltimore: Johns Hopkins University Press.

Hécaen, H., & Angelergues, R. (1961). Etude anatomo-clinique de 280 cas de lésions rétrorolandiques unilatérales des hémiphères cérébraux. *Encéphale*, *6*, 533–562.

Hécaen, H., Angelergues, R., & Houillier, S. (1961). Les variétés cliniques des acalculies au cours des lésions rétrorolandiques: Approche statistique du probléme. *Revue Neurologique*, *105*, 85–103.

Hediger, H. K. P. (1981). The Clever Hans phenomenon from an animal psychologist's point of view. *Annals of the New York Academy of Sciences*, *364*, 1–17.

Heilman, K. M., & Valenstein, E. (1972). Frontal lobe neglect in man. *Neurology*, *22*, 660–664.

Henschen, S. E. (1919). Über sprach-, musik- und rechenmechanismen und ihre lokalisation im großhirn." *Zeitschrift für die gesamte Neurologie und Psychiatrie*, *27*, 52–57.

Henschen, S. E. (1920). *Klinische und anatomische beiträge zu pathologie des gehirns*. Stockholm: Nordiska Bokhandeln.

Hinrichs, J. V., Yurko, D. S., & Hu, J. (1981). Two-digit number comparison: Use of place information. *Journal of Experimental Psychology: Human Perception and Performance*, *7*, 890–901.

Hittmair-Delazer, M., Semenza, C., & Denes, G. (1994). Concepts and facts in calculation. *Brain, 117,* 715–728.

Jackson, M., & Warrington, E. K. (1986). Arithmetic skills in patients with unilateral cerebral lesions. *Cortex, 22,* 611–620.

Jonides, J., Smith, E. E., Koeppe, R. A., Awh, E., Minoshima, S., & Mintun, M. A. (1993). Spatial working memory in humans as revealed by PET. *Nature, 363,* 623–625.

Kahn, H. J., & Whitaker, H. A. (1991). Acalculia: An historical review of localization. *Brain and Cognition, 17,* 102–115.

Koechlin, E., Basso, G., Pietrini, P., Panzer, S., & Grafman, J. (1999). The role of the anterior prefrontal cortex in human cognition. *Nature, 399,* 148–151.

Krapf, E. (1937). Ueber akalkulie. *Sweizerische Archiv für Neurologie und Psychiatrie, 39,* 330–334.

LaBar, K. S., Gitelman, D. R., Parrish, T. B., & Mesulam, M. M. (1999). Neuroanatomic overlap of working memory and spatial attention networks: A functional MRI comparison within subjects. *NeuroImage, 10,* 695–704.

Lampl, Y., Eshel, Y., Gilad, R., & Sarova-Pinhas, I. (1994). Selective acalculia with sparing of the subtraction process in a patient with left parietotemporal hemorrhage. *Neurology, 44,* 1759–1761.

Leonhard, K. (1939). Die bedeutung optisch-räumlicher vorstellungen für das elementaire rechnen. *Zeitschrift für die gesamte Neurologie und Psychiatrie, 164,* 321–351.

Levine, D. N., Mani, R. B., & Calvanio, R. (1988). Pure agraphia and Gerstmann's syndrome as a visuospatial-language dissociation: An experimental case study. *Brain & Language, 35,* 172–196.

Lewandowsky, M., & Stadelmann, E. (1908). Ueber einen bemerkenswerten fall von hirnbluntung und über rechenstörungen bei herderkrankung des gehirns. *Journal für Psychologie und Neurologie, 11,* 249–265.

Lucchelli, F., & DeRenzi, E. (1992). Primary dyscalculia after a medial frontal lesion of the left hemisphere. *Journal of Neurology, Neurosurgery and Psychiatry, 56,* 304–307.

McCloskey, M. (1992). Cognitive mechanisms in numerical processing: Evidence from acquired dyscalculia. *Cognition, 44,* 107–157.

McCloskey, M., Aliminosa, D., & Sokol, S. M. (1991). Facts, rules and procedures in normal calculation: Evidence from multiple single-patient studies of impaired arithmetic fact retrieval. *Brain and Cognition, 17,* 154–203.

McCloskey, M., Caramazza, A., & Basili, A. (1985). Cognitive mechanisms in number processing and calculation: Evidence from dyscalculia. *Brain and Cognition, 4,* 171–196.

McNeil, J. E., & Warrington, E. K. (1994). A dissociation between addition and subtraction with written calculation. *Neuropsychologia, 32,* 717–728.

Menon, V., Rivera, S. M., White, C. D., Glover, G. H., & Reiss, A. L. (2000). Dissociating prefrontal and parietal cortex activation during arithmetic processing. *NeuroImage, 12,* 357–365.

Mesulam, M.-M. (1981). A cortical network for directed attention and unilateral neglect. *Annals of Neurology, 10,* 309–325.

Mesulam, M.-M. (1990). Large-scale neurocognitive networks and distributed processing for attention, language, and memory. *Annals of Neurology, 28,* 598–613.

Mesulam, M.-M. (1998). From sensation to cognition. *Brain, 121,* 1013–1052.

Mesulam, M.-M. (1999). Spatial attention and neglect: Parietal, frontal, and cingulate contributions to the mental representation and attentional targeting of salient extrapersonal events. *Philosophical Transactions of the Royal Society of London, Ser B, 354,* 1325–1346.

Miller, K., Perlmutter, M., & Keating, D. (1984). Cognitive arithmetic: Comparison of operations. *Journal of Experimental Psychology: Learning, Memory, and Cognition, 10,* 46–60.

Moyer, R. S., & Landauer, T. K. (1967). Time required for judgments of numerical inequality. *Nature, 215,* 1519–1520.

Nobre, A. C., Sebestyen, G. N., Gitelman, D. R., Mesulam, M. M., Frackowiak, R. S., & Frith, C. D. (1997). Functional localisation of the neural network for visual spatial attention by positron-emission tomography. *Brain, 120,* 515–533.

Noël, M., & Seron, X. (1993). Arabic number reading deficit: A single case study or when 236 is read (2306) and judged superior to 1258. *Cognitive Neuropsychology, 10,* 317–339.

Parkman, J. M. (1972). Temporal aspects of simple multiplication and comparison. *Journal of Experimental Psychology, 95,* 437–444.

Parkman, J. M., & Groen, G. J. (1971). Temporal aspects of simple addition and comparison. *Journal of Experimental Psychology, 89,* 335–342.

Paus, T. (1996). Location and function of the human frontal eye-field: A selective review. *Neuropsychologia*, *34*, 475–483.

Peritz, G. (1918). Zur Pathopsychologie des rechnens. *Deutsche Zeitschrift für Nervenheilkunde*, *61*, 234–340.

Pesenti, M., Zago, L., Crivello, F., Mellet, E., Salmon, D., Duroux, B., Seron, X., Mazoyer, B., & Tzourio-Mazoyer, N. (2000). Mental calculation in a prodigy is sustained by right prefrontal and medial temporal areas. *Nature Neuroscience*, *4*, 103–107.

Pinel, P., Le Clec'h, G., van de Moortele, P. F., Naccache, L., Le Bihan, D., & Dehaene, S. (1999). Event-related fMRI analysis of the cerebral network for number comparison. *NeuroReport*, *10*, 1473–1479.

Poeck, K., & Orgass, B. (1966). Gerstmann's syndrome and aphasia. *Cortex*, *2*, 421–437.

Poeppel, D. (1996). A critical review of PET studies of phonological processing. *Brain and Language*, *55*, 317–385.

Polk, T. A., & Farah, M. J. (1998). The neural development and organization of letter recognition: Evidence from functional neuroimaging, computational modeling, and behavioral studies. *Proceedings of the National Academy of Sciences U.S.A.*, *95*, 847–852.

Poppelreuter, W. (1917). *Die psychischen schaedigungen durch kopfschuss im kriege 1914–1916*. Leipzig: Voss.

Posner, M. I. (1986). *Chronometric explorations of Mind*. New York: Oxford University Press.

Reuckert, L., Lange, L., Partlot, A., Appollonio, I., Lituan, I., Le Bihan, O., & Grafman, J. (1996). Visualizing cortical activation during mental calculation with functional MRI. *NeuroImage*, *3*, 97–103.

Roland, P. E., & Friberg, L. (1985). Localization of cortical areas activated by thinking. *Journal of Neurophysiology*, *53*, 1219–1243.

Romero, S. G., Granetz, J., Makale, M., Manly, C., & Grafman, J. (2000). Learning and memory in developmental dyscalculia. *Journal of Cognitive Neuroscience* (abstract) (Supplement): 104.

Rosselli, M., & Ardila, A. (1989). Calculation deficits in patients with right and left hemisphere damage. *Neuropsychologia*, *27*, 607–617.

Sakurai, Y., Momose, T., Iwata, M., Sasaki, Y., & Kanazawa, I. (1996). Activation of prefrontal and posterior superior temporal areas in visual calculation. *Journal of the Neurological Sciences*, *139*, 89–94.

Sathian, K., Simon, T. J., Peterson, S., Patel, G. A., Hofftman, J. M., & Grafton, S. T. (1999). Neural evidence linking visual object enumeration and attention. *Journal of Cognitive Neuroscience*, *11*, 36–51.

Sekuler, R., Rubin, E., & Armstrong, R. (1971). Processing numerical information: A choice time analysis. *Journal of Experimental Psychology*, *90*, 75–80.

Selemon, L. D., & Goldman-Rakic, P. D. (1988). Common cortical and subcortical targets of the dorsolateral prefrontal and posterior parietal cortices in the rhesus monkey: Evidence for a distributed neural network subserving spatially guided behavior. *Journal of Neuroscience*, *8*, 4049–4068.

Singer, H. D., & Low, A. A. (1933). Acalculia. *Archives of Neurology and Psychiatry*, *29*, 467–498.

Sittig, O. (1917). Uber störungen des ziffernschreibens bei aphasischen. *Zeitschrift für Pathopsychologie*, *3*, 298–306.

Sittig, O. (1921). Störungen des ziffernschreibens und rechnens. *Monatsschrift fuer Psychiatrie und Neurologie*, *49*, 299.

Sokol, S. M., McCloskey, M., Cohen, N. J., & Aliminosa, D. (1991). Cognitive representations and processes in arithmetic: Inferences from the performance of brain-damaged subjects. *Journal of Experimental Psychology: Learning, Memory and Cognition*, *17*, 355–376.

Spiers, P. A. (1987). Acalculia revisited: Current issues. In G. Deloche & X. Seron (Eds.), *Mathematical disabilities: A cognitive neuropsychological perspective* (pp. 1–25). Hillsdale, NJ: Lawrence Erlbaum Associates.

Starkey, P., Spelke, E. S., & Gelman, R. (1983). Detection of intermodal numerical correspondences by human infants. *Science*, *222*, 179–181.

Starkey, P., Spelke, E. S., & Gelman, R. (1990). Numerical abstraction by human infants. *Cognition*, *36*, 97–127.

Stazyk, E. H., Ashcraft, M. H., & Hamann, M. S. (1982). A network approach to mental multiplication. *Journal of Experimental Psychology: Learning, Memory, and Cognition*, *8*, 320–335.

Strub, R., & Geschwind, N. (1974). Gerstmann syndrome without aphasia. *Cortex*, *10*, 378–387.

Takahashi, A., & Green, D. (1983). Numerical judgments with kanji and kana. *Neuropsychologia*, *21*, 259–263.

Talairach, J., & Tournoux, P. (1988). *Co-planar stereotaxic atlas of the human brain*. New York: Thieme Medical.

Warrington, E. K. (1982). The fractionation of arithmetical skills: A single case study. *Quarterly Journal of Experimental Psychology, 34A*, 31–51.

Whetstone, T. (1998). The representation of arithmetic facts in memory: Results from retraining a brain damaged patient. *Brain and Cognition, 365*, 290–309.

Whitaker, H., Habinger, J., & Ivers, R. (1985). Acalculia from a lenticular-caudate lesion. *Neurology, 35*(suppl 1): 161.

Wojciulik, E., Kanwisher, N., & Driver, J. (1998). Covert visual attention modulates face-specific activity in the human fusiform gyrus: fMRI study. *Journal of Neurophysiology, 79*, 1574–1578.

Zago, L., Pesenti, M., Mellet, E., Crevello, F., Mazoyer, B., & Tzourio-Mazoyer, N. (2000). Neural correlates of simple and complex mental calculation. *NeuroImage, 13*, 314–327.

8 Transcortical Motor Aphasia: A Disorder of Language Production

Michael P. Alexander

The essential aphasia syndrome occurring after left frontal lobe lesions is not Broca's aphasia, it is transcortical motor aphasia (TCMA). TCMA has the following characteristics: (1) impoverished but grammatical utterances; (2) infrequent paraphasias that are usually semantic or perseverative; (3) preserved repetition, oral reading, and recitation; and (4) preserved comprehension (auditory and written).

At its mildest or most recovered limits, TCMA may not be apparent in conversation or even in clinical testing. At its most severe limits, output may be extremely reduced, perseverative, and echolalic, and response set impairments and perseveration may produce abnormalities in comprehension. This chapter summarizes the clinical and cognitive neuroscience of the full range of this disorder.

Case Reports

Patient G.D.: A 73-year-old right-handed man, high school educated, a retired office manager with a history of hypertension and coronary artery disease with mild exertional dyspnea, developed acute chest pain. He underwent coronary angioplasty and stenting and was given heparin for 1 day, then placed on aspirin and ticlopidine. At home 3 days later he became acutely "confused." When he was evaluated in the emergency room, he had no spontaneous or responsive speech, but could repeat sentences and read aloud with good articulation. Head computed tomography (CT) showed a large left frontal hemorrhage (figure 8.1). Aspirin and ticlopidine were discontinued. Two days later G.D. still had no spontaneous speech, but he could make one- to two-word responses to questions, limited by severe perseveration. There was echolalia, i.e., uninhibited repetition of the examiner's words, particularly for commands in testing. He had frequent disinhibited completions of questions and comments by others around him. Repetition was normal. Recitation required initial prompts but was then completely normal. In all testing he was, somewhat paradoxically, simultaneously stimulus bound and easily distracted.

Six days after onset he had occasional short spontaneous utterances, a wider range of accurate short responses, and could answer many questions about personal information and orientation accurately if the answers were one or two straightforward words. On the other hand, when asked what he had done for a living, he replied, "I did . . . I mean . . . what'd I do for a living . . . that. . . ." Comprehension was intact for word discrimination and brief commands. Oral reading was normal. He named three out of six common objects with primarily perseverative errors, but none of six lower-frequency objects, with no vocalized response at all. He named five animals in 60 seconds, but each required a general prompt ("think of a farm"). He did no spontaneous writing beyond his name. He wrote single words to dictation in all grammatical categories although with frequent perseveration within and across stimuli. Writing sentences to dictation, he produced the first one or two words and then stopped. There was no facial or limb apraxia. Drawing was perseverative.

Sixteen days after onset he was more fluent, but with long latencies, frequently with no responses at all; however, grammatical structure was normal when he did speak. He perseverated words and phrases. He named six out of six common objects, but only one of six low-frequency objects. Most naming errors were perseverations of the initial correct response, but he suppressed these responses after the initial phoneme. He could not generate a single sentence from a supplied verb (e.g., take, receive, applaud), usually just repeating the verb. He has been lost to follow-up since that examination.

Patient M.B.: An 86-year-old right-handed retired physician with no prior cerebral or cardiac history suddenly developed "confusion." Records of his initial hospitalization are not available. An initial, mild right hemiparesis rapidly cleared. He had an infarct on CT, but no definite etiology was established. He was reportedly mute for several days. The evolution of his language was not well described by the patient or his family. He returned home. He lived alone, supervised by family. He was independent in self-care, prepared light meals, and enjoyed cultural activities. Several months later he had a grand mal seizure while traveling outside the United States. According to his family, he was "confused" for a few days but returned to baseline. CT demonstrated no new lesions, just the residual of the earlier stroke (figure 8.2). Phenytoin was begun.

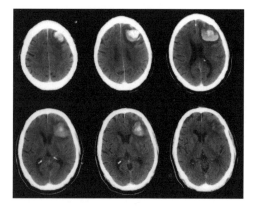

Figure 8.1
An acute-phase CT from patient G.D. shows a large hemorrhage above the frontal operculum, involving Brodmann areas 46, 9, 6, and 8. The final lesion site is speculative, but the center of mass of the blood (*upper right panel*) is in the middle frontal gyrus, areas 46 and 9.

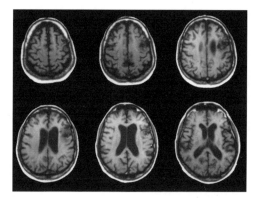

Figure 8.2
A chronic-phase MRI from patient M.B. shows a moderate infarction in the upper operculum, rising up in the middle frontal gyrus and involving Brodmann areas 46, 9, and 6.

Eight days after the seizure, the patient was alert and cooperative. Language output was fluent but anomic. Output was blocked on word-finding problems, followed by perseveration of the blocked phrase. He had frequent echolalia, sometimes partly suppressed. Comprehension at the word level of single words, descriptive phrases, and praxis commands was good. Repetition and oral reading were normal. He named all common objects, but only 60% of parts of objects. He named five animals in 60 seconds, but no words beginning with "b" despite prompting. When asked to produce a sentence given a verb, he quickly produced a pronoun subject and the verb (e.g., gave: "I give . . ."), but he could never progress further. Facial and limb praxis were normal.

A more detailed language assessment was completed 4 months later, 1 year post stroke. All measures of fluency, including grammatical form, were normal. The patient made no errors in syntax structure and no morphological errors. Speech was normal. He was severely anomic. Rare semantic paraphasias were all perseverative. He had fragments of echolalia. Comprehension was mildly impaired (eleven of fifteen commands and eight of twelve complex sentences or paragraphs). Word comprehension was normal or near normal for five of six categories, but poor for grammatical words, especially matching pictures with embedded sentence forms. Repetition and oral reading

were intact. His Boston Naming Test score was 46/60 (mildly impaired). He was very responsive to phonemic cues, but he could easily be cued to an incorrect answer. Writing showed good orthography and basically normal grammatical form, but anomia and perseveration of words.

Development of the Clinical Definition of TCMA

TCMA is one of the eight classical aphasia syndromes (Alexander, 1997). Initial characterizations by Lichtheim (1885) and Goldstein (1948) shared most features. Lichtheim fit the disorder into a theoretical schematic of aphasia that set the stage for "box-and-arrow" classification systems to come in the next hundred years. However, the placement of the arrows in Lichtheim's model indicated a belief that there was a disruption of the influence of nonlanguage mental capacities on preserved language.

Goldstein considered this disorder at length and provided good clinical descriptions and an extensive review of the postmortem correlations reported by many early investigators. His view is clear from the title of the relevant chapter from his 1948 text

(1971 edition): "Pictures of speech disturbances due to impairment of the non-language mental performances." He described two forms of TCMA. In one, partial injury to the "motor speech area" raised the threshold for speech. When speech was externally prompted (e.g., by answering short factual questions), it was normal or nearly so. When speech had to arise from internal intention (e.g., describing a personal experience), the elevated threshold could not be reliably reached. Whatever speech was produced had some articulatory impairment and "more or less motor agrammatism," but repetition, recitation, oral reading, and writing, were better. In modern models of aphasia (Goodglass, 1993), a combination of true agrammatism in speech with *no* other abnormality of spoken language or written language would be considered improbable, if not impossible, somewhere in the mildest Broca's aphasia domain. Goldstein suggested, however, that this disorder was always mild and transient. This characterization of mild Broca's aphasia as almost always transient received a new life in the 1970s from Mohr and colleagues with the description of "Broca's area aphasia," often called "Baby Broca's aphasia" (Mohr, Pessin et al., 1978).

The second variety of TCMA described by Goldstein (1948) was characterized as "an impairment of the impulse to speak at all." Patient descriptions fit the profile described in the introduction to this chapter. Goldstein also observed that patients often showed a "general akinesis" and that they often required prompts to generate any speech, even recitation. He concluded with the observation that TCMA was a disturbance of the "intention" to speak. Goldstein believed from the clinical reports available to him that echolalia was not a key element of TCMA because echolalia only occurred when the failure of intention was combined with impaired comprehension despite intact posterior perisylvian structures. His review of the literature at the time included some cases with echolalia with only a left frontal lesion and only modest comprehension deficits. The "comprehension impairment" that many of these patients showed may have been due to difficulty establishing a proper test set and avoiding perseveration, rather than actual loss of language competence, much as in the two patients described earlier.

Luria began the modern linguistically based description of the possible components of the "non-language mental processes" essential for connected, intentional language output (Luria, 1973). Luria's vocabulary and conceptual models were idiosyncratic, but he specified impairments that are readily recognized in modern cognitive neuropsychological terms. He described impairments in intention, in the formation of verbal plans, and in the assembly of a linear mental model (deep structure in modern terms). The intentional deficit suggests limbic disorders: deficient drive, arousal, motivation, etc. The planning deficit suggests supervisory executive impairment. The reduced capacity to produce linear structure suggests disturbed proceduralization of syntax and discourse. These three domains—intention, supervision, and planning—are the essence of modern theories about the frontal lobe's role in language, as well as many other complex cognitive operations.

Luria proposed that this constellation of deficits in language constituted "dynamic aphasia," as distinguished from TCMA, which he viewed as a more severe disorder with preservation of single word repetition but marked reduction of spontaneous language fluency, a characterization that suggests partial recovery from more typical Broca's aphasia (Luria & Tsevtkova, 1967). Luria also distinguished dynamic aphasia from the general lack of spontaneity and motivation seen in patients with major frontal lobe lesions. There is little specification of a precise lesion site causing dynamic aphasia other than the left inferior frontal lobe.

The role of the frontal lobes in language at the outset of the modern neuroimaging and neuroscience eras can be summarized. The fundamental processes of language can be utilized to achieve broad communication goals. Accomplishing these goals requires a variety of mental processes, including intention and planning, and narrative skills that can organize language structure and output. Deficits in this complex use of language are due to lesions in the left lateral frontal lobe. TCMA (or Luria's dynamic aphasia) represents the range of aphasic disorders in which the fundamental processes—semantics, phonology, articulation, grammar, and concatenation—are normal, but the utilization of them is impaired.

Clinical, imaging, and cognitive neuroscience investigations in the past 25 years have sharpened our understanding of TCMA and clarified its neural and psychological components, although Luria's basic characterizations remain fundamental even to modern concepts. Lesion specificity has been clarified. The roles of different regions of the frontal lobes in discrete aspects of language are better understood. Insights from other domains of cognitive neuroscience have illuminated the mechanisms of planning and intention in speech.

Lesion–Anatomy Correlations in TCMA

Any analysis of the language disorders due to frontal lesions must begin with Broca's aphasia. The eponymous area is usually marked with a "B" and lies over the frontal operculum, roughly Brodmann areas 44 and 45; sometimes it includes the lower motor cortex (area 4) and the anterior, superior insular cortex continuous with the inferior opercular surface. Damage restricted to these areas produces a somewhat variable clinical picture, sometimes called "Broca's area aphasia" (Mohr et al., 1978). In the acute phase, these patients have more similarities than differences. They are often briefly mute, then show effortful speech with articulation and prosody impairments, reduced phrase length, syntax errors, and mixed paraphasias, all variably but modestly benefited by repetition. Thus, Broca's area lesions produce acute Broca's aphasia.

In the chronic phase, these patients diverge along several paths (Alexander, Naeser, & Palumbo, 1990). Lesions centered in the posterior operculum and the lower motor cortex are likely to cause persistent articulation and prosody impairments, with rapid recovery of lengthy, grammatical utterances. Lesions centered in the anterior superior operculum

are likely to produce persistent truncation of utterances, although without much overt grammatical impairment, with rapid recovery of articulation and prosody and rapid normalization of repetition and recitation. Thus, viewed from the postacute perspective, Broca's area lesions damage two adjacent, perhaps overlapping, neural systems, one fundamentally for motor control of speech and one for realization of lengthy, complex utterances. Broca's area lesions do not produce lasting Broca's aphasia.

Freedman and colleagues (Freedman, Alexander, & Naeser, 1984) analyzed a large number of patients in the postacute stage that met a standard clinical definition of TCMA (Goodglass & Kaplan, 1983). More than one lesion site was identified. Some patients had damage to the frontal operculum, including the anterior portions of Broca's area. Some had damage to more dorsolateral midfrontal regions, which often projected into white matter. Some had damage only to the deep white matter including or adjacent to and above the head of the caudate nucleus. Some had large capsulostriatal lesions reaching up to the head of the caudate nucleus and the adjacent white matter. Some had medial frontal damage, including the supplementary motor area (SMA).

Earlier descriptions of aphasia after infarctions of the left anterior cerebral artery (ACA) territory or associated with parasagittal tumors had already established that large medial frontal lesions produced a speech and language impairment (Critchley, 1930). Mutism, paucity of speech, and repetitive utterances were described. Several reports in the 1970s (Von Stockert, 1974; Rubens, 1976) (Masdeu, Schoene, & Funkenstein, 1978) and 1980s (Alexander & Schmitt, 1980) defined the evolution of aphasia with left medial frontal lesions: initial mutism for hours to weeks and then gradual recovery of lengthy, fluent output, with preserved repetition and recitation.

In the report by Freedman and colleagues, a detailed assessment of the variation in postacute language impairment associated with left lateral frontal damage revealed the important anterior-posterior divergence of roles within the frontal cortex (Freedman et al., 1984). The posterior portions are essential for articulation; the anterior portions are essential for some aspect of generative language—complex sentences, narratives, etc.—but are unimportant for externally driven language—repetition, naming, oral reading, and short responses.

There is considerable controversy about the so-called "subcortical aphasias," particularly those associated with left capsulostriatal lesions. An analysis of absolute cortical perfusion and of the extent and location of carotid obstructive disease suggests to some investigators that aphasia is due to cortical hypoperfusion, causing microscopic cortical neuronal injury (Olsen, Bruhn, & Oberg, 1986) (Nadeau & Crosson, 1995). In this view, the subcortical lesion is irrelevant. With numerous collaborators, I have proposed a different mechanism for aphasia (Alexander, Naeser et al., 1987). Most structures within capsulostriatal lesions are, in fact, irrelevant to aphasia. Lesions in the putamen, the globus pallidus ventral anterior limb internal capsule (ALIC), or most of the paraventricular white matter (PVWM) do not appear to affect language. Lesions in the dorsal ALIC, the dorsal head of the caudate nucleus and the anterior PVWM, on the other hand, are associated with a mild generative aphasia, i.e., TCMA, in the postacute period (Mega & Alexander, 1994). These patients also often have severe articulatory impairment (descending corticobulbar pathways), hypophonia (putamen), and hemiparesis (corticospinal pathways). None of these are pertinent to aphasia; the aphasia diagnosis is independent of the neurological findings (Alexander et al., 1987). Spontaneous (hypertensive) hemorrhages in capsulostriatal territories produce a more severe initial aphasia and a broader range of aphasias in the postacute period because a dissection of a hemorrhage can produce idiosyncratic lesion extensions (D'Esposito & Alexander, 1995). The "core syndrome" of mild TCMA after lesions in caudate or anterior white matter is maintained.

Consolidation of these disparate observations is possible. Damage to the medial frontal cortex, including the SMA and anterior cingulate gyrus (ACG), produces akinetic mutism (Freemon, 1971). The akinesia, including akinesia of the speech apparatus (i.e., mutism), is due to the loss of ascending cortical dopaminergic input (Lindvall, Bjorkland, Moorc, Steneui, 1974). Thus, the progressive aphasia commonly associated with progressive supranuclear palsy (PSP) is dynamic aphasia or TCMA, although it is often embedded in more pervasive activation and executive impairments (Esmonde, Giles et al., 1996).

The SMA (Jürgens, 1984) and ACG (Baleydier & Mauguiere, 1980) have interesting connectivity principles. Afferents are received from all sensory association cortices and potently from dopaminergic brainstem nuclei, but efferents are bilateral to all frontal regions and to the striatum. Thus, processed sensory information converges with subcortical drive and activation mechanisms. The resultant output from the SMA and ACG is the activation transformer of the brain. Medial structures provide the drive for continued sustained movement and cognition. Projections through anterior PVWM regions and to the caudate nucleus carry this activation to the lateral frontal regions, converging on the left frontal operculum for speech (Alexander et al., 1987). Lesions anywhere in this system will damage drive, activation, and generative capacities, producing truncated, unelaborated language. Thus, damage to this efferent, bilateral medial to left lateral frontal system is the foundation for the impairment observed in "intention" to speak. Simple responses, recitation, repetition, even naming require much less generative effort; thus they are preserved. The posterior operculum, in turn, organizes motor programs of speech.

Modern Notions of Dynamic Aphasia

Recent investigators have analyzed the cognitive and linguistic impairments that might underlie the planning and supervisory deficits in TCMA by focusing on dynamic aphasia, the cleanest exemplar of TCMA. Some extrapolation from functional neuroimaging studies in normal subjects also illuminates this issue. These investigations have attempted to specify more precisely the testable deficits that make up the generality of "planning."

The most carefully analyzed single case reports of dynamic aphasia meet clinical criteria for TCMA with left frontal lesions. Costello and Warrington (1989) demonstrated that their patient was unable to produce a conceptual structure for an utterance prior to any implementation of syntactic options for expression and prior to actual sentence production. Robinson et al. observed that their patient was unable to select propositional language when the communication context provided little constraint or prompting (Robinson, Blair, & Cipolotti, 1998). When there were numerous possible utterances and constructions, the patient was impaired. When context defined a response, language was normal.

Thompson-Schill et al. have shown the same type of deficit at the single-word level in patients with lesions that included the left posterior frontal regions (Thompson-Schill, Swick, Farah, D'Esposito, Kan, & Knight, 1998). Language activation studies with positron emission tomography (PET) (Petersen, Fox, Posner, Mintun, & Raichle, 1989) or functional magnetic resonance imaging (fMRI) (Desmond, 1995) have long demonstrated that the left frontal opercular area is activated in tasks of semantic generation, such as naming a verb that is associated with a given noun. This activation is not just associated with semantic retrieval, but depends as much on selection of an item from a range of retrieved choices (Thompson-Schill, D'Esposito, Aguirre, & Farah, 1997). Patients with posterior frontal lesions have difficulty with verb generation in proportion to the number of choices available to them (Thompson-Schill et al., 1998). Nadeau (1988) analyzed the syntactic constructions of two patients with large left lateral frontal lesions. He demonstrated that word choice and grammar within a sentence can be intact when the syntactic frame selected for the overall response is defective.

In a PET study of memory retrieval in normal subjects, Fletcher et al. observed a distinction in left frontal activation, depending on the relationship of word pairs to be retrieved. Thus, retrieval and production of verbal material that was highly probably linked, whether imageable (arm-muscle) or not (happiness-love), produced little left frontal activation. When retrieval required construction of novel links between unrelated word pairs, even if they were highly imageable individually (hurricane-puppy), there was marked left lateral frontal activation (Fletcher, Shallice, Frith, Frackowiak, & Dolan, 1996). The authors remarked on the similarity of this finding to the difficulty that patients with left frontal lesions and dynamic aphasia have producing responses that are not highly connected semantically.

All of these potential explanations for dynamic aphasia revolve around impaired language planning when the context of the utterance does not immediately guide output. Whether at the word or sentence level (or even at the discourse level; see the following discussion), this planning and selection problem appears fundamental to frontal aphasias. When numerous responses are possible, when word and syntax selections are not constrained, when social context does not restrict the form that utterances might take, the left frontal region is critical for selection and execution of a particular response strategy. This is action planning in the domain of language.

Discourse

Discourse is the production of structured complex output (Chapman, Culhane et al. 1992). During development, humans learn rules and accepted procedures for discourse and in parallel, they learn how and when to use these procedures (Chapman, Culhane et al., 1992). They learn a "theory of mind," that is, the capacity to place themselves in a listener's mind to estimate what knowledge or expectations or emotions the listener might bring to an interaction (Stone, Baron-Cohen, & Knight, 1998; Gallagher, Happe, Brunswick, Fletcher, Frith, & Frith, 2000). They learn the context and constraints for the use of discourse. They learn their culture's rules, styles, and strategies for discourse.

Some forms of discourse are highly rule bound: pleading a court case, structuring a medical report, writing a book chapter, and telling some types of jokes. Discourse can be narrative (telling a story) or procedural (relating a recipe, teaching car repair) or a mixture of both (teaching biology). The forms of discourse have rules of construction (story grammar), rules of coherence (using intelligible references), rules of indirection, etc.

Prefrontal lesions produce impairments in discourse (Kaczmarek, 1984; Chapman et al., 1992). The discourse errors of left prefrontal lesions are mostly simplifications (Novoa & Ardila, 1987). There is a reduction in variation of sentence structure and a tendency to repeat sentence forms. There is a reduction in the number of relevant themes and concepts recruited to fill out a narrative; thus reference within a narrative is often incomplete. The boundary between dynamic aphasia and defective discourse is not fixed. Patients with dynamic aphasia use simple and unelaborated sentence forms and tend to repeat a few sentence structures. There are clearly nested levels of impairment in the recruitment of the elements of complex language.

Thus far this review has only dealt with left frontal lesions. At the level of discourse, right prefrontal injury may also disrupt communication (Novoa & Ardila, 1987). The limited evidence suggests that right prefrontal lesions reduce organization and monitoring, allowing the tangential, unrelated, and at times inappropriate and in some cases, frankly confabulatory narratives characteristic of right frontal damage.

Production of complex language presupposes intact fundamental language processes—phonetics, phonology, semantics, and grammar. Using those preserved functions, a large group of interrelated operations must unfold to produce complex language. The operations include selection of discourse intention and form, allowing for shared knowledge with the listener; selection of syntactic procedures that fit the intended communication; and selection from the many options of the precise lexical elements that express the intentions and fit the syntax. How all of this unfolds online is beyond the abili-

ties of this writer and is a complex, vital issue in cognitive science (Levelt, 1989), but at the "offline" level of impairments due to frontal injury, we return to action planning.

Action Planning

Action planning has been evaluated in patients with neurological damage. The models for action planning vary somewhat (Shallice, 1982; Schwartz, Reed, Montgomery, Palmer, & Mayer, 1991). All appear to suppose that experience has taught everyone a wide variety of simple actions (pouring, cutting, untwisting, etc.) and of possible assemblies of those actions to achieve certain goals (fixing coffee, making a sandwich, etc.). When some actions are frequently combined in an unvarying manner, then the resulting practiced complex action may become a unit of action of its own (eating breakfast, getting dressed). Across life's experiences, a large repertoire of simple and combined actions become proceduralized, that is, produced as a whole without explicit conscious direction. As the complexity of action increases and as the possible order of recruitment of subparts of the action (schemas) becomes less fixed, more explicit conscious direction is required to select and assemble the parts into an intended whole, delaying or holding some actions, inhibiting others, and monitoring progress to the goal (intention). Deficits in action planning have been studied with simple everyday behaviors, such as eating breakfast (Schwartz et al., 1991), and with more complex behaviors, such as shopping (Shallice & Burgess, 1991).

TCMA, at least dynamic aphasia, and discourse deficits are action planning failures in language. Patients cannot generate a plan or subplans, select from among alternative plans, or maintain an initial selection without contamination from other activated possible plans; nor can they keep track of how the several selected plans are progressing. This assembly and planning function operates at numerous levels that appear to have anterior-posterior arrangements in the left frontal lobe (Sirigu, Cohen et al. 1998). In the posterior ventrolateral frontal lobe, deficits may be at the level of word activation and selection (Thompson-Schill et al., 1998). Thus, language is quite restricted whenever the response is not prompted by words in the question or some other externality. With lesions of the dorsolateral frontal lobe, deficits may be at the level of syntactic selection (Costello & Warrington, 1989). Language is restricted whenever a novel sentence structure must be generated and, in default, any provided sentence may be pirated, at least in part, to carry the response; thus echolalia and perseveration. With prefrontal lesions, deficits may be at the discourse level. Language is produced and word selection proceeds, but the organization of plans for complex action (discourse) is impaired. There may be reliance on a few syntactic forms to carry the communication load and great difficulty generating new syntactic or narrative structures.

Conclusions and Future Directions

Dynamic aphasia appears to be an ideal substrate for analyzing the elements of action planning. Mapping the conceptual framework of action plans on to language production should be a path to a clearer understanding of both. If the elements of TCMA or dynamic aphasia are well defined now, methodologies for treatments are not. Is it possible to re-train the use of complex syntax or discourse? Can patients learn substitutions and compensatory rules or must complex language be rehearsed and practiced in a natural context? Can planning be taught offline with picture and story arrangement tasks or can it only be relearned in the process of speaking? Does dopaminergic deficiency actually underlie any component of the language deficit (Sabe, Salvarezza, Garcia Cuerva, Leiguarda, & Starkstein, 1995) or is it only relevant to the more pervasive akinetic mutism syndromes (Ross & Stewart, 1981)? The progress from Goldstein to Shallice is palpable, but as yet of little benefit to patients.

There are embedded impairments in action planning for language that in their interactions make up

the frontal language disorders. The essential frontal language disorder is TCMA. The deficits in TCMA are a mixture of delayed initiation (even mutism), impaired lexical selection, and reduced capacity to generate unconstrained syntactic forms. The prototypical lesions are in the left lateral frontal cortex, including much of the classic Broca's area, or in subcortical structures, including white matter projections and dorsal caudate nucleus.

The two fundamental factors that underlie defective language production after a left frontal lobe injury are intention and planning. Intention deficits are due to damage to medial frontal structures, their afferent projections, or their efferent convergence in left lateral frontal regions, probably quite diffusely. Planning deficits are due to damage to the left lateral frontal lobe, again rather diffusely, with interleaved impairments in planning extending from the level of word selection to syntax selection to discourse construction roughly correlating with a posterior-to-polar progression of frontal lesions.

References

Alexander, M. P. (1997). Aphasia: Clinical and anatomic aspects. In T. E. Feinberg, & M. J. Farah (Eds.), *Behavioral neurology and neuropsychology* (pp. 133–149). New York: McGraw-Hill.

Alexander, M. P., Naeser, M. A., & Palumbo, C. L. (1987). Correlations of subcortical CT lesion sites and aphasia profiles. *Brain*, *110*, 961–991.

Alexander, M. P., Naeser, M. A. et al. (1990). Broca's area aphasia. *Neurology*, *40*, 353–362.

Alexander, M. P., & Schmitt, M. A. (1980). The aphasia syndrome of stroke in the left anterior cerebral artery territory. *Archives of Neurology*, *37*, 97–100.

Baleydier, C., & Mauguiere, F. (1980). The duality of the cingulate gyrus in monkey: Neuroanatomical study and functional hypothesis. *Brain*, *103*, 525–554.

Chapman, S. B., Culhane, K. A., Levin, H. S., Harward, H., Mendelsohn, D., Ewing-Cobbs, L., Fletcher, J. M., & Bruce, D. (1992). Narrative discourse after closed head injury in children and adolescents. *Brain and Language*, *43*, 42–65.

Costello, A. L., & Warrington, E. K. (1989). Dynamic aphasia. The selective impairment of verbal planning. *Cortex, 25*, 103–114.

Critchley, M. (1930). Anterior cerebral artery and its syndromes. *Brain, 53*, 120–165.

D'Esposito, M., & Alexander, M. P. (1995). Subcortical aphasia: Distinct profiles following left putaminal hemorrhages. *Neurology, 45*, 33–37.

Desmond, J. E., Sum, J. M., Wagner, A. D., Demb, J. B., Shear, P. K., Glover, G. H., Gabrieli, J. D., & Morrell, M. J. (1995). Functional MRI measurement of language lateralization in Wada-tested patients. *Brain, 118*, 1411–1419.

Esmonde, T., Giles, E., Xuereb, J., & Hodges, J. (1996). Progressive supranuclear palsy presenting with dynamic aphasia. *Journal of Neurology, Neurosurgery and Psychiatry, 60*, 403–410.

Fletcher, P. C., Shallice, T., Frith, C. D., Frackowiak, R. S., & Dolan, R. J. (1996). Brain activity during memory retrieval: The influence of imagery and semantic cueing. *Brain, 119*, 1587–1596.

Freedman, M., Alexander, M. P., & Naeser, M. A. (1984). Anatomic basis of transcortical motor aphasia. *Neurology, 34*, 409–417.

Freemon, F. R. (1971). Akinetic mutism and bilateral anterior cerebral artery occlusion. *Journal of Neurology, Neurosurgery and Psychiatry, 34*, 693–698.

Gallagher, H. L., Happe, F., Brunswick, N., Fletcher, P. C., Frith, U., & Frith, C. D. (2000). Reading the mind in cartoons and stories: An fMRI study of "theory of mind" in verbal and nonverbal tasks. *Neuropsychologia, 38*, 11–21.

Goldstein, K. (1948). *Language and language disorders.* New York: Grune & Stratton.

Goodglass, H. (1993). *Understanding aphasia.* San Diego: Academic Press.

Goodglass, H., & Kaplan, E. (1983). *The assessment of aphasia and related disorders.* Philadelphia: Lea & Febiger.

Jürgens, U. (1984). The efferent and afferent connections of the supplementary motor area. *Brain Research, 300*, 63–81.

Kaczmarek, B. L. J. (1984). Neurolinguistic analysis of verbal utterances in patients with focal lesions of frontal lobes. *Brain and Language, 21*, 52–58.

Levelt, W. J. M. (1989). *Speaking: From intention to articulation.* Cambridge, MA: MIT Press.

Lichtheim, L. (1885). On aphasia. *Brain, 7*, 433–484.

Lindvall, O., Bjorkland, A., Moore, R. Y., & Stenevi, U. (1974). Mesencephalic dopamine neurons projecting to neocortex. *Brain Research, 81*, 325–331.

Luria, A. R. (1973). *The working brain.* New York: Basic Books.

Luria, A. R., & Tsevtkova, L. S. (1967). Towards the mechanism of "dynamic aphasia". *Acta Neurologica Psychiatrica Belgica, 67*, 1045–1067.

Masdeu, J. C., Schoene, W. C., & Funkenstein, H. (1978). Aphasia following infarction of the left supplementary motor area. *Neurology, 28*, 1220–1223.

Mega, M. S., & Alexander, M. P. (1994). The core profile of subcortical aphasia. *Neurology, 44*, 1824–1829.

Mohr, J. P., Pessin, M. et al. (1978). Broca aphasia: Pathologic and clinical aspects. *Neurology, 28*, 311–324.

Nadeau, S. (1988). Impaired grammar with normal fluency and phonology. *Brain, 111*, 1111–1137.

Nadeau, S., & Crosson, B. (1995). Subcortical aphasia. *Brain and Language, 58*, 355–402.

Novoa, O. P., & Ardila, A. (1987). Linguistic abilities in patients with prefrontal damage. *Brain and Language, 30*, 206–225.

Petersen, S. E., Fox, P. T., Posner, M. I., Mintun, M., & Raichle, M. E. (1989). Positron emission tomographic studies of the processing of single words. *Journal of Cognitive Neuroscience, 1*, 153–170.

Robinson, G., Blair, J., & Cipolotti, L. (1998). Dynamic aphasia: An inability to select between competing verbal responses? *Brain, 121*, 77–89.

Ross, E. D., & Stewart, R. M. (1981). Akinetic mutism from hypothalamic damage: Successful treatment with dopamine agonists. *Neurology, 31*, 1435–1439.

Rubens, A. B. (1976). Transcortical motor aphasia. *Studies in Neurolinguistics, 1*, 293–306.

Sabe, L., Salvarezza, F., Garcia Cuerva, A., Leiguarda, R., & Starkstein, S. (1995). A randomized, double-blind, placebo-controlled study of bromocriptine in nonfluent aphasia. *Neurology, 45*, 2272–2274.

Schwartz, M. F., Reed, E. S., Montgomerv, M., Palmer, C., & Mayer, N. H. (1991). The quantitative description of action disorganization after brain damage: A case study. *Cognitive Neuropsychology, 8*, 381–414.

Shallice, T. (1982). Specific impairments of planning. *Philosophical Transactions of the Royal Society of London, 298*, 199–209.

Shallice, T., & Burgess, P. W. (1991). Deficits in strategy application following frontal lobe damage in man. *Brain, 114*, 727–741.

Sirigu, A., Cohen, L., Zalla, T., Pradat-Diehl, P., Van Eechout, P., Grafman, J., & Agid, Y. (1998). Distinct frontal regions for processing sentence syntax and story grammar. *Cortex, 34*, 771–778.

Olsen, T. S., Bruhn, P., & Oberg, R. G. (1986). Cortical hypoperfusion as a possible cause of "subcortical aphasia." *Brain, 109*, 393–410.

Stone, V. E., Baron-Cohen, S., & Knight, R. T. (1998). Frontal lobe contributions to theory of mind. *Journal of Cognitive Neuroscience, 10*, 640–656.

Thompson-Schill, S. L., D'Esposito, M., Aguirre, G. K., & Farah, M. J. (1997). Role of left inferior prefrontal cortex in retrieval of semantic knowledge: A reevaluation. *Proceedings of the National Academy of Sciences U.S.A., 94*, 14792–14797.

Thompson-Schill, S. L., Swick, D., Farah, M. J., D'Esposito, M., Kan, I. P., & Knight, R. T. (1998). Verb generation in patients with focal frontal lesions: A neuropsychological test of neuroimaging findings. *Proceedings of the National Academy of Sciences U.S.A., 95*, 15855–15860.

Von Stockert, T. R. (1974). Aphasia sine aphasie. *Brain and Language, 1*, 277–282.

9 Wernicke Aphasia: A Disorder of Central Language Processing

Jeffrey R. Binder

Case Report

Patient H.K. is a 75-year-old, right-handed woman with mild hypertension who suddenly developed language difficulty and right hemiparesis. Prior to this, she had been healthy, living alone and managing her own affairs. Hemiparesis was confined to the right face and hand and resolved within 24 hours. Persistent language deficits observed during the acute hospitalization included poor naming of objects, difficulty producing understandable words in speech, and impaired understanding of commands and questions. A computed tomography (CT) scan obtained on the third day after onset showed an acute infarction in the territory of the left middle cerebral artery, affecting posterior temporal and parietal regions. She was discharged home after 1 week. Although she was able to perform all necessary activities such as shopping, cooking, and cleaning, persistent communication deficits made social interactions difficult and embarassing.

Initial Examination

When examined in more detail 4 weeks after onset, the patient was alert and able to write her name, the date, and the name of the hospital. She was calm and attentive, always attempting to understand and comply with what was requested of her. She spoke frequently and with fluent, well-articulated production of phonemes. Her sentences were of normal length and prosody. Spontaneously uttered words were mostly recognizable except for occasional neologisms (nonwords). Her word output consisted almost entirely of familiar combinations of closed-class words (articles, prepositions, pronouns) and common verbs, with relatively little noun content. The following is a transcription of her description of the Cookie Theft Picture from the Boston Diagnostic Aphasia Evaluation (BDAE) (Goodglass & Kaplan, 1972):

"What has he got here? That . . . that's coming right over there, I'll tell you that. This is the . . . the conner? . . . the bonner falling down here. And that's the boy going to getting with it over there. She's got this washering it's upside, and down. She'd doing the . . . the fixing it, the plape? . . . the plate, that she's got it there. And on it, the girl's sort of upside. Is that about? Anything else I'm missing, if it's down, that I wouldn't know?"

Verbal and phonemic paraphasias were more common in tasks requiring production of specific words, such as naming, repeating, and reading. She was unable to name correctly any presented objects, pictures, or colors, but produced neologistic utterances for many of these ("hudder" for hammer, "remp" for red), as well as occasional semantically related words ("dog" for horse). Her responses were characterized by repeated attempts and successively closer phonemic approximations to the target word ("fleeth, fleth, fleether, fleather" for feather). Naming of numbers and letters was sometimes correct, and more often than with objects resulted in semantic substitution of other items in the same category. Strikingly, she was often able to write correctly the names of objects she was unable to pronounce. After failing to name orally six object pictures from the BDAE (glove, key, cactus, chair, feather, hammock), she succeeded in writing four of these correctly (cactus, chair, feather, hammock) and wrote a semantically related word for the others ("hand" for glove and "lock" for key).

Repetition was severely defective for all stimuli. Even after correctly writing the names for objects, she was unable to repeat these names aloud after hearing the examiner and simultaneously looking at the name she had just written. Errors in repetition and reading aloud were almost entirely phonemic paraphasias. She was often able to write to dictation familiar nouns she could not repeat aloud (dog, cat, horse, hand, ear, nose), but was unable to do this with less common words (sheep, goat, trout, jaw, chin, knee). She was unable to write a simple sentence to dictation (For "A boy had a dog," she wrote with some hesitation "He and aswer").

She followed simple oral commands given without accompanying gestures ("close eyes," "open mouth," "smile," "stand up") in approximately half of the trials, possibly inferring some of the meaning from context. She was unable to follow less likely commands ("look left," "lick lips," "clench jaw," "lean back") or multicomponent commands. Simple questions containing five to seven words ("Did you eat lunch today?" "How did you get here?") evoked fluent, empty responses with no apparent relationship to the question. On auditory-visual matching tasks using six to eight-item visual arrays, she was able to point to named objects, words, and letters with 100% accuracy, indicating preservation of some auditory comprehension for single words. She understood written commands and questions no better than the auditory versions. The remainder of the neurological examination was normal, including tests for visual neglect, visual field, and other cranial nerve tests, motor and sensory examination, and cerebellar and gait testing.

Structural Magnetic Resonance Imaging

High-resolution, T1-weighted magnetic resonance images (MRI) (voxel size = 1 mm^3) were obtained 14 months postonset (figure 9.1). A large region of

encephalomalacia was observed in the posterior left hemisphere. Damaged areas included most of Heschl's gyrus (HG) and the planum temporale (PT), the superior temporal gyrus (STG) and superior temporal sulcus (STS) lateral and ventral to HG, and the dorsal aspect of the posterior middle temporal gyrus (MTG). Left parietal lobe damage affected the entire supramarginal gyrus (SMG) except for a thin ribbon of preserved cortex along the intraparietal sulcus, and approximately the anterior two-thirds of the angular gyrus (AG). Subcortical white matter was destroyed in these gyri, while deep periventricular white matter was spared.

Subsequent Course

Severe aphasic deficits have persisted over 6 years of follow-up, although the patient remains able to manage all daily necessities of living. Spontaneous speech remains fluent, with relatively little noun or adjective content. Oral confrontation naming has improved modestly, so that the patient succeeds in a small proportion of trials, but with frequent phonemic paraphasias and successive approximations to the target ("coxis, caxis, coctis, cactus" for cactus). Written naming is consistently superior to

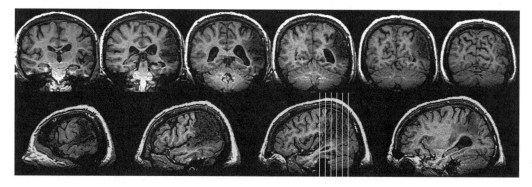

Figure 9.1
A T1-weighted MRI in patient H.K. In the top row are serial coronal slices through the posterior perisylvian region, taken at 10-mm intervals and arranged anterior to posterior. The left hemisphere is on the reader's right. The bottom row shows serial sagittal slices through the left hemisphere at 7-mm intervals. The position of the coronal slices is indicated by the vertical lines in the third image.

oral naming, and writing to dictation remains notably better than oral repetition. The patient has spontaneously developed a strategy of writing down or spelling aloud what she is trying to say when listeners do not appear to understand. At 8 months postonset, she produced the following transcription of several simple sentences she was unable to repeat orally:

Auditory Stimulus (Patient's Transcription)

A boy had a dog. (A boy and girl found dog.)

The dog ran into the woods. (The dogs run into the woods.)

The boy ran after the dog. (The boy ran away the dog.)

He wanted the dog to go home. (The boys run and the dog is all home.)

But the dog would not go home. (The bog isn't home.)

The little boy said. (The little boy was).

I cannot go home without my dog. (The boy werit that the I home.)

Then the boy began to cry. (He carire cried.)

The ability to carry out simple oral commands is now more consistent, whereas comprehension of multistep commands and simple questions not related to the immediate context remains severely deficient in both auditory and visual modalities.

Clinical Description of Wernicke Aphasia

Like the other aphasias, Wernicke aphasia is a syndrome complex composed of several distinct signs (table 9.1). The central characteristic is a disturbance of language comprehension, manifested by incorrect or unexpected responses to spoken commands and other language stimuli. In the acute stage, this deficit may be so severe as to seem to involve more than language alone, the patient often appearing to show no reaction to verbal input from

Table 9.1
Characteristic clinical features of Wernicke aphasia and several related syndromes

Tasks	Clinical Syndromes			
	Wernicke aphasia	Transcortical sensory aphasia	Pure word deafness	Conduction aphasia
Comprehension				
Auditory verbal	Impaired	Impaired	Impaired	Normal
Written	Impaired	Impaired	Normal	Normal
Production				
Error type	Phonemic + verbal	Verbal > phonemic	Phonemic	Phonemic
Speech				
Propositional	Paraphasic and/or anomic	Paraphasic and/or anomic	± Paraphasic	Paraphasic
Naming	Paraphasic and/or anomic	Paraphasic and/or anomic	± Paraphasic	Paraphasic
Repetition	Paraphasic	Normal	Paraphasic	Paraphasic
Reading aloud	Paraphasic	Paraphasic or alexic	± Paraphasic	Paraphasic
Writing				
Propositional	Paragraphic/anomic	Paragraphic/anomic	Normal	Normal
Naming	Paragraphic/anomic	Paragraphic/anomic	Normal	Normal
Dictation	Paragraphic	± Lexical agraphia	Paragraphic	± Phonological agraphia

others and no interest in comprehending what is said. He or she may be very difficult to engage in language testing procedures and may show only the briefest interest in the test materials, as if entirely missing the point of the examiner–patient interaction. It has often been said that this type of behavior indicates an unawareness of the deficit (anosognosia) on the part of the patient (Kinsbourne & Warrington, 1963; Lebrun, 1987; Maher, Gonzalez Rothi, & Heilman, 1994; Wernicke, 1874/1968), although in the absence of verbal confirmation, such claims are difficult to substantiate.

Over the ensuing days to weeks, there is gradually increasing attentiveness of the patient to spoken input from others and an increasing relation between this input and the patient's subsequent responses. Eventually, the patient is able to comply with simple test procedures, at which point it can be shown that there are deficits in such tasks as pointing to named objects, carrying out motor commands, and responding accurately to questions. Care must be taken that these procedures actually measure language comprehension; patients often respond correctly by inference based on context, minute gestures made by the examiner, or familiarity with the test routine. A patient who learns to protrude the tongue in response to the first command from a particular examiner, for example, or when the examiner directs his gaze to the patient's mouth, is demonstrating inferential skill rather than language comprehension. Inference of this kind can be ubiquitous and unnoticed, causing significant underestimation of the deficit in language comprehension during casual encounters.

In keeping with Wernicke's original cases and neuroanatomical formulation, it is universally agreed that patients with the syndrome must demonstrate a comprehension disturbance for auditory verbal input. Somewhat surprisingly, there is no such agreement on whether the syndrome necessarily includes a disturbance of reading comprehension as well. Although most authorities have described the comprehension problem as multimodal (Alexander & Benson, 1993; Geschwind, 1971; Goodglass & Kaplan, 1972; Hécaen & Albert,

1978), a few have focused relatively exclusively on the auditory component (Kleist, 1962; Naeser, Helm-Estabrooks, Haas, Auerbach, & Srinivasan, 1987; Pick, 1931). Wernicke was rather vague on this point from a theoretical perspective, stating that in his view the "center for word-sound images" was critically needed by unskilled readers, who must mentally sound out words before comprehension can occur, but it is not needed by skilled readers.[1] Wernicke in fact did not report tests of reading comprehension for any of the patients described in his original monograph. Many subsequent theorists have, perhaps unfortunately, simplified Wernicke's model by claiming that all written material must first be transformed into an auditory image and then recognized by Wernicke's center in the STG (Geschwind, 1971; Lichtheim, 1885). Damage to Wernicke's center would, according to this view, necessarily disrupt both auditory and visual language comprehension. Insistence on an accompanying reading comprehension deficit is probably necessary to clearly distinguish Wernicke's syndrome from "pure word deafness," in which auditory verbal comprehension is disturbed, but reading comprehension is intact (table 9.1). Nevertheless, it is not rare to find Wernicke aphasics who understand written material better than auditory material, or who produce words better by writing than by speaking (Alexander & Benson, 1993; Hécaen & Albert, 1978; Hier & Mohr, 1977; Kirschner, Webb, & Duncan, 1981).

Another chief characteristic of the syndrome is the appearance of *paraphasia* in spoken and written output. This term refers to a range of output errors, including substitution, addition, duplication, omission, and transposition of linguistic units. Paraphasia may affect letters within words, syllables within words, or words within sentences. A relatively standardized nomenclature has been developed to describe and categorize paraphasic errors, and a number of detailed analyses of actual utterances by Wernicke aphasics have been published (Buckingham & Kertesz, 1976; Lecour & Rouillon, 1976). Paraphasic errors typically affect all output regardless of the task being performed by the patient, including naming, repetition, reading aloud, writing, and spontaneous speech. Paraphasic errors appearing in written output are also called "paragraphia."

Phonemic (or *literal*) paraphasia refers to errors involving individual phonemes (consonant or vowel sounds) within words. For example, the utterance "stuke" in reference to a picture of a stool constitutes a substitution of the final phoneme /k/ for the intended /l/. More complex errors involving transposition, omission, addition, or duplication of phonemes also occur, as in "castuck" produced in response to a picture of a cactus. Nonwords such as these resulting from phonemic paraphasia are also referred to as *neologisms*, and when these are frequent, the speech of such aphasics has been called "neologistic jargon" (Alajouanine, 1956; Buckingham & Kertesz, 1976; Kertesz & Benson, 1970).

Of course, not all phonemic paraphasias result in nonwords, as in this example, in which a patient attempted to repeat a sentence: (Examiner): "The spy fled to Greece." (Patient): "The sly fed to geese." These are examples of *formal paraphasias*, errors in which the target word has been replaced by another word that is phonemically similar to it (Blanken, 1990). Although these errors are real words, the phonemic resemblance to the intended word in formal paraphasia has suggested to many observers that the errors arise during the process of phoneme selection rather than word selection. These theoretically important errors are discussed in more detail in the next section. The example just given also vividly illustrates how even minor phonemic errors can completely disrupt an utterance. Without knowledge of the intended target words in this example, the utterance would almost certainly have been deemed incoherent. It seems reasonable to assume, then, that the paraphasic errors made by Wernicke aphasics may in some cases make them appear much less coherent than they truly are.

Morphemic paraphasia refers to errors involving word stems, suffixes, prefixes, inflections, and other parts of words (Lecour & Rouillon, 1976). These are not uncommon and are clinically underappreciated. Several examples occur in the following: (Patient, describing the Cookie Theft Picture from the BDAE): "The mommer is overing the sink, and it's not good to. Over that one the boy is there, on toppening it, and fallering." Here "mommer" is a morphemic paraphasia in which the related stem "mom" has been inserted into the target word "mother." The preposition "over," the phrase "on top," and the word "falling" have been altered by the addition of morphemic suffixes such as "ing" and "er." Such inflectional and derivational additions are not random, but rather are restricted to those that commonly occur in the patient's language.

Verbal paraphasia refers to errors involving whole words. These may be related in meaning to the intended word, in which case the term *semantic paraphasia* is applied (Buckingham & Rekart, 1979). Semantic paraphasias may involve substitution of a different exemplar from the same category (as in boy for girl or dog for cat), referred to as a *paradigmatic error*, or they may involve substitution of a thematically related word (as in sit for chair or fork for food), referred to as a *syntagmatic error*. Whole-word substitutions may have no discernible semantic relationship to the intended word; many of these are formal errors that phonemically resemble the target (see the repetition example above). Other verbal paraphasias show both semantic and phonemic resemblance to the target word and are thus referred to as *mixed errors*, as in the substitution of skirt for shirt or train for plane. Many other verbal paraphasias reflect perseveration on a particular word or theme that recurs from one utterance to the next, as in the following example from a Wernicke patient interviewed several months after onset (from Lecour & Rouillon, 1976, p. 118):

I talk with difficulty. You know, I worked easily in the old days for the work that I worked, the . . . very well the . . . English—not the English—the . . . to work in the . . . and thus, now, I do not talk of anything. Absolutely of that: nothing, nothing, nothing, nothing! I worked because I worked in the old days . . . (etc.)

Several authors have remarked on a typical pattern of paraphasia evolution with time after onset of the injury (Butterworth, 1979; Dell, Schwartz, Martin, Saffran, & Gagnon, 1997; Kertesz & Benson, 1970; Kohn & Smith, 1994; Lecour & Rouillon, 1976). The acute period is marked by severe, continuous phonemic paraphasia and frequent neologisms. With time there is lessening of phonemic errors and neologisms, and verbal paraphasias become more noticeable. Whether it is the case that phonemic paraphasias are replaced by verbal paraphasias or, alternatively, that the decrease in phonemic errors allows the verbal paraphasias to be identifiable, is unclear. The mix of paraphasia types may also depend partly on lesion location (see the section on lesion localization). In the chronic, partially recovered phase, phonemic errors may be almost absent, while the anomic disorder becomes more obvious in the form of word-finding pauses, circumlocutions, and repeated words (as in the example just cited).

In addition to paraphasia, speech output in Wernicke aphasia has several other salient characteristics. The speech is fluent and clearly articulated. There may be, particularly during the acute phase, an abnormal number of words produced during each utterance, described by the colorful term *logorrhea*. Despite this ease of production, there is a relative lack of content words, particularly nouns and adjectives, resulting in semantically empty speech that conveys little information, even after phonemic paraphasia has lessened and real words can be recognized (see the preceding case report). In place of content words, there is excessive use of high-frequency, nonspecific nouns and pronouns (thing, he, she, they, this, that, it), low-content adjectives (good, bad, big, little), and auxiliary verbs (is, has, does, goes). A typical patient describing a woman washing dishes while the sink overflows, for example, might say, "She's got it like that, but it's going and she's not doing it." Because the production of such sentences is fluent and seemingly effortless, a casual observer may not notice the underlying impairment of word retrieval, which is usually severe in Wernicke aphasia. This deficit is more obvious during confrontation naming, which is characterized typically by paraphasic neologisms in the acute period, empty circumlocutions ("That's a thing you have and you go do it if you need that . . .") in the subacute stage, and finally omissions and word-finding pauses in the chronic, partially recovered phase.

Certain earlier writers emphasized the spoken and receptive grammatical errors made by Wernicke aphasics (Head, 1926; Kleist, 1962; Pick, 1913). These include the morphemic paraphasic errors described earlier; incorrect selection of pronouns, auxillary verbs, prepositions, and other closed-class words; errors involving word order; and particular difficulty understanding complex sentence structures. Many of these errors can be explained as either morphemic or verbal paraphasias, and the degree to which syntax processing per se is impaired in Wernicke aphasia is still a matter of some uncertainty (Shapiro, Gordon, Hack, & Killackey, 1993; Zurif, Swinney, Prather, Solomon, & Bushell, 1993).

In contrast to these disturbances related to word and phoneme selection and sequencing, motor control of speech articulators is conventionally held to be normal in Wernicke's aphasia. Recent acoustic analysis studies, however, have identified clinically imperceptible abnormalities believed to be related to subtly impaired motor control. For example, Wernicke aphasics show increased variability in vowel duration and formant frequency position during vowel production (Gandour et al., 1992; Ryalls, 1986).

Processing Models of Wernicke Aphasia

Modern students of neurology are indoctrinated in the view that Wernicke's aphasia reflects damage to the brain's "comprehension center" (Bogen & Bogen, 1976), yet this model is an unacceptable oversimplification for several reasons. First, comprehension is not a unitary process in the brain, but rather a complex cascade of interacting events involving sensory processing, pattern recognition, mapping of sensory patterns to more abstract word representations, and retrieval of semantic and syntactic information. Comprehension may be disturbed only for speech sounds, as in pure word deafness, or only for written language, as in isolated alexia. Comprehension can be disturbed together with speech production, as in Wernicke aphasia, or with sparing of speech production, as in transcortical sensory aphasia. These considerations make it improbable in the extreme that there is anything like a unitary "comprehension" module in the brain.

A second objection to equating Wernicke's area with comprehension is that Wernicke aphasia includes other key components in addition to comprehension disturbance, notably paraphasic and paragraphic output. Wernicke explained the co-occurrence of these symptoms by postulating a center for "word-sound images" (*Wortklangsbilder*) that is necessary for both word recognition and production. These images were thought of as stored memories of the sound of each word in the vocabulary. Auditory and written input would excite the corresponding auditory word image, which would then activate a corresponding concept, resulting in comprehension. Far from postulating a unitary comprehension center, Wernicke's original model thus makes a clear distinction between the word-sound center, which contains information only about the sound of words, and a later stage at which meaning is accessed. Production of speech and writing was dependent on the interactive cooperation of the concept area, the word-sound center, and the motor speech area. Paraphasia and paragraphia were the result of a breakdown in this interactive link, and so could result from a lesion in the word-sound center or at any of the connecting pathways between the three centers (Lichtheim, 1885; Wernicke, 1874/1968).

Even as the relative complexity of Wernicke's theory has been lost to generations of neurologists, other developments have made it clear that the original theory is itself a vast oversimplification. In the past several decades, experimental studies of normal and aphasic individuals, together with the rise of modular "information-processing" accounts

of cognition, have contributed to an ever more fractionated view of language processes. One recent review, for example, concluded that the classic Wernicke aphasia syndrome reflects damage to no less than nine distinct language-processing modules (Margolin, 1991). As if this proliferation of language modules was not enough to confuse both the twentieth- and twenty-first-century student of aphasia, there has also appeared on the scene in recent decades a serious effort to account for language processes at the level of neural networks. While these modular and microstructural approaches have produced nothing less than a revolution in our understanding of language processing in the brain, little or none of this information has found its way into the educational curriculum of clinical neuroscientists or had an impact on the care of patients with language disturbances. In this section, an attempt is made to summarize some of this information in a comprehensible way, with an emphasis on the language processing systems most closely associated with Wernicke aphasia. Because of space limitations, detailed discussion will be confined to the auditory comprehension and paraphasic components of the syndrome. Some of the same principles apply to comprehension and production of written text, and a thorough review of aphasic reading impairments is provided in chapter 6 of this volume.

General Architecture of the Language Processing System

Much of what follows will be made clearer by first sketching a basic architecture of the central language processing system and by defining some of its principal components (figure 9.2). Of some importance is the distinction between representations and mappings, symbolized in figure 9.2 by boxes and arrows, respectively. A representation (or code) is any pattern of neural activity that corresponds to information being processed by the system. For example, the input phoneme representations in figure 9.2 correspond to patterns of neural activity accompanying the perception of vowel and consonant speech sounds presented to the auditory

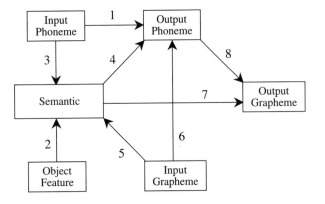

Figure 9.2
A minimal central processing architecture for describing language behavior. For example, speech comprehension requires pathway 3; speech repetition, pathway 1; propositional speech, pathway 4; confrontation naming, pathways 2 and 4; reading comprehension, pathway 5; reading aloud, pathways 6 or 5 and 4 (or both); writing to dictation, pathways 1 and 8 or 3 and 7 (or both), etc.

system, the input grapheme representations correspond to letters perceived by the visual system, and the semantic representations correspond to functional and perceptual features of concepts. Input representations are activated by appropriate input from lower sensory systems and pass their activation on to neighboring representational levels. Mappings are the means by which representations at one level produce activation of appropriate representations in adjacent levels, as occurs, for example, when particular combinations of input phonemes activate particular semantic representations, resulting in comprehension of spoken words.

The representational levels (boxes) included in the diagram are the minimal set needed to begin an account of such language acts as repetition, comprehension, and naming. They are, that is, the starting points and end points for these processes, excluding earlier sensory and later motor processes with which we are not concerned. Their prominence in the diagram should not, however, detract from the importance of the mappings (arrows) that connect the starting and ending points, which are best viewed as complex processing streams, often

involving intermediary representational levels not shown in figure 9.2. The field of generative linguistics, for example, is concerned with pathway 4 in the figure (semantics to output phonemes), virtually to the exclusion of all other parts of the model. This mapping, which involves sentence construction (syntax) mechanisms as well as word and phoneme selection, illustrates the enormous complexity typical of many of the mappings underlying language behavior.

Mappings are acquired as a result of experience. The numbers in figure 9.2 suggest a developmental order of acquisition of the pathways, although this is a crude approximation given that many pathways develop simultaneously with others. The mapping from input phonemes to output phonemes is an early acquisition, represented by the infant's capacity to repeat simple phonemes. Mapping 2 develops simultaneously with mapping 1 as the child experiences objects and associates these with particular physical, emotional, and contextual phenomena. Mappings 3 and 4 result from hearing words used in reference to objects and are reflected in the ability to understand spoken words and use these words to refer to concepts. Mappings 5 and 6 develop as we learn to read, enabling reading comprehension and reading aloud. Pathway 6, though not strictly necessary for reading comprehension, probably develops because of the quasi-regular correspondence between graphemes and phonemes and may be encouraged by teaching methods that emphasize "sounding out" and reading aloud. Finally, mappings 7 and 8 permit concepts (as in propositional writing) or heard phonemes (as in writing to dictation) to be translated into written form.

One important class of intermediary code postulated to play a role in these mapping processes is the whole-word or lexical representation. For example, the mapping from input phonemes to semantics is often envisioned as involving an intermediate "phonological input lexicon" composed of whole-word representations that become active as a result of input from appropriate representations in the input phoneme level and send activation, in turn, to the semantic level. Such whole-word representations correspond closely to Wernicke's concept of word-sound images. In Wernicke's model, the same center for word-sound images participates in the mappings marked 1, 3, 4, 5, 6, and 7 in figure 9.2. As we will see, modern neurolinguistic studies provide evidence for at least a partial separation of these pathways. As a result of this evidence, there has flourished the idea of a separate phonological input lexicon mediating mapping 3, a phonological output lexicon mediating mapping 4, an orthographic input lexicon mediating mapping 5, and an orthographic output lexicon mediating mapping 7.

Precisely how these mappings are actually accomplished is another question, one not addressed at all by the classic Wernicke–Lichtheim model of language processing nor by many recent modular models composed entirely of boxes and arrows. How, for example, can there be transformations between entities so dissimilar as phonemes and concepts? At the root of this problem is the fact that there exists no regular relationship between a word's sounds and its meaning (e.g., words as different in meaning as cat, cot, coat, and cut nevertheless sound very similar); the mapping between phonemes and semantics is essentially arbitrary. The idea that a lexicon of word representations links phonemes to meanings reflects our intuition that something is needed to mediate between these very different kinds of information. Explicit neural network simulations of these same mappings, explored in some detail over the past 20 years, support this intuition by demonstrating that arbitrary mappings of this sort can only be accomplished by adding an intermediary (or hidden) representational level between the input and output levels.[2] As we will see, the notion of intermediate representational levels is central to understanding both the pathophysiology of aphasia and the nature of the activations observed in functional imaging experiments.

Figure 9.3 shows a somewhat more realistic language-processing architecture complete with intermediate representational levels supporting arbitrary and quasi-regular mappings. The figure makes clear the parallel between these intermediate representations and the "lexicons" of cognitive neuropsychology. The implication of this comparison is that models postulating lexicons with whole-word representations are but one possible version of a more general architecture based on intermediate representations. In contrast to the whole-word model, neural network simulations of grapheme-to-semantic and grapheme-to-phoneme mappings have been described in which intermediate representations do not correspond to words (Hinton & Shallice, 1991; Plaut, McClelland, Seidenberg, & Patterson, 1996; Seidenberg & McClelland, 1989), leaving uncertain the theoretical need for whole-word codes in language processing (Besner, Twilley, McCann, & Seergobin, 1990; Coltheart, Curtis, Atkins, & Haller, 1993; Seidenberg & McClelland, 1990). With this brief exposition of a general language processing architecture, we now proceed to a discussion of the processing impairments underlying auditory comprehension and speaking disorders in Wernicke's aphasia.

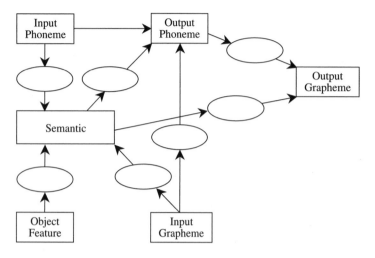

Figure 9.3
A language-processing architecture with intermediate representational levels (ovals). Unidirectional arrows show the typical directions in which information spreads during language tasks. At a local level, however, these connections are probably bidirectional, allowing continuous interactions between adjacent representational levels.

Auditory Comprehension Disturbance

Because comprehension of spoken words depends on the auditory system, speech comprehension deficits in Wernicke's aphasia could be due to underlying abnormalities of auditory processing. Luria, for example, theorized that speech comprehension deficits reflect an inability to discriminate subtle differences between similar speech sounds (Luria, 1966; Luria & Hutton, 1977). Although a discussion of acoustic phenomena in speech sounds is beyond the scope of this chapter, a few examples might serve to illustrate this point (the interested reader is referred to excellent reviews on this important and relatively neglected topic in clinical neuroscience: Klatt, 1989; Liberman, Cooper, Shankweiler, & Studdert-Kennedy, 1967; Oden & Massaro, 1978; Stevens & Blumstein, 1981).

Speech contains both periodic sounds produced by vocal cord vibrations (exemplified by the vowels) and nonperiodic noises produced by turbulence at constriction points like the lips, teeth, and palate (exemplified by sounds like /s/ and /f/). The distribution of energy across the acoustic frequency spectrum (i.e., the relative loudness of low or high frequencies) at any point in time depends on the shape of the vocal tract (e.g., the position of the tongue, the shape of the lips, the position of the soft palate), which creates resonances that amplify or dampen particular frequencies. Accentuated frequencies are referred to as *formants*; vowels are distinguished on the basis of the frequency position of the lowest three or four of these formants, which typically occupy frequencies in the range from 300 to 4000 Hz. With rapid changes in vocal tract shape, such as those that occur during production of consonants like /b/ and /d/, the formants rapidly change position; this is referred to as *formant transition*.

One cue for distinguishing between consonants is the direction of movement (i.e., up, down, or straight) of these transitions. In some consonants, such as /p/ and /t/, a very brief noise burst precedes the onset of vocal cord vibration. Thus, /b/ and /p/, which are both produced by opening the lips and therefore have very similar formant transitions, are distinguished largely on the basis of this burst-toperiodicity onset asynchrony, referred to as *voice onset time*. The inability to detect acoustic cues such as those distinguishing /b/ from /d/ or /b/ from /p/ might lead to misinterpretation of bay as day or bye as pie, for example, causing severe comprehension disturbance. Because acoustic events in speech occur rapidly, other investigators have proposed an underlying problem with rapid processing in the auditory system, leading to the inability to discriminate phoneme order (e.g., hearing cast as cats or task as tax) or impaired perception specifically involving rapid dynamic phenomena such as formant transitions and differences in voice onset time (Brookshire, 1972; Efron, 1963; Tallal & Newcombe, 1978; Tallal & Piercy, 1973).

The hypothesis that auditory processing deficits underlie the speech comprehension problem in Wernicke's aphasia has been tested in several ways. One task paradigm involves explicit identification or labeling of speech sounds. For example, subjects hear a word or nonword (e.g., ba) and must select a matching visual word or nonword in an array containing phonologically similar items (e.g., BA, DA, PA). Patients with Wernicke's aphasia perform poorly in such tests (Basso, Casati, & Vignolo, 1977; Blumstein, Cooper, Zurif, & Caramazza, 1977; Blumstein, Tartter, Nigro, & Statlender, 1984; Goldblum & Albert, 1972; Reidl & Studdert-Kennedy, 1985). It is critically important to note, however, that this type of task requires the integrity of two possibly distinct processes. That is, the identification task not only requires auditory processing but also the ability to match the auditory percept to another, nonidentical stimulus (the visual form).

In an effort to disentangle these components, investigators have employed sensory discrimination paradigms that do not require such cross-modal association. In a typical experiment of this type, the subject hears two speech sounds and must merely decide if these are identical or different. Deficits in this discrimination task are much less pronounced than in the identification task, with some Wernicke aphasics performing within the normal range (Blumstein, Baker, & Goodglass, 1977; Blumstein et al., 1984; Reidl & Studdert-Kennedy, 1985).

Many patients tested with both paradigms are found to be deficient in the identification task, but not in the discrimination task, demonstrating the essentially independent nature of these deficits. Most important, there does not appear to be a necessary correspondence between deficits in either of these tasks and measures of speech comprehension: Patients are found who show severe comprehension disturbances and normal discrimination, and others are found who have marked identification and discrimination deficits, but relatively normal comprehension (Basso et al., 1977; Blumstein et al., 1977; Blumstein et al., 1984; Jauhiainen & Nuutila, 1977; Miceli, Gainotti, Caltagirone, & Masullo, 1980).

The fact that Wernicke aphasics often perform normally on phoneme discrimination tests even when they are unable to identify phonemes explicitly suggests that their speech comprehension deficit is unlikely to be due to impaired auditory processing alone. Rather, the deficit elicited in these studies reflects an inability to use auditory information to access associated linguistic representations. Having adequately perceived a speech sound, the Wernicke aphasic is typically unable to retrieve associated information, such as its written form, picture equivalent, or meaning. A similar dissociation between sensory and associative processing in patients with fluent aphasia was documented by Faglioni et al. using nonspeech auditory stimuli (Faglioni, Spinnler, & Vignolo, 1969), further illustrating the independence of comprehension deficits from auditory perception. Patients with left hemisphere lesions in this study showed an intact ability to discriminate between two meaningless nonspeech sounds, but were impaired in a task requiring matching meaningful nonspeech sounds (animal noises, machine noises, etc.) to pictures. Deficits in the latter task were significantly correlated with speech comprehension deficits as measured by the Token Test.

Recent research has further explored this difficulty in retrieving information associated with speech stimuli in Wernicke aphasia. This problem could be explained in any of three ways: (1) as an impairment in activating the information, (2) as a loss or corruption of the information itself, or (3) as an impairment in using the information once it is activated. These possible scenarios are not mutually exclusive, and in fact there is evidence supporting all three, suggesting that variable combinations of these deficits might occur in different patients. Before embarking on an assessment of this evidence, it would be useful to review briefly some current ideas about how information associated with words and concepts might be organized and represented in the brain.

We store information about words internally as a result of encountering the words in various contexts throughout life. This information collectively provides the meaning (or meanings, literal and figurative, verbal and nonverbal) of the word. The study of word meaning is referred to as *semantics*, and the processes by which word meanings are stored, retrieved, and used are collectively called "semantic processes." A great deal of theoretical and empirical work has expanded our conception of such processes since Wernicke articulated his simple notion of word meaning as a connection linking sensory memories of an object. Most notable is the recognition that in addition to sensory attributes associated with objects, semantic processing concerns the learning and retrieval of conceptual categories and the hierarchical relationships between different categories.

To take a simple example, we learn by visual-auditory association that an object with four legs of a certain length range, a squarish platform resting on the legs, and a panel rising from one end of the platform, is called CHAIR. We learn that a chair has other typical sensory attributes such as being inanimate, quiet, and able to support weight. We discover the functions of a chair by seeing it used and by using it ourselves. The concept of CHAIR is said to be a *basic-level* concept, because all objects possessing these simple structural and functional attributes are similarly categorized as CHAIR (Rosch, Mervis, Gray, Johnson, & Boyes-Braem, 1976).

In addition to associating these direct sensory impressions with the word CHAIR, however, we learn about abstract attributes of chairs, such as the fact that they are nonliving, often contain wood, and are made by people. Using this information, we learn to associate chairs to varying degrees with other types of objects that share some of the same sensory, functional, or abstract attributes, resulting in the formation of hierarchical relationships between words. Reference to these relationships enables the formation of *superordinate categories* that include objects with similar attributes. For example, based on the knowledge that it is man-made, useful in a home, can be moved from place to place, and is not mechanical, CHAIR becomes a member of the superordinate category FURNITURE. Other members of this category (e.g., TABLE, DESK, COUCH) differ from CHAIR in terms of specific sensory or functional attributes; these are the *basic-level neighbors* of CHAIR.

Finally, a large number of words become associated with CHAIR as a result of how chairs are used in daily life and in larger social contexts; these are the *function associates* of CHAIR. The facts concerning where and how chairs are typically used, for example, create function associations between CHAIR and HOME, CHAIR and RELAX, and CHAIR and READ. Facts concerning society and chairs create function associations between CHAIR and EXECUTION, CHAIR and COMMITTEE, and CHAIR and BARBER. The sheer number and complexity of such relations stored in the human brain are staggering, and they are an essential base on which the comprehension and formulation of language depend.

Some studies suggest that this network of semantic representations is altered or defectively activated in Wernicke's aphasia. In most of these studies, patients were required to judge the degree of relatedness between words or pictures. In an experiment by Zurif et al. (Zurif, Caramazza, Myerson, & Galvin, 1974), for example, fluent aphasics, most of whom had mild Wernicke's aphasia, were shown groups of three words and asked to pick the two that "go best together." Unlike the nonfluent aphasia patients and normal control subjects, fluent aphasics showed very poorly defined categorization schemes, with maintenance of only the most broad category distinctions (e.g., human versus nonhuman).

Goodglass and Baker (1976) presented subjects with a picture followed by a series of spoken words; for each word, the subjects indicated whether the word was related to the picture. The types of word–picture relations tested included identity (e.g., ORANGE and picture of orange), sensory attribute (JUICY and picture of orange), function (EAT and picture of orange), superordinate category (FRUIT and picture of orange), basic-level neighbor (APPLE and picture of orange), and function associate (BREAKFAST and picture of orange). As anticipated, Wernicke aphasics performed poorly in this task relative to normal controls and aphasics with good comprehension. In addition to this quantitative difference, however, qualitative differences were notable. Subjects with good comprehension had relative difficulty recognizing the basic-level neighbor relations, while the Wernicke patients recognized (that is, responded affirmatively to) this type of relation more easily than other relations. Unlike the other patients, Wernicke patients had particular difficulty recognizing function relations. When performance in this task was compared with performance in confrontation naming of the same pictures, it was found that patients had more difficulty making relatedness judgments for items they were unable to name. These performance patterns have been largely replicated in other studies (Chenery, Ingram, & Murdoch, 1990; McCleary, 1988; McCleary & Hirst, 1986).

Several studies focused specifically on the integrity of superordinate–basic level relations. Grossman (1980, 1981) used a task in which aphasics were given a superordinate category (e.g., FURNITURE) and had to generate basic-level examples of the category. Responses were scored using published prototypicality ratings (Rosch et al., 1976) that indicate the degree to which an item is a typical or central example of the category (e.g., DESK is a central example of the category FURNITURE, while LAMP is a more peripheral member). Nonfluent aphasics produced exemplars with high prototypicality ratings, whereas fluent

aphasics produced more peripheral items and often violated the category boundaries altogether. Grober et al. (Grober, Perecman, Kellar, & Brown, 1980) assessed the integrity of superordinate category boundaries using a picture–word relatedness judgment task like that employed by Goodglass and Baker. The degree of relatedness to the target category was manipulated so that word items included central members of the category, peripheral members, semantically related nonmembers (e.g., WINDOW for the category FURNITURE), and semantically unrelated nonmembers (e.g., HORSE for the category FURNITURE). Anterior aphasics accurately classified peripheral members and semantically related nonmembers, suggesting intact category boundaries, while Wernicke aphasics often misclassified these items, indicating impaired discrimination near category boundaries. Similar conclusions were reached by Kudo (1987), who used a task in which patients judged whether depicted objects were members of hierarchical superordinate categories (domestic animal, beast, animal, and living thing). Aphasics showed abnormally diffuse categorization schemes, in that they frequently included semantically related nonmembers in categories (e.g., they included GIRAFFE as a domestic animal). This abnormality was strongest in severe fluent aphasics.

Despite this evidence, other investigators have questioned whether these findings necessarily indicate a defect in the structural organization of the semantic system itself. Claims to the contrary are based on a series of studies measuring semantic priming effects during word recognition tasks. Normal subjects take less time to decide if a stimulus is a word (the lexical decision task) if the stimulus is preceded by a semantically related word (Meyer & Schvaneveldt, 1971). The preceding word, or prime, is thought to activate semantic information shared by the two words, resulting in a partial spread of activation that lowers the recognition threshold for the second word (Collins & Loftus, 1975; Neely, 1977). Milberg and colleagues showed in several studies that patients with Wernicke's aphasia demonstrate semantic priming effects that are as robust as those in normal persons (Blumstein, Milberg, & Shrier, 1982; Milberg & Blumstein, 1981; Milberg, Blumstein, & Dworetzky, 1987; Milberg, Blumstein, Saffran, Hourihan, & Brown, 1995). These basic results were replicated by several investigators (Chenery et al., 1990; Hagoort, 1993). Moreover, when the same patients were presented with word pairs and asked to judge explicitly whether the words were semantically related, they showed deficits like those observed in other studies using explicit semantic judgment tasks (Blumstein et al., 1982; Chenery et al., 1990). Thus, the patients showed normal semantic priming for word pairs, but they were impaired when asked to explicitly identify the semantic relationships that underlie the priming effect. These findings have led a number of investigators to conclude that the network of stored semantic representations is largely intact in Wernicke's aphasia, and that the deficit underlying the language comprehension and naming deficits shown by these patients consists of an inability to explicitly retrieve and manipulate this information.

The presence of semantic priming, however, does not necessarily indicate that semantic representations are intact. The past two decades have witnessed the development of neural network models of semantic information retrieval that could explain preserved semantic priming even within a defective semantic system. A full explanation of these models is beyond the scope of this chapter, and the reader is referred to several excellent reviews (Hinton, McClelland, & Rumelhart, 1986; Hinton & Shallice, 1991; McClelland & Rumelhart, 1986). In these models, perceptual features of words (i.e., letter shapes and phonemes) and semantic features associated with words are represented by large numbers of units in an interconnected network. Connections exist between units of the same level (e.g., between representations of different phonemes) and between levels. These connections may be excitatory or inhibitory, and the strength of each connection is defined by a numerical weight. Through real-world experience, the network learns to associate combinations of graphemes or phone-

mes with appropriate semantic features by incremental adjustment of the connection weights.

Knowledge about words in such models is said to be distributed because the network can learn to correctly associate a large number of different words with a large number of semantic features using the same sets of units and connection weights. It is the precise tuning of these excitatory and inhibitory weights that allows similar words like cat and cot to activate entirely different semantic features, very different words like cot and bed to activate very similar semantic features, and reliable behavioral distinctions to be made between words with very similar meanings. Such networks exhibit many characteristic phenomena shown by human semantic systems, including automatic formation of categories and prototypes (pattern generalization), word frequency and context effects in recognition tasks, and semantic priming (Becker, Moscovitch, Behrmann, & Joordens, 1997; Masson, 1995; McClelland & Rumelhart, 1986; Moss, Hare, Day, & Tyler, 1994). When "lesioned" by random removal of units or connections, or by random changes in connection weights, such networks exhibit characteristic phenomena shown by neurological patients, including mixtures of correct and incorrect performance on different items (rather than absolute loss of function), a graded decrease in performance that is dependent on lesion extent, phonemic and semantic paraphasias, and semantic retrieval deficits that may be category specific (Farah & McClelland, 1991; Hinton & Shallice, 1991; McRae, de Sa, & Seidenberg, 1997; Plaut & Shallice, 1993).

To gain an intuitive feeling for how semantic priming might be preserved after damage to such a network, consider the schematic example in figure 9.4, which is similar to one of the models tested by Plaut and Shallice (1993). Small boxes indicate individual featural units in the network. Such units are not strictly analogous to individual neurons; rather, each unit can be thought of as representing a smaller module that is itself composed of interconnected units. Thus, there is no implied one-to-one relationship between features (such as "has four legs") and individual neurons. Units in the left column represent the phoneme or grapheme units that encode features of the word name, such as the graphemes C, A, and T for cat. Units in the right column represent semantic features associated with the word, such as "eats mice" or "has four legs." The middle column represents intermediate units, which provide the network with sufficient computational power to learn arbitrary mappings between patterns represented on the perceptual and semantic units.[2] The lines between units represent excitatory connections (for display purposes, the connections between units of the same level are not shown).

After suitable training accompanied by incremental adjustments of the weights on all connections, the presentation of any word pattern (e.g., CAT) to the perceptual layer at left results in activation of the correct associated semantic pattern (figure 9.4A). Semantic priming is due to the fact that the semantic pattern of a following semantically related word (e.g., DOG) partially overlaps that of the priming word (figure 9.4B), and this second pattern will be activated more easily because of residual activation from the priming word.

Lesioning of the network at any location results in a loss of precision in the mapping between perceptual and semantic patterns (figure 9.4C). Input words activate semantic patterns that resemble the target pattern, but with omissions or inappropriately included units. As a result of this imprecision, words may be associated with incorrect semantic information and assigned incorrectly to superordinate categories; category boundaries and prototypes themselves lose definition, and subjects lack the precise information needed to judge semantic relatedness. Because the activated semantic pattern partially resembles the target pattern, however, semantic priming, which is an imprecise phenomenon that depends only on partial overlap between semantic patterns, will be preserved because of the large number of semantic units contained within each pattern.

A number of other observations from studies of Wernicke's aphasia are consistent with such an account. Goodglass and Baker (1976) and Chenery

et al. (1990) documented one such phenomenon during relatedness judgment tasks performed by normal persons and aphasics. When asked to decide if two words were related, normal subjects and aphasics with good comprehension were slower to respond and made more errors when the two words were basic-level neighbors of the same superordinate category (e.g., CAT and DOG) than when the words were associated in other ways, such as object-superordinate (CAT and ANIMAL) or object-attribute (CAT and FURRY). In contrast, Wernicke aphasics paradoxically did not show this relative difficulty with basic-level neighbor relations. This difference can be explained by a loss of distinctiveness of the semantic patterns activated by different basic-level neighbors. In the normal state, basic-level neighbors such as CAT and DOG activate highly overlapping but distinguishable patterns of semantic units. Inhibitory connections, which suppress activation of DOG semantic units when CAT is presented, for example, are particularly important in this regard, and allow normal subjects to respond appropriately when asked questions like "Does a cat growl at strangers?" In responding affirmatively to word pairs such as CAT-DOG during a relatedness judgment task, subjects must overcome this inhibition between basic-level neighbors. In the lesioned state, such distinctions are blurred, and patterns of semantic unit activity for basic-level neighbors of the same category become more similar. As a result, there is less inhibition between basic-level neighbors, and subjects with damage to the network paradoxically recognize the relationship between such neighbors more accurately and quickly than in the normal state.

Milberg et al. documented another interesting phenomenon in studies of semantic priming using nonwords (Milberg, Blumstein, & Dworetzky, 1988b). As in previous semantic priming studies, the subjects were presented with stimulus pairs (in this case, auditory stimuli) and were asked to perform a lexical decision task on the second stimulus of the pair. The initial phoneme of the first stimulus in the pair was manipulated to produce primes that were either semantically related words

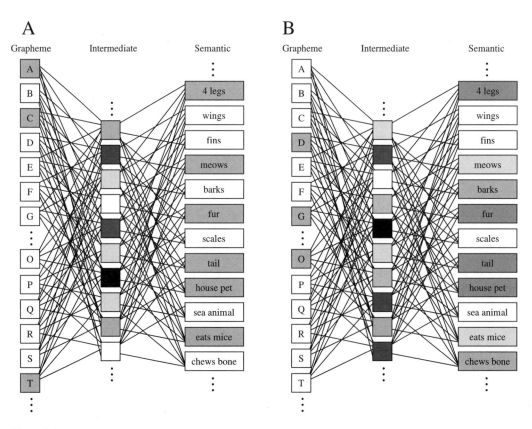

Figure 9.4

A schematic representation of part of the pathway from input graphemes to semantics (pathway 5 in figure 9.2), illustrating the effects of semantic priming and structural damage. The diagram has been greatly simplified for the sake of clarity, in that the grapheme layer contains no representation of letter position; less than half of the possible connections are drawn; no representation of the connection strengths is given; and only a very small portion of the total set of semantic units is shown. (*A*) Presentation of "cat" to the grapheme layer, represented in the left column by shading of the appropriate graphemes, produces patterns of activation in the intermediate and semantic units determined by the set of connection strengths between each of the layers, which have been adjusted through experience with cats and the letter sequence "cat." (*B*) If presentation of "dog" quickly follows, as in a semantic priming experiment, activation of the semantic units appropriate to dogs is facilitated by residual activation from those units that were activated by "cat" and that are shared by dogs and cats (four legs, fur, tail, house pet), while activation of those features specific to cats (meows, eats mice) decays. (*C*) Damage to a portion of the network, represented here by the removal of several intermediate units and their connections, disrupts the pattern of activation input to semantic units, resulting in activation of inappropriate units (barks, scales) or failure to activate appropriate units (fur). The activation of an incorrect pattern of semantic units disrupts performance on semantic tasks, but semantic priming of "dog" may still be possible because of the preserved activation of a sufficient number of shared semantic units (four legs, tail, house pet). Semantic priming may even be exaggerated in some cases if incorrect activation results in falsely "shared" features (barks).

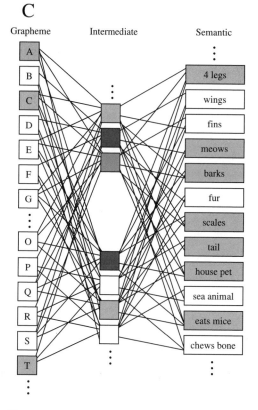

C

Grapheme	Intermediate	Semantic

A
B
C
D
E
F
G
⋮
O
P
Q
R
S
T
⋮

4 legs
wings
fins
meows
barks
fur
scales
tail
house pet
sea animal
eats mice
chews bone

Figure 9.4
Continued

(e.g., CAT before DOG), nonwords differing from the semantic prime by one phonetic feature (GAT before DOG), or nonwords differing from the semantic prime by two phonetic features (WAT before DOG). The baseline condition used unrelated primes (NURSE before DOG). Unlike nonfluent aphasics, who showed priming effects only for the undistorted real-word prime, fluent aphasics showed priming effects for all phonetically distorted nonword conditions relative to the unrelated word baseline.

These results suggest that in fluent aphasia, nonwords more easily activate semantic patterns associated with phonetically similar real words. To understand this phenomenon, recall that in the normal state the semantic network is able to accurately distinguish phonetically similar words such as CAT and COT and to associate each with an appropriate pattern of activation on the semantic units. This feat is accomplished despite the fact that because the phonetic inputs for CAT and COT are similar, the initial activity across the set of semantic units is relatively similar after presentation of CAT and COT (figure 9.5). The separation of CAT and COT is possible because of recurrent interactions between units in the network, which cause the semantic units to gradually settle into a steady state that is very different for CAT and COT (figure 9.5A). Networks that behave in this way are known as *attractor networks*, and the patterns toward which the units gradually settle (the black dots in figure 9.5) are the attractor states. Just as perceptually similar words like CAT and COT move gradually toward different attractor states, nonwords that are perceptually similar to words may move toward the attractor states for those words, resulting in partial activation of the semantic pattern of the word (figure 9.5). In normal subjects, this phenomonon depends on the degree of perceptual similarity between the nonword and the word associated with the attractor state; nonwords that differ by a greater number of phonetic features are less likely to move toward the attractor state (Milberg, Blumstein, & Dworetzky, 1988a). After the network is lesioned, the area of semantic space dominated by a given attractor state (called the "attractor basin") becomes distorted and less sharply defined (Hinton & Shallice, 1991), with the result that activation patterns elicited by words and nonwords are more likely to move toward attractor states of phonetically similar words, resulting in enhanced semantic priming of these words (figure 9.5B). The general effect of such lesions is thus to blur the distinctions between words and phonetically related (or graphemically related) nonwords. This loosening of phoneme-to-semantic mapping may also explain the observation by Blumstein et al. that patients with Wernicke aphasia do not show the usual lexical

A

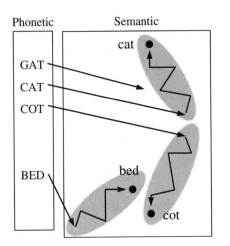

B

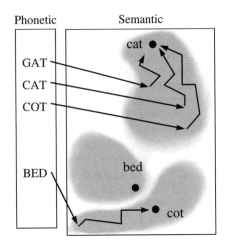

Figure 9.5
The role of attractor states in phoneme-to-semantic (or grapheme-to-semantic) mapping. The box on the left of each figure represents spoken word or nonword input. The larger box on the right represents semantic space. Points in this semantic space represent patterns of activation across a set of semantic units (activation states). Three such states are marked by black dots and correspond to the concepts cat, cot, and bed. Lines and arrows show the initial state of the semantic network when it is presented with a given input and subsequent changes as the network settles into an attractor state. Shaded regions are the attractor basins for each attractor state. Any input that initially produces an activation state that falls within an attractor basin will eventually reach the attractor state for that basin. (A) In the normal state, attractor dynamics allow similar inputs, such as cat and cot, which produce similar initial activation states, to eventually activate very different states in semantic space. Conversely, very different inputs, such as cot and bed, may nevertheless reach relatively similar states in semantic space. (B) Damage to the network causes distortion and loss of definition of the attractor basins. As a result, semantic states resulting from a given input word may gravitate toward incorrect (phonologically or semantically related) attractors (cot → cat, bed → cot), and attractor states may be reached more easily from nonword inputs. (Based on Hinton & Shallice, 1991.)

effect on placement of perceptual boundaries during phoneme categorization (Blumstein, Burton, Baum, Waldstein, & Katz, 1994).

In summary, the speech comprehension disturbance in Wernicke aphasia is not well explained by a phoneme perceptual disturbance. The input phoneme representations in figure 9.3 appear to be, for the most part, intact. In contrast, there is a deficit either in the pathway from input phonemes to semantics or within semantic representations (or both), as demonstrated by the inability of Wernicke aphasics to match perceived phonemes with their associated visual forms or meanings. Several lines of evidence suggest that semantic representations are activated inaccurately, causing blurring of category boundaries, loss of distinctiveness between basic-level neighbors, inability to judge semantic relatedness, and abnormal activation of semantic representations by wordlike nonwords. Although preserved semantic priming in Wernicke's aphasia has been interpreted as indicating intact semantic representations, an alternative explanation is that priming merely reflects partial overlap of semantic activation between word pairs and does not require that this activation be precise or accurate.

Paraphasia

As described earlier, Wernicke aphasics produce a variety of speech output errors involving sound elements within words (phonemic paraphasia), grammatical units such as word stems or suffixes (morphemic paraphasia), and whole words (verbal paraphasia). At least since Freud's claim that "paraphasia in aphasic patients does not differ from the incorrect use and distortion of words which the healthy person can observe in himself in states of fatigue or divided attention" (Freud, 1891/1953, p. 13), it has been recognized that speech errors made by aphasic patients share many features with those made by normal speakers (Blumstein, 1973; Buckingham, 1980; Dell et al., 1997; Garrett, 1984; Schwartz, Saffran, Bloch, & Dell, 1994). In recent years, quantitative techniques and theoretical models arising from the study of normal "slips of the tongue" have been applied productively to the analysis of speech errors made by aphasics. This section briefly recounts some of the important findings from these studies as well as a computational model that explains many of the basic paraphasic phenomena exhibited by fluent aphasics.

It is clear that paraphasic errors are not entirely random. One example of a general rule operating at the phoneme level is the frequent occurrence of *contextual errors*—phoneme errors that are influenced by other nearby phonemes. Examples include anticipations, in which a later sound is duplicated in an earlier utterance ("park bench" → "bark bench"); perseverations, in which an earlier sound is duplicated in a later utterance ("beef noodle" → "beef needle"); and exchanges, in which two sounds exchange places ("big deal" → "dig beal"). Contextual errors are the principal type of phoneme error in normal slips of the tongue (Nooteboom, 1969), and imply a speech production mechanism in which the selection of each phoneme to be uttered is partly influenced by preceding and following phonemes. A related finding is that phonemes interacting in this way tend to be those that are similar to each other. That is, phonemes are more likely to be switched with other phonemes if they share similar phonetic features (e.g., /b/ and /d/ share the same manner and voicing features) and if they occupy the same position within their respective syllables (e.g., the /b/ and /d/ in "big deal" are both syllable onset phonemes) (Blumstein, 1973; Lecour & Rouillon, 1976; MacKay, 1970; Shattuck-Hufnagel & Klatt, 1979; Stemberger, 1982). Thus, the mechanism that selects phonemes appears to be influenced by other surrounding phonemes, particularly if these are easily confused with the target phoneme.

Analogous contextual phenomena are observed for words within multiword phrases. Thus, there occur contextual word anticipations ("The sun is in the sky" → "The sky is in the sky"), perseverations ("The boy is reaching for the cookies" → "The boy is reaching for the boy"), and exchanges ("writing a letter to my mother" → "writing a mother to my letter") in both aphasic and normal speech (Dell & Reich, 1981; Fromkin, 1971; Garrett, 1975; Lecour & Rouillon, 1976). Analogous to the confusability effects seen with phoneme errors, word substitutions show effects of semantic and grammatical class similarity. That is, for both normal and aphasic speakers, substituted words are more likely to be semantically related to the target word (Buckingham & Rekart, 1979; Dell & Reich, 1981; Fay & Cutler, 1977; Fromkin, 1971; Garrett, 1992) and are more likely to be from the same grammatical class (i.e., noun, verb, adjective) as the target word (Fay & Cutler, 1977; Gagnon, Schwartz, Martin, Dell, & Saffran, 1997; Garrett, 1975) than would be expected by chance alone. Thus, the mechanism used for selecting words appears to be influenced by other nearby words in the planned utterance, particularly those that are from the same grammatical class as the target word, and by the possible "semantic neighbors" of the target word.

These examples involving phoneme and word-level substitutions by no means capture all of the error patterns observed in fluent aphasia. Of particular theoretical interest are errors that appear to indicate interactions between word and phoneme information. One example of this is the *formal paraphasia*, a real-word error that is phonologically but not semantically similar to the intended target word ("horse" → "house"). Although formal paraphasias are real words, the question of whether they represent phoneme or word-level errors has been controversial, for several reasons. First, these errors are not common in most patients. Second, patients who produce formal paraphasias also utter nonwords (neologisms) that are phonologically related to targets. These data have usually been accepted as evidence that formal paraphasias represent phoneme-level errors that happen by chance to result in real words (Buckingham, 1980; Butterworth, 1979; Ellis, Miller, & Sin, 1983; Lecour & Rouillon, 1976; Nickels & Howard, 1995).

In contrast, several investigators have recently provided evidence for a greater-than-chance incidence of formal paraphasias in some aphasics. That is, in producing errors that sound similar to the intended target, some patients appear to produce real words (as opposed to nonwords) at a higher rate than would be predicted by chance (Best, 1996; Blanken, 1990; Gagnon et al., 1997; Martin, Dell, Saffran, & Schwartz, 1994). The same phenomenon has been observed in studies of normal slips of the tongue, which typically show a higher than chance rate of word compared with nonword errors (Baars, Motley, & MacKay, 1975; Dell & Reich, 1981). If these errors truly represent incorrect word selection rather than phoneme errors that happen to have resulted in words, we might expect the errors to be in the same grammatical word class as the intended target. Evidence suggests that this is the case (Dell et al., 1997; Fay & Cutler, 1977; Gagnon et al., 1997). These findings are important because they suggest a production mechanism in which selection at the word level is partly constrained by information about the sound of the word, possibly through feedback from phoneme to word-level representations.

Other evidence for interaction between phoneme and word information during speech production comes from the observation of *mixed paraphasias*, in which a real-word error response is related both phonologically and semantically to the intended target ("skirt" → "shirt"). While such errors comprise only a small proportion of the total errors made by aphasic patients, the issue again is whether this proportion is small enough to be explained as coincidence. Studies of both normal and fluent aphasic subjects show that the incidence of mixed errors is significantly greater than would be expected by chance alone (Dell & Reich, 1981; Dell et al., 1997; Harley, 1984; Martin, Gagnon, Schwartz, Dell, & Saffran, 1996). As with formal paraphasias, the higher than expected incidence of mixed paraphasias suggests that phonological resemblance to a target word is somehow enhancing the selection of an error word. In the case of the mixed error, this phonological resemblance between target and error words is acting in concert with a semantic resemblance.

Many of the basic error phenomena observed in normal slips of the tongue and aphasic paraphasia—contextual effects, similarity effects, and phoneme–word interactions—can be seen as the natural product of a neural network in which word selection and phoneme selection partly overlap in time and influence each other through an interactive spreading activation mechanism. Models of this kind have been presented by Dell and colleagues (Dell, 1986; Dell & O'Seaghdha, 1992; Dell et al., 1997) and by others (Harley, 1984; Roelofs, 1992; Stemberger, 1985). Figure 9.6 shows a simplified diagram of a hypothetical portion of such a network.

A central starting point of the model is that speech production involves two distinct processes or stages of information access that partly overlap in time. The first of these is a translation from the abstract concept the speaker wishes to express (the semantic representation) to a word or ordered string of words that express the concept. This process is referred to as *lemma access*. "Lemma" refers to a type of representation in the brain similar to a word, but with some important differences.[3] The lemma representation of a word contains information about its syntactic role (noun, verb, etc.), and the lemma

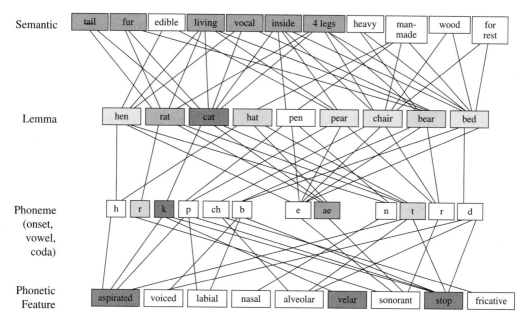

Figure 9.6
Schematic representation of an interactive, spreading activation model of speech production. The network is shown at a moment in time during production of *cat*. A set of semantic units have produced activation of the target lemma as well as several semantically related lemmas (*rat*, *bear*). Position-specific (onset, vowel, and coda) phonemes are activated as a result of the spread of activation from the lemma to the phoneme level. The network has just selected the onset phoneme /k/, resulting in increased activation of the phonetic feature nodes (aspirated, velar, stop) associated with /k/. Note weak activation of the lemma *hat* despite lack of input from the semantic level, owing to feedback from the phoneme units for /ae/ and /t/. This feedback is postulated to be the main source of formal (i.e., semantically unrelated but phonologically related) paraphasic errors. The lemma *rat* also receives phoneme-level feedback, and is more strongly activated than *hat* because of combined input from semantic and phoneme levels, increasing the likelihood of a mixed (semantic + phonological) error. Finally, note that activation of the phonetic feature nodes, aspirated and stop, feed back to phoneme nodes, such as /t/, that share these features, increasing the likelihood of selection errors involving phonemes similar to the target phoneme.

is a more abstract entity than a word in that it contains no information about the sound of the word, its phonological representation (Dell, 1986; Dell & O'Seaghdha, 1992; Kempen & Huijbers, 1983; Levelt et al., 1991). In this sense, the lemma differs from Wernicke's notion of a word-sound image— a kind of memory of a word stored in auditory format—and it differs from the phonological lexicon found in many contemporary models of language processing (Allport & Funnell, 1981; Morton & Patterson, 1980), which is composed of phonological word forms. In the second stage of the two-stage model, the sounds of the word are computed by translating the lemma into a string of ordered phonemes, a process referred to as *phonological access.*

As shown schematically in figure 9.6, the component nodes of the network are organized into semantic, lemma, phoneme, and phonetic feature levels.[4] Each level contains a large number of nodes that represent, in a distributed manner, the individual's fund of information about concepts, words, and phonemes. Connections between nodes in adjacent levels represent relationships between concepts, words, phonemes, and phonetic features, which have been learned over time as a result of experience. A key feature of the model is that connections between adjacent levels are reciprocal, permitting activation to flow in both top-down and bottom-up directions. As with other models of this type, the activation state of each node in the network is computed at discrete points in time as a weighted sum of all the inputs to the node, plus the activation level at the immediately preceding point in time modified by a decay term, e.g.:

$$A_i(t) = A_i(t-1) \times (1-d) + \sum_j a_j(t-1) \times w_{ij} + \text{noise}$$

where $A_i(t)$ is the activation of node i at the current time step t, $A_i(t-1)$ is the activation at the immediately preceding time point, d is a decay parameter, $a_j(t-1)$ is the activation at the immediately preceding time point of a node j sending input to node i, and w_{ij} is the strength, or weight, of the connection between the sending node j and receiving node i.

Speech production in the model begins with activation of semantic nodes representing the concept that the subject wishes to express. Semantic nodes are usually envisioned as representations of physical, functional, or associative properties (e.g., "has fur") that collectively define a word, although the specific format in which semantic information is encoded is probably not critical for the model. The active semantic nodes then send activation to all lemma nodes to which they are connected. An important point is that a given semantic node is connected to all lemmas that share that semantic feature; thus activation of a given semantic node results in some degree of activation of all lemmas to which it is connected. Lemma nodes, in turn, send activation to all phoneme nodes to which they are connected, and these phoneme nodes send activation on to all phonetic feature nodes to which they are connected. Because of the reciprocal connections between layers, activation is also returned from the lemma to semantic level, from the phoneme to lemma level, and from the phonetic feature to phoneme level.

Similarity effects—the occurrence of word errors that resemble the target semantically (semantic paraphasia) and phoneme errors that resemble the target phoneme—are readily explained by such a model. Because semantic nodes send activation to all lemmas to which they are connected, lemmas that strongly resemble the target will be activated nearly as much as the target itself. For example, because chair and couch share many semantic features, activation of the semantic representation for chair will necessarily activate the lemmas of both chair and couch (and many other related items).

Under normal conditions, the network is able to select the correct lemma on the basis of its activation being slightly higher than that of its semantic neighbors (adding to the model inhibitory connections between lemma nodes also helps to suppress activation of these neighbors), but adding noise to the system by partial damage to nodes or to connections can easily cause this fidelity to be compromised, resulting in lemma selection errors of a semantic nature.

Phoneme similarity effects happen by a similar mechanism, but are due to feedback from the phonetic feature level. Because phonetic features have reciprocal connections to all phonemes that share that feature, activation of a given set of phonetic features by a phoneme node will cause reciprocal activation of other phoneme nodes that share those features. Again, adding noise to the system can occasionally cause one of these phonetic neighbors to become more active than the target phoneme, resulting in a phoneme selection error on the basis of similarity.

Interactive effects—the occurrence of formal paraphasias and mixed semantic-phonological errors—are also a natural consequence of the model. Recall that a higher-than-chance incidence of formal paraphasias means that errors that resemble the target phonologically are more likely than chance to form real words. In the network model, this phenomenon is accounted for by feedback from phoneme to lemma levels. When the target lemma (e.g., train) becomes activated, this produces activation of the phoneme nodes connected to the target lemma (e.g., /t/, /r/, /e/ and /n/). Reciprocal connections allow these phoneme nodes to feed back on all other lemmas to which they are connected, producing particularly significant activation of lemma nodes that share several phonemes in common with the target lemma (e.g., crane and trait). If selected, such a lemma will in turn increase the activation level of its phonemes, increasing their likelihood of being selected. Although small, these effects increase the likelihood that a phonological neighbor of the target lemma will be produced, rather than a randomly generated nonword (e.g., prain).

Mixed errors have a similar explanation, except that here the error results from a combination of semantic and phoneme influences at the lemma level. That is, shared semantic features result in the activation of semantic neighbors of the target lemma, while shared phonemes cause the activation of phonological neighbors. These influences add together to increase the likelihood that a mixed semantic-phonological neighbor of the target, if one exists (e.g., plane), will be selected at the lemma level.

Because contextual errors (anticipations, perseverations, exchanges) typically involve words that are near each other in time, an account of these phenomena requires a look at how the model handles multiword utterances. A complete description is beyond the scope of this review, but the main point is that words within multiword sequences are, to a large degree, selected in parallel. That is, as activation is accumulating in the lemma and phoneme nodes related to the first word in the string, activation also begins to accumulate in the nodes pertaining to the second word. After reaching maximum levels, activation also takes time to decay back to baseline levels; there is thus residual activation in the nodes for a preceding word even as the nodes for a following word are being selected. Moreover, because selection at the lemma level occurs earlier than selection at the phoneme level, activation at the lemma level for a following word may be occurring almost simultaneously with activation at the phoneme level for a preceding word. This considerable temporal overlap occasionally creates selection of a lemma or phoneme node that is actually a target lemma or phoneme for a preceding or following word, resulting in contextual errors.

Specifically, anticipations are due to selection of a phoneme or lemma from a later word, which happened by chance to have been more activated than the target phoneme or lemma. Perseverations are due to selection of a phoneme or lemma from an earlier word, which happened by chance to have been more activated than the target phoneme or lemma. Exchanges are believed to reflect a mechanism that transiently suppresses the activation of a node after it has been selected. For example, during phonological translation of the lemma for cat, the network transiently suppresses or inhibits the activation level of the phoneme node for /k/ after this is selected. Although the mechanism by which this occurs is not clear, some sort of suppression appears necessary to prevent, for example, the /k/ phoneme from being chosen again and again for subsequent phoneme positions. Exchanges thus occur when an anticipation error causes a phoneme from a following word to be selected prematurely, and the node for this phoneme is transiently suppressed. The target phoneme, which had not been selected because of the anticipation error, then achieves an activation level higher than the previously selected, now suppressed phoneme, resulting in an exchange.

Other aspects of the paraphasic errors made by fluent aphasics can also be accommodated by the model if certain assumptions are accepted. For example, as mentioned earlier, contextual phoneme errors usually involve pairs of phonemes that occupy the same position in their respective syllables (e.g., onset, vowel, or final position). This can be explained by assuming that phoneme nodes are position specific. Thus, an exchange such as "spy fled" → "fly sped" is possible, but the exchange "spy fled" → "dye flesp" is highly unlikely because the /sp/ target node of the first word is represented in the network specifically as an onset phoneme. An analogous phenomenon at the lemma level is the observation that contextual errors nearly always occur between words of the same grammatical class. For example, an exchange involving two nouns, such as "writing a mother to my letter," is possible, whereas exchange of a noun for a possessive pronoun, such as "writing a my to letter mother," is highly unlikely. This preservation of grammatical class follows from the assumption that lemmas contain information about grammatical class, which constrains the set of lemmas that are candidates for selection at any given position in an utterance.

What kinds of "lesions" in the network lead to an increased incidence of paraphasic errors, and do different kinds of lesions produce different error patterns? Do such lesions have any meaning in terms of real brain lesions? These questions are just beginning to be addressed, but preliminary reports are interesting (Dell et al., 1997; Hillis, Boatman, Hart, & Gordon, 1999; Martin et al., 1994; Schwartz et al., 1994). Martin et al. (1994) proposed the idea of modeling their patient's paraphasic errors by increasing the decay parameter of the network. This produces an overall dampening effect on activation levels, essentially weakening the ability of the network to maintain a given pattern of activation.

The target lemma and its semantic neighbors, which are activated early during the selection process by direct input from semantic nodes, experience abnormally large activation decay prior to lemma selection. In contrast, lemmas that are activated at a later stage, primarily by feedback from phoneme nodes (i.e., phonological neighbors and mixed phonological-semantic neighbors of the target) have less time to be affected by the decay and so end up with more activation relative to the target at the time of lemma selection. The result is an increase in the incidence of formal and mixed paraphasias relative to other types. This class of lesion has been referred to as a *representational defect* because the network nodes themselves, which represent the lemmas, phonemes, and phonetic features, have difficulty remaining activated and so are unable to faithfully represent the pattern of information being retrieved. A similar kind of defect could as well be modeled by randomly removing a proportion of the nodes, or by adding random noise to the activation values.

A qualitatively different kind of lesion, referred to as a *transmission defect*, results from decreasing the connection weights between nodes (Dell et al., 1997). This impairs the spread of activation back and forth between adjacent levels, decreasing interactivity. As a result, selection at the lemma level is less guided by phoneme-to-lemma feedback, producing a lower incidence of formal and mixed errors, and selection at the phoneme level is less governed by lemma input, resulting in a relatively higher proportion of nonword and unrelated errors.

For both types of lesions, the overall accuracy rate and the proportion of errors that are nonwords increase as the parameter being manipulated (decay or connectivity) is moved further from the normal value. This reflects the fact that defects in either representational integrity or connectivity, if severe enough, can interfere with the proper spread of activation through the network, allowing random noise to have a larger effect on phoneme selection. Because there are many more nonwords than words that can result from random combinations of phonemes, an increase in the randomness of selection necessarily produces an increase in the rate of nonwords. This natural consequence of the model is consistent with the general correlation between severity of paraphasia and the rate of nonword errors observed in many studies (Butterworth, 1979; Dell et al., 1997; Kertesz & Benson, 1970; Kohn & Smith, 1994; Mitchum, Ritgert, Sandson, & Berndt, 1990; Moerman, Corluy, & Meersman, 1983).

Dell et al. (1997) used these two kinds of lesions to individually model the pattern of paraphasic errors produced by twenty-one fluent aphasic patients (seven Wernicke, five conduction, eight anomic, and one transcortical sensory) during a picture-naming task. Naming was simulated in the model by activating a set of semantic features associated with the pictured object from each trial and recording the string of phonemes selected by the network. Errors produced by the patients and by the network were categorized as semantic, formal, mixed, unrelated words, and nonwords. The decay and connection weight parameters were altered until the best fit was obtained for each patient between the error pattern produced by the patient and by the network. Good fits were obtained, and patients fell into distinct groups based on whether the decay parameter or the connection weight parameter was most affected.

Patients with representational lesions (increases in the decay rate parameter) showed relatively more formal and mixed errors, while patients with transmission lesions (decreases in the connection weight parameter) showed relatively more nonword and unrelated word errors. Particularly interesting was the finding that the formal paraphasias made by the decay lesion group were much more likely to be nouns (the target grammatical class) than were the formal errors made by the connection lesion group. This suggests that the formal errors made by the decay group were more likely to be errors of lemma selection, as the model predicts, while those made by the connection lesion group were more likely to have resulted from selection errors at the phoneme level that happened by chance to form real words.

An important aspect of the simulation by Dell et al. is that the "lesions" to the decay rate and connection weight parameters were made globally, i.e., uniformly to every node in every layer of the network. Consequently, the simulation does not attempt to model lesions that might be more localized, affecting, for example, the connections between lemma and phoneme levels. Despite this simplification, it is notable that all five of the conduction aphasics were modeled best using transmission lesions, while the Wernicke and anomic groups included both representational and transmission types. A tempting conclusion is that the conduction syndrome, which features a high incidence of nonwords relative to formal and mixed errors, may represent a transmission defect that weakens the connections between lemma and phoneme levels.

Another interesting aspect of the Dell et al. results is that anomic patients often showed a lower incidence of nonword errors than that predicted by the model and a lower incidence than would be expected on the basis of the severity of their naming deficits. Instead, these patients tended to make more semantic errors than predicted. Other patients have been reported who make almost exclusively semantic errors on naming tasks, without nonwords or other phonological errors (Caramazza & Hillis, 1990; Hillis & Caramazza, 1995). This pattern is difficult to explain on the basis of a global lesion, but might be accounted for using a representational lesion localized to the semantic level or a transmission lesion affecting connections between semantic and lemma levels.

In Wernicke's original model, the center for word-sound images was thought to play a role in both comprehension and production of words. It is therefore noteworthy that the interactive, bidirectional nature of the connections in the production model just described permits information to flow in either direction, from semantics to phonemes or phonemes to semantics. An ongoing debate among language scientists is the extent to which reception and production systems overlap, particularly with regard to transformations between phonemes and semantics. Psychological models of language that employ discrete processing modules often include a "phonological lexicon" that stores representations of individual words in a kind of auditory format. Early versions of the theory assumed that a single phonological lexicon was used for both input (comprehension) and output (production) tasks (Allport & Funnell, 1981). It is clear, however, that some aphasic patients have markedly disparate input and output abilities. For example, conduction aphasia is characterized by frequent phonemic paraphasias in all speech output tasks, whereas speech comprehension is intact (table 9.1), indicating a lesion localized at some point in the production pathway but sparing the input pathway. Conversely, patients with pure word deafness typically have only minimal paraphasia in spontaneous speech and naming tasks (repetition is paraphasic in pure word deafness owing to the input deficit; see table 9.1), indicating relative sparing of the production pathway. A variety of evidence from patients and normal subjects supports the general notion of some degree of independence between speech perception and production processes (Allport, MacKay, & Prinz, 1987; Allport, 1984; Kirschner & Webb, 1982; Nickels & Howard, 1995).

These and other observations led to proposals that there are separate input and output phonological lexicons, i.e., distinct input and output pathways linking phonology with semantics (Allport, 1984; Caramazza, 1988; Monsell, 1987; Morton & Patterson, 1980). Preliminary data from neural network simulations also support this thesis. For example, Dell et al. (1997) were unable to predict the performance levels of their patients in a repetition task, which involves both input and output, using model parameters derived from performance in a naming (output) task. Scores for repetition were consistently better than would have been predicted if the same (lesioned) network was used for both input and output, whereas the repetition performances were generally well accounted for by assuming a separate, intact, speech perceptual system.

The main objection to the idea of separate systems is the apparently needless duplication of the phonological lexicon that it entails. The lexicon is presumably a huge database that includes structural and grammatical information about the entire stored vocabulary, so this duplication seems like an inefficient use of neural resources. The model in figure 9.6, however, contains no phonological lexicon; in

its place are the interconnected lemma, phoneme, and phonetic feature levels. Such an arrangement permits an even larger set of possible relationships between input and output speech pathways, some of which would avoid duplication of word-level information. For example, it may be that the pathways share only a common lemma level, or share common lemma and phoneme levels, but use separate phoneme feature levels. Further careful study of patients with isolated speech perception or production syndromes will be needed to more clearly define the relationships between input and output speech pathways.

Dissociated Oral and Written Language Deficits

Although most Wernicke aphasics have impairments of reading and writing that roughly parallel those observed with auditory comprehension and speech, many show disparate abilities on tasks performed in the auditory and visual modalities. Because Wernicke's aphasia is classically considered to involve deficits in both modalities (Goodglass & Kaplan, 1972), such patients strain the definition of the syndrome and the classification scheme on which it is based. For example, many patients described as having "atypical Wernicke's aphasia" with superior comprehension of written compared with spoken language (Caramazza, Berndt, & Basili, 1983; Ellis et al., 1983; Heilman, Rothi, Campanella, & Wolfson, 1979; Hier & Mohr, 1977; Kirschner et al., 1981; Marshall, Rappaport, & Garcia-Bunuel, 1985; Sevush, Roeltgen, Campanella, & Heilman, 1983) could as readily be classified as variants of pure word deafness (Alexander & Benson, 1993; Metz-Lutz & Dahl, 1984). On the other hand, these patients exhibited aphasic signs such as neologistic paraphasia, anomia, or mild reading comprehension deficits that are atypical of pure word deafness. Similarly, patients with relatively intact auditory comprehension together with severe reading and writing disturbances have been considered to be atypical Wernicke cases by some (Kirschner & Webb, 1982),

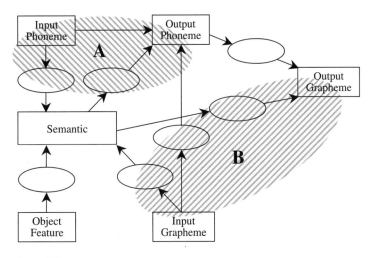

Figure 9.7
Theoretical lesion loci underlying modality-specific language deficits. Lesion A impairs tasks involving input and output phonemes, including auditory verbal comprehension, repetition, propositional speech, naming, reading aloud, and writing to dictation. Lesion B impairs tasks involving input and output graphemes, including reading comprehension, proposi- tional writing, written naming, reading aloud, and writing to dictation.

but as having "alexia and agraphia with conduc- tion aphasia" by others (Selnes & Niccum, 1983). Regardless of how these patients are categorized within the traditional aphasiology nomenclature, their deficit patterns provide additional information about how language perception and production systems might be organized according to the modal- ity of stimulus or response.

Patients with superior written compared with spoken language processing can be explained by postulating damage to phoneme systems or path- ways between phoneme and semantic representa- tions (lesion A in figure 9.7). Such damage would disrupt not only speech comprehension, but any task dependent on recognition of speech sounds (re- petition and writing to dictation) and any task in- volving production of speech (spontaneous speech, reading aloud, naming objects, and repetition). Be- cause pathways from visual input to semantics are spared, such patients retain the ability to com- prehend written words, match written words with pictures, and name objects using written responses

(Caramazza et al., 1983; Ellis et al., 1983; Heilman et al., 1979; Hier & Mohr, 1977; Hillis et al., 1999; Howard & Franklin, 1987; Ingles, Mate-Kole, & Connolly, 1996; Kirschner et al., 1981; Marshall et al., 1985; Semenza, Cipolotti, & Denes, 1992; Sevush et al., 1983). The preserved written naming ability shown by these patients despite severely impaired auditory comprehension and paraphasic speech is very clearly at odds with Wernicke's belief that word-sound images are essential for writing.[5]

Errors of speech comprehension in these patients reflect problems with phonemes rather than with words or word meanings. For example, in writing to dictation, patients make phonemic errors (e.g., they write "cap" after hearing "cat"), and in match- ing spoken words with pictures, they select incor- rect items with names that sound similar to the target. Such errors could result either from damage to the input phoneme system or to the pathway between phoneme and semantic levels. The patient studied in detail by Hillis et al. (1999) made typical errors of this kind on dictation and word–picture matching tasks, but could readily discriminate between similar-sounding spoken words like cap and cat on a same-different decision task. This pattern suggests that the patient was able to analyze the constituent phonemes and to compare a sequence of phonemes with another sequence, but was unable to translate correctly from the phoneme to the semantic level.

Similarly, the errors of speech production made by these patients are overwhelmingly of the phonemic type, including phonemic paraphasias, neologisms, and formal paraphasias, with only infrequent semantic or mixed errors. Hillis et al. (1999) modeled their patient's neologistic speech by lesioning Dell's spreading activation speech production network. Unlike the global lesions used by Dell et al. (1997), Hillis et al. postulated a local transmission lesion affecting connections between the lemma (intermediate) and output phoneme levels. When the lemma–phoneme connection strength was lowered sufficiently to produce the same overall error rate as that made by the patient during object naming, the model network reproduced the patient's pattern of errors with remarkable precision, including high proportions of phonologically related nonwords (patient 53%, model 52.5%), a smaller number of formal errors (patient 6%, model 6.5%), and infrequent semantic or mixed errors (patient 3%, model 2.7%). These results provide further evidence not only for the processing locus of the lesion causing superior written over oral language processing in this patient but also for the concept that a focal transmission lesion can cause a characteristic error pattern that depends on the lesion's locus.

Patients with this auditory variant of Wernicke aphasia vary in terms of the extent to which speech output is impaired. Most patients had severely paraphasic speech (Caramazza et al., 1983; Ellis et al., 1983; Hier & Mohr, 1977; Hillis et al., 1999; Ingles et al., 1996; Kirschner et al., 1981; Marshall et al., 1985), but others made relatively few errors in reading aloud (Heilman et al., 1979; Howard & Franklin, 1987; Semenza et al., 1992; Sevush et al., 1983). Even among the severely paraphasic patients, reading aloud was generally less paraphasic than

spontaneous speech or object naming (Caramazza et al., 1983; Ellis et al., 1983; Hillis et al., 1999).

The fact that some patients showed relatively spared reading aloud despite severe auditory comprehension disturbance provides further evidence for the existence of at least partially independent input and output phoneme systems, as depicted in the model presented here. This observation also provides evidence for a direct grapheme-to-phoneme translation mechanism that bypasses the presumably lesioned semantic-to-phoneme output pathway. Because patients with this pattern are relying on the grapheme-to-phoneme pathway for reading aloud, we might expect worse performance on exception words, which depend relatively more on input from the semantic pathway, and better reading of nonwords (see chapter 6 in this volume). These predictions have yet to be fully tested, although the patient described by Hillis et al. (1999) clearly showed superior reading of nonwords.

Patients with superior oral over written language processing have also been reported (Déjerine, 1891; Kirschner & Webb, 1982). A processing lesion affecting input and output grapheme levels or their connections (lesion B in figure 9.7) would produce a modality-specific impairment of reading comprehension and written output directly analogous to the oral language impairments discussed earlier. Such a lesion would not, however, affect speech output or speech comprehension. It is perhaps because a disturbance in auditory-verbal comprehension is considered the sine qua non of Wernicke aphasia that patients with relatively isolated reading and writing impairments of this kind have usually been referred to as having "alexia with agraphia" rather than a visual variant of Wernicke aphasia (Benson & Geschwind, 1969; Déjerine, 1891; Goodglass & Kaplan, 1972; Nielsen, 1946).

These dissociations between oral and written language processes also offer important clues concerning the neuroanatomical organization of language comprehension and production systems. For example, they suggest that input and output phoneme systems are segregated anatomically from input and output grapheme systems. The observation that input and output phoneme systems are often involved together, but that output may be relatively spared, suggests that these systems lie close together in the brain, but are not entirely overlapping. The co-occurrence, in a few patients, of paraphasic speech output with reading and writing disturbance and spared speech comprehension (Kirschner & Webb, 1982) suggests a smaller anatomical distance between speech output and grapheme systems than between speech input and grapheme systems. These and other data regarding lesion localization in Wernicke aphasia are taken up in the next section.

Neuroanatomical Correlates of Wernicke Aphasia

Wernicke's aphasia has been recognized for well over a century and has been a subject of great interest to neurologists and neuropsychologists, so it is not surprising that the lesion correlation literature concerning this syndrome is vast. The neuroanatomical basis of sensory aphasia was a central issue for many German-speaking neurologists of the late nineteenth and early twentieth century who followed after Wernicke, including Lichtheim, Bonhoefer, Liepmann, Heilbronner, Pick, Pötzl, Henschen, Goldstein, and Kleist. French neurologists of the time who presented data on the topic included Charcot, Pitres, Dejerine, Marie, and others. Early contributions in English were made by Bastian, Mills, Bramwell, Head, Wilson, Nielsen, and others. In the last half of the twentieth century, important investigations were reported by Penfield, Russell, Hécaen, Luria, Goodglass, Benson, Naeser, Kertesz, Selnes, Warrington, Damasio, and many others. It is well beyond the scope of this chapter to review even a small portion of this information in detail. Our aim here is rather to sketch the origins of some of the neuroanatomical models that have been proposed and to evaluate, admittedly briefly, their relation to the actual data.

Patients with Wernicke aphasia have lesions in the lateral temporal and parietal lobes, so a review of the anatomy of this region is a useful starting point for discussion (figure 9.8). The lesions involve brain tissue on the lateral convex surface of these lobes and almost never involve areas on the ventral or medial surfaces. The lesion area typically includes cortex in and around the posterior sylvian (lateral) fissure, giving rise to the term *posterior perisylvian* to describe their general location. These predictable locations result from the fact that in most cases the lesions are due to arterial occlusion, and that the vascular supply to the affected region– the lower division of the middle cerebral artery– follows a similar, characteristic pattern across individuals (Mohr, Gautier, & Hier, 1992).

Temporal lobe structures within this vascular territory include the superior temporal gyrus (Brodmann areas 41, 42, and 22), the middle temporal gyrus (Brodmann areas 21 and 37), and variable (usually small) portions of the inferior temporal gyrus (ITG; Brodmann areas 20 and 37). Parietal lobe structures within the territory include the angular gyrus (Brodmann area 39) and variable portions of the supramarginal gyrus (Brodmann area 40). In addition, the lesion almost always damages the posterior third of the insula (the cortex buried at the fundus of the sylvian fissure) and may extend back to involve anterior aspects of the lateral occipital lobe (figure 9.8).

Near the origin of this large vascular territory is the posterior half of the STG, which studies in human and nonhuman primates have shown to contain portions of the cortical auditory system. The superior surface of the STG in humans includes a small, anterolaterally oriented convolution called "Heschl's gyrus" and, behind HG, the posterior superior temporal plane or planum temporale. These structures, located at the posterior-medial aspect of the dorsal STG and buried in the sylvian fissure, receive auditory projections from the medial geniculate body and are believed to represent the primary auditory cortex (Galaburda & Sanides, 1980; Liègeois-Chauvel, Musolino, & Chauvel, 1991; Mesulam & Pandya, 1973; Rademacher, Caviness, Steinmetz, & Galaburda, 1993).

Studies in nonhuman primates of the anatomical connections and unit activity of neurons in the STG suggest that these primary areas then relay auditory information to cortical association areas located

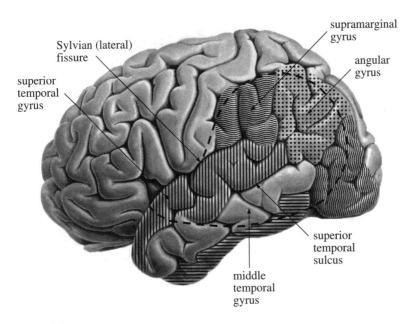

superior temporal gyrus

Sylvian (lateral) fissure

supramarginal gyrus

angular gyrus

superior temporal sulcus

middle temporal gyrus

Figure 9.8
Gross anatomy of the lateral temporal and parietal lobes. Gyri are indicated as follows: superior temporal = vertical lines; middle temporal = unmarked; inferior temporal = horizontal lines; angular = dots; supramarginal = horizontal waves; and lateral occipital lobe = vertical waves. The approximate vascular territory of the lower division of the middle cerebral artery is indicated with a dashed line.

more laterally on the superior surface and on the outer surface of the STG (Galaburda & Pandya, 1983; Kaas & Hackett, 1998; Morel, Garraghty, & Kaas, 1993; Rauschecker, 1998). It thus appears, on the basis of these comparative studies, that the superior and lateral surfaces of the STG contain unimodal auditory cortex (Baylis, Rolls, & Leonard, 1987; Creutzfeld, Ojemann, & Lettich, 1989; Galaburda & Sanides, 1980; Kaas & Hackett, 1998; Leinonen, Hyvärinen, & Sovijärvi, 1980; Rauschecker, 1998), whereas the superior temporal sulcus and more caudal-ventral structures (MTG, ITG, AG) contain polymodal cortex that receives input from auditory, visual, and somatosensory sources (Baylis et al., 1987; Desimone & Gross, 1979; Hikosawa, Iwai, Saito, & Tanaka, 1988; Jones & Powell, 1970; Seltzer & Pandya, 1978, 1994). For regions caudal and ventral to the STG and STS,

however, inference about function in humans on the basis of nonhuman primate data is perilous owing to a lack of structural similarity across species. The MTG and AG, in particular, appear to have developed much more extensively in humans than in monkeys, so it is difficult to say whether data from comparative studies shed much direct light on the function of these areas in humans.

Like the STG and MTG, the AG is frequently damaged in patients with Wernicke aphasia. Although its borders are somewhat indistinct, the AG consists of cortex surrounding the posterior parietal extension of the STS and is approximately the region Brodmann designated area 39. The SMG (Brodmann area 40) lies just anterior to the AG within the inferior parietal lobe and surrounds the parietal extension of the sylvian fissure. The SMG is frequently damaged in Wernicke aphasia, although its anterior aspect is often spared because of blood supply from more anterior sources.

It hardly, needs mentioning that Wernicke attributed his sensory aphasia syndrome to a lesion of the STG (Wernicke, 1874, 1881), but the actual motivations behind this view are less than obvious. Wernicke's case material was rather slim: ten patients in all, only three of whom showed a combination of auditory comprehension disturbance and paraphasic speech (reading comprehension was not mentioned). Two of these patients, Rother and Funke, came to autopsy. In these two cases there were large left hemisphere lesions reaching well beyond the STG, including in the patient Rother (who also had shown signs of advanced dementia clinically and had diffuse cerebral atrophy at autopsy), the posterior MTG and the AG (described as "the anastomosis of the first and second temporal convolution") and in Funke including the inferior frontal lobe, SMG, AG, MTG, and inferior temporal lobe.

In emphasizing the STG component of these large lesions, Wernicke was influenced in part by the views of his mentor, Theodor Meynert, who had described the subcortical auditory pathway as leading to the general region of the sylvian fissure. Even more important, however, was Wernicke's concept of the STG as the lower branch of a single gyrus supporting speech functions (his "first primitive gyrus"), which encircles the sylvian fissure and includes Broca's area in the inferior frontal lobe. Inferring from Meynert's view that the frontal lobe is involved in motor functions and the temporal lobe in sensory functions, Wernicke assumed that the STG must be the sensory analog of Broca's motor speech area.

Although subsequent researchers were strongly influenced by Wernicke's model, views regarding the exact lesion correlate of Wernicke's aphasia have varied considerably (Bogen & Bogen, 1976). As early as 1888, Charcot and his student Marie included the left AG and MTG in the region associated with Wernicke's aphasia (Marie, 1888/ 1971). Marie later included the SMG as well (Marie & Foix, 1917). In 1889, Starr reviewed fifty cases

of sensory aphasia published in the literature with autopsy correlation, twenty-seven of whom had Wernicke's aphasia (Starr, 1889). None of these patients had lesions restricted to the STG, and Starr concluded that "in these cases the lesion was wide in extent, involving the temporal, parietal and occipital convolutions" (Starr, 1889, p. 87). Similar views were expressed by Henschen, Nielsen, and Goldstein, among others (Goldstein, 1948; Henschen, 1920–1922; Nielsen, 1946).

Much of modern thinking on this topic is influenced by the work of Geschwind, who followed Wernicke, Liepmann, Pick, Kleist, and others in emphasizing the role of the left STG in Wernicke's aphasia (Geschwind, 1971). Geschwind and his students drew attention to left-right asymmetries in the size of the planum temporale, that is, the cortex posterior to Heschl's gyrus on the dorsal STG. This cortical region is larger on the left side in approximately two-thirds of right-handed people (Geschwind & Levitsky, 1968; Steinmetz, Volkmann, Jäncke, & Freund, 1991; Wada, Clarke, & Hamm, 1975). Recent studies have made it clear that this asymmetry is due to interhemispheric differences in the shape of the posterior sylvian fissure, which angles upward into the parietal lobe more anteriorly in the right hemisphere (Binder, Frost, Hammeke, Rao, & Cox, 1996; Rubens, Mahowald, & Hutton, 1976; Steinmetz et al., 1990; Westbury, Zatorre, & Evans, 1999). Geschwind and others interpreted this asymmetry as confirming a central role for the PT and the posterior half of the STG in language functions (Foundas, Leonard, Gilmore, Fennell, & Heilman, 1994; Galaburda, LeMay, Kemper, & Geschwind, 1978; Witelson & Kigar, 1992) and argued that lesions in this area are responsible for Wernicke aphasia. Many late twentieth-century textbooks and review articles thus equate the posterior STG with "Wernicke's area" (Benson, 1979; Geschwind, 1971; Mayeux & Kandel, 1985; Mesulam, 1990).

The advent of brain imaging using computed tomography and magnetic resonance imaging allowed aphasia localization to be investigated with much larger subject samples and systematic, standardized protocols (Caplan, Gow, & Makris, 1995; Damasio, 1981; Damasio, 1989; Damasio & Damasio, 1989; Kertesz, Harlock, & Coates, 1979; Kertesz, Lau, & Polk, 1993; Naeser, Hayward, Laughlin, & Zatz, 1981; Selnes, Niccum, Knopman, & Rubens, 1984). The aim of most of these studies was to identify brain regions that are lesioned in common across the majority of cases. This was typically accomplished by drawing or tracing the lesion on a standard brain template and finding areas of lesion overlap across individuals. Several of these studies showed the region of most consistent overlap in Wernicke aphasia to be the posterior left STG or STG and MTG (Damasio, 1981; Kertesz et al., 1979), providing considerable support for Wernicke's original model and its refinements by Geschwind and colleagues.

A potential problem with the lesion overlap technique is that it emphasizes overlap across individuals in the pattern of vascular supply, which may or may not be related to the cognitive deficits in question. As already noted, Wernicke's aphasia is due to occlusion of the lower division of the middle cerebral artery. The proximal trunk of this arterial tree lies in the posterior sylvian fissure, near the PT and posterior STG, with its branches directed posteriorly and ventrally. The territory supplied by these branches is somewhat variable, however, in some cases including more or less of the anterior parietal or ventral temporal regions shown in figure 9.8. Because of this variability, and because retrograde collateral flow arising from other major arteries commonly causes variable sparing of the territory supplied by the more distal branches, regions supplied by the trunk and proximal branches (i.e., the STG and PT) are the most likely to be consistently damaged (Mohr et al., 1992). Thus the region of maximal overlap is determined largely by the vascular anatomy pattern and is not necessarily the region in which damage leads to Wernicke's aphasia (figure 9.9).

Given the critical role assigned by Wernicke and others to the STG, it is reasonable to ask whether lesions confined solely to the left STG actually cause

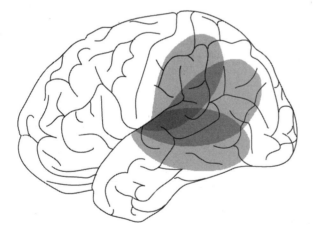

Figure 9.9
Diagram of three hypothetical ischemic lesions in the lower division of the middle cerebral artery territory, illustrating typical patterns of lesion overlap (dark shading). Because the vascular tree in question arises from a trunk overlying the posterior STG, this region is the most consistently damaged. Wernicke aphasia, on the other hand, might result from injury to a more distributed system that includes middle temporal, angular, and supramarginal gyri, which are outside the area of common overlap.

Wernicke's aphasia. Henschen was perhaps the first to seriously test this prediction and offer evidence to the contrary (Henschen, 1920–1922). In his meticulous review of 109 autopsied cases with temporal lobe lesions reported in the literature, 19 cases had damage confined to the left STG. None of these patients had the syndrome of Wernicke's aphasia; 5 were reported to have some degree of disturbance in auditory comprehension, but all had intact reading comprehension and writing. Henschen pointed out that this pattern was inconsistent with Wernicke's model of the STG as a center for language comprehension and concluded that the STG is involved in perception of spoken sounds.

Some later authors similarly disputed the claim that lesions restricted to the posterior left STG ever cause Wernicke's aphasia (Foix, 1928; Mohr et al., 1992), while several others have emphasized that large lesions involving the STG, MTG, SMG, and AG are typical (Damasio, 1989; Henschen, 1920–1922; Starr, 1889). Nielsen (1938) reviewed several cases that purportedly had Wernicke's aphasia from an isolated posterior STG injury. Of these, however, most had lesions clearly extending into the MTG and the inferior parietal lobe, and several cases were most likely caused by hematomas, which are known to produce relatively nonlocalized neural dysfunction owing to pressure effects from the hematoma mass.

Perhaps the best-documented case was Kleist's patient Papp, who presented with impaired auditory comprehension and paraphasia (Kleist, 1962). Reading comprehension was, unfortunately, not tested. At autopsy there was a lesion centered in the posterior left STG, with only minimal involvement of the posterior MTG. Unfortunately, there was also a large right perisylvian lesion that would, in conjunction with the left STG lesion, explain the case as one of pure word deafness caused by bilateral STG lesions. Kleist dismissed the importance of the right hemisphere lesion, however, relating it to the appearance of left hemiparesis well after the onset of aphasia.

In contrast to this rather scant evidence in support of the original Wernicke model, many instances of

isolated left STG lesion with completely normal auditory and written comprehension have been documented (Basso, Lecours, Moraschini, & Vanier, 1985; Benson et al., 1973; Boller, 1973; Damasio & Damasio, 1980; Henschen, 1920–1922; Hoeft, 1957; Kleist, 1962; Liepmann & Pappenheim, 1914; Stengel, 1933). Most of these were extensive lesions that involved Heschl's gyrus, the PT, the posterior lateral STG, and underlying white matter. Many of these patients had the syndrome of conduction aphasia, consisting of paraphasia (with primarily phonemic errors) during speech, repetition, and naming; variable degrees of anomia; and otherwise normal language functions, including normal auditory and reading comprehension. Kleist's patients are particularly clear examples because of the meticulous detail with which they were studied at autopsy (Kleist, 1962). Believing as he did that the posterior left STG (and particularly the PT) was critical for auditory comprehension, Kleist viewed these patients' preserved comprehension as evidence that they must have had comprehension functions in the right STG, even though two of the three were right-handed. Others have echoed this view (Boller, 1973), although the explanation seems quite unlikely given the rarity of aphasic deficits after right hemisphere injury (Faglia, Rottoli, & Vignolo, 1990; Gloning, Gloning, Haub, & Quatember, 1969) and recent functional imaging studies showing that right hemisphere language dominance is exceedingly rare in healthy right-handed people (Pujol, Deus, Losilla, & Capdevila, 1999; Springer et al., 1999). Recognizing this problem, Benson et al. postulated instead that "the right hemisphere can rapidly assume the functions of comprehension after destruction of the Wernicke area" despite the fact that "comprehension of spoken language was always at a high level" in their patient with left posterior STG infarction (Benson et al., 1973, pp. 344–345).

A review of Kleist's patients, however, suggests another, much simpler explanation. The autopsy figures and brief clinical descriptions provided by Kleist make it clear that the patients' comprehension deficits tended to increase as the lesion extended beyond the STG, either ventrally into the MTG or posteriorly into the AG. Subsequent CT correlation studies provide other evidence for a critical role of the MTG and AG in auditory comprehension. Investigators in these studies rated the degree of damage in selected brain regions and correlated this information with patterns of recovery.

Several studies showed a correspondence between poor recovery of auditory comprehension and greater damage to the MTG, the AG, or both (Dronkers, Redfern, & Ludy, 1995; Kertesz et al., 1993; Naeser et al., 1987; Selnes et al., 1983). Total infarct size was predictive of both degree of recovery and initial severity (Kertesz et al., 1993; Naeser et al., 1987; Selnes et al., 1983; Selnes et al., 1984). Moreover, even extensive damage to the STG did not preclude a good recovery in some patients (Kertesz et al., 1993; Naeser et al., 1987; Selnes et al., 1984). One interpretation of these findings is that they indicate a reorganization process by which neighboring regions take over functions originally performed by the STG (Kertesz et al., 1993). On the other hand, Dronkers et al. (1995) presented evidence that patients with lesions centered in the MTG have more lasting deficits, even when the STG is relatively spared, implying a primary rather than a secondary role for the MTG in comprehension.

Given the lack of reported cases with comprehension deficits from isolated STG damage, a parsimonious account of these data is that the MTG and other areas surrounding the STG play a more critical role in auditory comprehension than the STG does itself, and that both initial severity and degree of recovery are determined by the extent of acute dysfunction in these neighboring regions. In general, the data suggest that lesions centered in the STG tend to produce either no comprehension disturbance or a transient deficit that improves, whereas MTG and AG lesions tend to produce a more permanent deficit, with or without STG involvement.

Further supporting this model is evidence that the MTG and more ventral areas of the left temporal lobe play a critical role in accessing and storing semantic representations. For example, the syndrome of transcortical sensory aphasia, which is characterized by impairments of spoken and written language comprehension without phonemic paraphasia, has been consistently linked to lesions in the ventral and ventrolateral temporal lobe that involve the fusiform gyrus and the ITG, and to posterior convexity lesions that involve the posterior MTG and the temporo-occipital junction (Alexander, Hiltbrunner, & Fischer, 1989; Damasio, 1989; Kertesz, Sheppard, & MacKenzie, 1982; Rapcsak & Rubens, 1994).

Many aphasic patients (most of whom fit the classic syndromes of anomic aphasia or transcortical sensory aphasia) have now been described who show comprehension or naming deficits that are relatively restricted to particular object categories (Forde & Humphreys, 1999). Such patients may make more errors with living than nonliving items, more errors with animals than tools, more errors with fruits and vegetables than other objects, and so on. The category-specific nature of these deficits suggests damage at the level of semantic representations, and nearly all the cases have been associated with lesions involving left temporal lobe regions outside the STG. Perhaps the first such patient was Nielsen's case, C.H.C., who developed severe impairment of auditory comprehension after focal infarction of the left MTG and ITG (Nielsen, 1946). C.H.C. had marked anomia, but was able to recognize and name living things much better than nonliving objects. Similar cases have been associated with focal infarctions of the left MTG or ITG (Hart & Gordon, 1990; Hillis & Caramazza, 1991) or with herpes encephalitis that caused anterior ventral temporal lobe damage (Laiacona, Capitani, & Barbarotto, 1997; Silveri & Gainotti, 1988; Sirigu, Duhamel, & Poncet, 1991; Warrington & Shallice, 1984).

Other evidence for the importance of the left MTG in semantic processing comes from a report by Chertkow and colleagues (Chertkow, Bub, Deaudon, & Whitehead, 1997), who studied eight aphasic patients with comprehension deficits following posterior perisylvian lesions (two Wernicke's aphasia, six global aphasia). Five of the patients showed comprehension deficits in associative matching tasks, even when the test materials consisted entirely of pictures, which suggested damage to semantic information stores. In these patients, the lesions extended further ventrally than in the other three patients, with the largest area of overlap in the middle and posterior MTG.

Finally, several studies show that aphasic patients who make primarily semantic paraphasias have lesions restricted to ventral temporal regions, particularly the posterior MTG and ITG (Cappa, Cavallotti, & Vignolo, 1981; Gainotti, Silveri, & Villa, 1986). In contrast, patients who make primarily phonemic paraphasias have posterior STG, insula, or inferior parietal lesions (Benson et al., 1973; Cappa et al., 1981; Damasio & Damasio, 1980; Palumbo, Alexander, & Naeser, 1992). A similar dorsal-ventral dissociation between areas associated with phonemic and semantic paraphasia has been observed during electrical interference stimulation studies (Ojemann, 1983).

Some authors have disputed the importance of the left MTG in word comprehension. In particular, a case reported by Pick in 1909 (Pick, 1909) and later cited by Nielsen and others (Henschen, 1920–1922; Hickok & Poeppel, 2000; Nielsen, 1946) has been used as evidence to the contrary. At autopsy the patient had cysts in the white matter of both temporal lobes, the remnants of intracerebral hemorrhages, which affected much of the middle portion of the MTG bilaterally, and on the left also involved the white matter of the posterior MTG, portions of the STG, and a small amount of the angular gyrus. The patient was apparently able to understand spoken words, although his own speech was paraphasic and unintelligible, consisting of "disconnected nonsense," and he was completely unable to write. The case provides some negative evidence, although this is tempered by the knowledge that subcortical hematomas are known to produce rather unpredictable deficits relative to cortical lesions, and by the fact that the patient was not examined until 3 weeks after the onset of the stroke,

during which time considerable recovery may have occurred.

Against this single case are several examples, from the same time period, of patients with small left MTG cortical lesions who showed profound comprehension disturbances (Henschen, 1920–1922). The patient of Hammond, for example, had complete loss of comprehension for spoken and written material as a result of a focal lesion that involved the midportion of the left MTG (Hammond, 1900). Nielsen's patient, C.H.C., who developed severe comprehension disturbance after a posterior MTG and ITG lesion, has already been mentioned (Nielsen, 1946). Although ischemic lesions restricted to the MTG are rather rare owing to the anatomical characteristics of the vascular supply, the modern literature also contains several examples (Chertkow et al., 1997; Dronkers et al., 1995; Hart & Gordon, 1990). These patients uniformly demonstrated deficits in spoken and written word comprehension.

If the STG and PT do not play a primary role in language comprehension, damage to these regions almost certainly contributes to the paraphasic component of Wernicke's aphasia. As noted earlier, isolated posterior STG lesions have frequently been observed in association with phonemic paraphasia (Benson et al., 1973; Damasio & Damasio, 1980; Kleist, 1962; Liepmann & Pappenheim, 1914), as have lesions in nearby posterior perisylvian areas also frequently damaged in Wernicke's aphasia, such as the SMG and posterior insula (Benson et al., 1973; Damasio & Damasio, 1980; Palumbo et al., 1992). This functional–anatomical correlation has been further corroborated by cortical stimulation studies demonstrating the appearance of phonemic paraphasia and other speech errors during electrical interference stimulation of the posterior STG (Anderson et al., 1999; Quigg & Fountain, 1999). It thus appears that the posterior STG (including the PT), the SMG, and the posterior insula play a critical role in the selection and production of ordered phoneme sequences. In addition to the selection of output phonemes, this complex process requires mapping from output phoneme to articulatory codes, sensory feedback mechanisms that help guide movements of the vocal tract, and short-term memory mechanisms for maintaining a phoneme sequence as it is being produced (Caplan & Waters, 1992).

To summarize some of this extensive material, there seems to be little evidence that lesions of the STG and/or PT produce the profound, multimodal comprehension disturbance typical of Wernicke's aphasia, but such lesions do regularly cause paraphasic production, particularly phonemic paraphasia. In contrast to the effects of isolated STG lesions, lesions in more ventral areas of the temporal lobe and in the angular gyrus may produce profound disturbances in comprehension. The clear double dissociation between phonemic paraphasia and comprehension impairment observed in patients with posterior STG lesions and in patients with lesions beyond the STG, respectively, is strong evidence that these two components of Wernicke's aphasia syndrome have no necessary functional or anatomical link. Their co-occurrence in Wernicke's aphasia, according to the model being developed here, results from the fact that the typical lesion in Wernicke's aphasia includes the STG but spreads beyond it into surrounding areas ventral and posterior to the STG that are critical for word comprehension.

As discussed earlier, patients with fluent aphasia do not always have equivalent impairment in comprehending spoken and written words. This is to be expected given the very different pathways to semantic representations that are engaged as a result of phonemic versus graphemic input. The available anatomical data suggest that patients with relatively worse speech comprehension and better reading comprehension characteristically have lesions in the left temporal lobe (Hier & Mohr, 1977; Hillis et al., 1999; Ingles et al., 1996; Kirschner et al., 1981; Roeltgen, Sevush, & Heilman, 1983). It is important to note that when the lesions are unilateral, the deficits nearly always involve both modalities, i.e., the differences between spoken and written comprehension are relative rather than absolute. Relative sparing of reading comprehension seems to be

most pronounced when the lesion is restricted to the dorsal temporal lobe, involving only the STG and MTG (Kirschner et al., 1981), or to the anterior aspect of the temporal lobe.

The patient of Hillis et al. (1999), who presented with speech comprehension deficit and phonemic paraphasia after a small hemorrhage in the posterior left sylvian fissure, is an extreme example in that reading comprehension (as assessed by word–picture matching and synonym matching) was entirely normal. This patient, however, had encephalomalacia in the contralateral anterior perisylvian region, the result of a previous meningioma resection, and so probably had disturbed speech comprehension as a result of bilateral superior temporal lobe damage, as occurs in the syndrome of pure word deafness (Barrett, 1910; Buchman, Garron, Trost-Cardamone, Wichter, & Schwartz, 1986; Goldstein, 1974; Henschen, 1918–1919; Tanaka, Yamadori, & Mori, 1987).

Two similar recent cases are well documented, both of whom had severe disturbance of speech comprehension, phonemic paraphasia, sparing of reading comprehension, and bilateral perisylvian lesions sparing the MTG and more ventral temporal areas (Marshall et al., 1985; Semenza et al., 1992). It is notable that the patient of Semenza et al. presented with language deficits only after a right hemisphere lesion, an earlier left unilateral lesion having caused no comprehension or production deficits. These three patients are by no means unique: many, if not most, of the reported cases of pure word deafness from bilateral superior temporal lesions also had varying degrees of phonemic paraphasia, sometimes with mild anomia (Buchman et al., 1986; Goldstein, 1974).

Thus there appear to be two distinct syndromes of preserved comprehension for written over spoken language. In cases with multimodal deficits and relative sparing of reading, the lesion is unilateral and affects multiple regions in the left temporal lobe. This lesion damages some part of the pathway leading from input phoneme representations to semantics, with relatively less involvement of the grapheme-to-semantics pathway. In patients with complete sparing of reading comprehension, the lesion affects the STG bilaterally, affecting only the phoneme pathway. The complete sparing of reading comprehension in the latter syndrome suggests that the functional impairment lies at a relatively early stage in the phoneme-to-semantics pathway, such as at the input phoneme level or its connections to the intermediate level (Hillis et al., 1999). The anatomical data, then, suggest that this early component is bilaterally organized in the STG, in contrast to later components of the phoneme-to-semantics pathway, such as the intermediate level or its connections to the semantic level, which are more unilaterally represented and partially overlap the grapheme-to-semantics pathway.

Patients with this auditory variant of Wernicke aphasia also have relatively greater impairment of speech production compared with writing (Hier & Mohr, 1977; Hillis et al., 1999; Kirschner et al., 1981; Marshall et al., 1985; Roeltgen et al., 1983; Semenza et al., 1992). In keeping with the studies cited previously, the mix of speech errors depends on the location of the lesion along the dorsal-ventral axis of the temporal lobe. Lesions involving ventral temporal regions produce empty speech with few phonemic errors (Hier & Mohr, 1977), while temporal lobe lesions confined to the STG or involving the STG and SMG produce marked phonemic paraphasia with frequent neologisms (Hillis et al., 1999; Semenza et al., 1992). Naming errors consist primarily of omissions (inability to produce a word) in the larger lesions and phonemic paraphasia or neologism in the STG and SMG cases. Analogous to reading comprehension, writing performance in these patients is impaired but relatively better than speaking if the lesion is large (Hier & Mohr, 1977; Kirschner et al., 1981; Roeltgen et al., 1983) and is almost completely preserved if the lesion is confined to the STG and SMG (Hillis et al., 1999; Marshall et al., 1985; Semenza et al., 1992). These data indicate that, as with the input pathways, the phoneme and grapheme production pathways are to some extent functionally and anatomically independent. In particular, the phoneme output pathway is strongly associated with the left STG and SMG,

which appear not to be involved much at all in the grapheme ouput pathway. Although large left temporal lobe lesions produce impairments in both modalities, writing production is relatively less dependent on the temporal lobe than is speech production.

The converse syndrome involves relative impairment of reading comprehension and writing compared with speech comprehension. Evidence exists in the early aphasia literature (Déjerine, 1892; Henschen, 1920–1922; Nielsen, 1946) as well as in more recent studies (Basso, Taborelli, & Vignolo, 1978; Kirschner & Webb, 1982) localizing this syndrome to the posterior parietal lobe or parietotemporo-occipital junction, including the angular gyrus. Such cases further illustrate the relative independence of grapheme input from phoneme input pathways as well as writing from speech production mechanisms.

It should be noted that cases exist of patients with speech comprehension deficits from lesions in the vicinity of the angular gyrus (Chertkow et al., 1997; Henschen, 1920–1922), so it remains unclear why some patients with lesions in this region have relatively preserved speech comprehension. It may be that speech comprehension is more likely to be preserved as the lesion focus moves posteriorly in the parietal lobe, or that the variability from case to case merely reflects individual variability in the functional anatomy of this region. The patients described by Kirschner and Webb (1982) are somewhat intermediate in this regard, in that they presented initially with speech comprehension deficits that later cleared, leaving predominantly reading comprehension and writing impairments. These patients also showed persistent paraphasic errors in speech, as well as naming difficulty, prompting Kirschner and Webb to classify them as atypical cases of Wernicke's aphasia rather than "alexia with agraphia."

From the point of view of the model developed here, the paraphasic speech of the patients described by Kirschner and Webb can be attributed to involvement of the posterior STG and/or the SMG, which was documented in two of the three cases (the third patient was not scanned). Thus, the co-occurrence of alexia, agraphia, and paraphasic speech in these patients may simply reflect the anatomical proximity of the angular gyrus, which appears to be critical to both the grapheme-to-semantics pathway activated during reading and the semantics-to-grapheme pathway activated during writing, to the output phoneme pathway in the STG and SMG.

More detailed studies of agraphia have uncovered patients in whom there appear to be writing deficits related specifically to damage in the phoneme-to-grapheme pathway. This syndrome, known as *phonological agraphia*, is characterized by particular difficulty writing or spelling nonwords (e.g., slithy) compared with real words. The spelling of nonwords is thought to depend particularly on a direct translation from output phonemes to output graphemes because these items have no representation at the semantic level. The spelling of actual words, in contrast, can be accomplished by either the phoneme-to-grapheme pathway or by a less direct phoneme-to-semantic-to-grapheme route.

One functional lesion that could produce phonological agraphia would be damage to the output phoneme level, which would be expected to produce co-occurring phonemic paraphasia. This prediction is well supported by the available lesion data, which show that most patients with phonological agraphia have SMG lesions, often with accompanying posterior STG damage, and are also severely paraphasic (Alexander, Friedman, Loverso, & Fischer, 1992; Roeltgen et al., 1983). The phoneme-to-grapheme mapping process is certain to be rather complex, however, probably involving an intermediate representational level as well as short-term memory systems to keep both the phoneme string and the grapheme string available while the writing process unfolds. At present it is unclear precisely which process or combination of processes is impaired by the posterior perisylvian lesions producing phonological agraphia.

Figure 9.10 summarizes some of the functional–anatomical correlations observed in patients with lateral convexity temporal and/or parietal lobe lesions. Such correlations can only be approximate

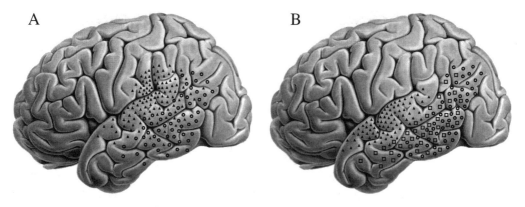

Figure 9.10

Summary of some lesion-deficit correlations in fluent aphasia. The figures are approximations only and represent the author's interpretation of a large body of published data. (*A*) Patterns of paraphasia. Triangles mark areas in which damage produces phonemic errors, and circles mark areas associated with verbal errors. (*B*) Comprehension deficits. Triangles indicate regions in which bilateral lesions cause an auditory verbal comprehension deficit without impairment of reading comprehension. Squares indicate regions associated with auditory verbal deficit, and circles indicate areas associated with impaired reading comprehension. Auditory verbal and reading areas overlap through much of the posterior temporal lobe and segregate to some degree in anterior temporal and posterior parietal regions.

owing to the great variability present in naturally occurring lesions, the often incomplete anatomical and/or behavioral descriptions of the data, and the underlying intersubject variability in functional organization. Clinical signs also depend greatly on the amount of time elapsed since the initial injury. As mentioned, for example, the mixture of phonemic and verbal paraphasias observed in Wernicke aphasia evolves to some extent over time, so part A of the figure is nothing more than a general outline. Other data concerning the functional anatomy of Wernicke's aphasia and related syndromes come from functional neuroimaging studies of normal language processing, which are summarized in the next section.

Functional Neuroimaging Studies

As should be clear from the previous section, studies of lesion location are performed with two general aims in mind. The first of these is the more modest: to describe the lesion that produces a clinical syndrome. Like the other aphasias, Wernicke aphasia can be viewed simply as a syndrome—a collection of deficits that tend to occur together—without reference to an underlying theoretical model of how damage produces the syndrome. Research along these lines has focused, for example, on defining the average lesion characteristics associated with the syndrome and how variations from the average are associated with variations in the syndrome. The second aim, a natural outgrowth of the first, involves formulation and testing of an underlying processing model that describes the functional role of each brain region involved in the lesion area. Such models are interesting in their own right and, more important, can lead to a deeper understanding of the syndrome, permitting predictions to be made about the location of a lesion in newly encountered patients, factors that produce variations in the syndrome, and the manner and time course of recovery.

Although much has been learned about underlying brain processes from studying lesions, this approach also has important limitations. The overall

size and exact location of lesions vary considerably across individuals, creating a large number of lesion variables that may or may not be related to the behavioral deficits. As noted earlier, commonly shared features of the vascular supply result in areas of lesion overlap across subjects, independently of any shared deficits. The detection of deficits varies with the method and timing of testing, and with the a priori aims of the researcher. Finally, damage to one subsystem in a distributed processing network may interfere with a wide assortment of behaviors, leading to overlocalization through false attribution of these behaviors to the lesioned area.

Functional imaging of intact human brains provides useful complementary information for the development of neuroanatomically oriented processing models. In contrast to lesion techniques, these methods provide a picture of the full, intact system at work. By experimentally manipulating aspects of the task performed during scanning and recording the regional changes in activation correlated with these manipulations, inferences can be made about the processes carried out in each brain region. By integrating this information with that obtained from lesion studies, it is hoped that a more complete and explicit theory will emerge to account for how damage in specific regions or combinations of regions leads to specific deficits. This section presents a brief overview of PET and fMRI studies of speech and language processing that are relevant to an account of Wernicke aphasia. Where possible, the data are compared and contrasted with information from lesion-deficit correlation studies.

Perception of Speech Sounds

Many PET and functional MRI (fMRI) studies have focused on the neural basis of processing speech sounds. In most such studies, brain activation states were measured during the presentation of speech sounds in contrast to no sounds, a comparison that consistently and robustly activates the STG bilaterally (Binder et al., 2000; Binder et al., 1994b; Dhankhar et al., 1997; Fiez, Raichle, Balota, Tallal, & Petersen, 1996a; Fiez et al., 1995; Hirano et al., 1997; Howard et al., 1992; Jäncke, Shah, Posse,

Grosse-Ryuken, & Müller-Gärtner, 1998; Mazoyer et al., 1993; O'Leary et al., 1996; Petersen, Fox, Posner, Mintun, & Raichle, 1988; Price et al., 1996b; Warburton et al., 1996; Wise et al., 1991). The stimuli used in these experiments included syllables, single words, pseudowords, reversed speech, foreign words, and sentences. Activated areas included Heschl's gyrus, the PT, the dorsal STG anterior to HG (the planum polare and the dorsal temporal pole), the lateral STG, and the superior temporal sulcus. These results fit very well in the long tradition linking speech comprehension with the STG, and many investigators have simply viewed these experiments as revealing activation of "Wernicke's area."

What has sometimes been forgotten in interpreting such results is that speech is a very complex and nuanced acoustic signal, containing a variety of simultaneous and sequential auditory patterns that must be analyzed prior to phoneme or word recognition (Klatt, 1989; Liberman et al., 1967; Oden & Massaro, 1978; Stevens & Blumstein, 1981). These auditory operations include not only the well-known spectral analysis performed by the cochlea and reflected in tonotopic organization of the primary auditory cortex, but also analysis of static spectral shapes and changes in spectral configurations over time, and analysis of temporal asynchronies (see the section on comprehension disturbance). The possibility that considerable neural activity might be required for analysis of these acoustic features has often been overlooked in neuroimaging studies of speech perception, although such neural activity could explain much of the STG activation observed in such studies. More important, it seems likely that such prephonemic auditory analysis constitutes an important and conceptually distinct processing level between primary auditory and word recognition levels. A proposal of this kind was first put forward clearly by Henschen in 1918, although he has received almost no credit for it.[6]

In addition to these purely theoretical concerns, there are aspects of the STG activation results themselves that suggest a prelinguistic, auditory basis

for at least some of the activation. For example, although language functions are believed to be lateralized to the left hemisphere in most people, STG activation by speech sounds occurs bilaterally. Many investigators reported no asymmetry in the degree of left versus right STG activation (Fiez et al., 1995; Hirano et al., 1997; Howard et al., 1992; Jäncke et al., 1998; O'Leary et al., 1996; Warburton et al., 1996; Wise et al., 1991). Others found slightly stronger activation on the left side, although the degree of asymmetry was small (Binder et al., 2000; Mazoyer et al., 1993). Many of the studies examined only passive listening, which might not be expected to fully engage the language system and therefore might explain the lack of leftward lateralization. However, in several studies, adding a language task did not produce greater asymmetry than passive listening (Fiez et al., 1995; Grady et al., 1997; Wise et al., 1991).

The consistent finding of bilateral, symmetrical activation is consistent with an account based on general auditory processing, which would be expected to occur bilaterally. Another observation consistent with this view is that the degree of STG activation is very closely correlated with the amount of auditory information presented, i.e., the number of sounds presented per unit of time (Binder et al., 1994a; Dhankhar et al., 1997; Mummery, Ashburner, Scott, & Wise, 1999; Price et al., 1992; Price et al., 1996b; Wise et al., 1991) and is usually neglible during silent language tasks involving purely visual stimulation (e.g., silent word reading) (Howard et al., 1992; Petersen et al., 1988; Price et al., 1994; Rumsey et al., 1997).

Finally, anatomical studies (Flechsig, 1908; Galaburda & Pandya, 1983; Jones & Burton, 1976; Kaas & Hackett, 1998; Mesulam & Pandya, 1973; Rademacher et al., 1993; von Economo & Horn, 1930) and electrophysiological data from human and nonhuman primates (Baylis et al., 1987; Creutzfeld et al., 1989; Leinonen et al., 1980; Liégeois-Chauvel et al., 1991; Merzenich & Brugge, 1973; Morel et al., 1993; Rauschecker, 1998) are consistent with a unimodal, auditory processing role for most of the STG, particularly the dorsal (HG and PT) and lateral aspects of the gyrus. These observations suggest that much of the STG activation observed during auditory presentation of speech arises from processing the complex auditory information present in these stimuli rather than from engagement of linguistic (phonemic, lexical, or semantic) processes.

In an effort to directly assess the contribution of early auditory processes to STG activation, several research groups have compared activation of the STG by speech sounds with activation by simpler, nonspeech sounds such as noise and tones. These experiments included both passive listening and active, target detection tasks. The consistent finding is that speech and nonspeech sounds produce roughly equivalent activation of the dorsal STG, including HG and PT, in both hemispheres (Belin, Zatorre, Lafaille, Ahad, & Pike, 2000; Binder et al., 2000; Binder et al., 1997; Binder et al., 1996; Démonet et al., 1992; Mummery et al., 1999; Zatorre, Evans, Meyer, & Gjedde, 1992). Indeed, in several studies, tones produced stronger

activation of the PT than speech sounds, particularly when active decision tasks were performed (Binder et al., 1997; Binder et al., 1996; Démonet et al., 1992). These data strongly support the idea that neural activity in the dorsal STG (HG and PT) has more to do with processing acoustic information than linguistic information. Confirmatory support comes from a recent fMRI study of acoustic complexity, in which it was shown that the PT responds more strongly to frequency-modulated tones than to unorganized noise, suggesting that this region plays a role in the analysis of temporally organized acoustic patterns (Binder et al., 2000).

In contrast to these findings for the dorsal STG, more ventral areas, located on the anterolateral STG and within the adjacent superior temporal sulcus, are preferentially activated by speech sounds (figure 9.11). Although bilateral, this activation shows a modest degree of leftward lateralization (Binder et al., 2000; Binder et al., 1997; Démonet et al., 1992; Mummery et al., 1999; Zatorre et al., 1992). The relatively anterior and ventral location of this "speech

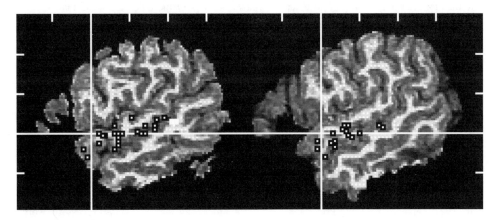

Figure 9.11
Brain locations associated with stronger activation to speech sounds than to non-speech sounds (tones or noise) in five imaging studies (Binder, Frost, Hammeke, Bellgowan, Springer, Kaufman, Possing, 2000; Binder, Frost, Hammeke, Cox, Rao, Prieto, 1997; Demonet et al., 1992; Mummery, Ashbumer, Scott, & Wise, 1999; Zatorre, Evans, Meyer, & Gjedde, 1992). The squares represent activation peaks in standard stereotaxic space. The anterior-posterior (y) and inferior-superior (z) axes of the stereotaxic grid are shown with tick marks at 20-mm intervals. All left and right peaks have been collapsed onto common left and right sagittal planes at x = ±55.

sound region" was initially surprising given the traditional emphasis on the PT and posterior STG as centers for speech comprehension. In contrast to this traditional model, the functional imaging data thus suggest that projections from primary to secondary auditory cortex enabling speech recognition follow an anteroventral rather than a posterior course. Recent anatomical studies in monkeys provide further support for this model by showing two distinct projection systems within the auditory system, one anteriorly directed and presumably supporting the recognition of complex sounds, and the other posteriorly directed and presumably involved in sound localization (Romanski et al., 1999). Also of note, the STS location of these speech sound-processing areas neatly explains several previously documented cases of pure word deafness in which the lesion involved the STS bilaterally while sparing the dorsal STG (Barrett, 1910; Henschen, 1918–1919).

The nature of the processes carried out by this speech sound region, however, remains somewhat uncertain. The fact that speech sounds activate the region more than tones or noise does not necessarily mean that this activation is related to language processing. Because the tone and noise stimuli used in these studies were much less complex from an acoustic standpoint than the speech stimuli, it may be that the increased activation for speech sounds simply represents a more complex level of auditory pattern analysis. This is underscored by the fact that stronger activation is observed in the STS for speech sounds irrespective of whether the sounds are words or nonwords (Binder et al., 2000; Démonet et al., 1992). In fact, activation in this region is not even different for speech and reversed speech (Binder et al., 2000; Dehaene et al., 1997; Hirano et al., 1997; Perani et al., 1996; Price et al., 1996b). Scott et al. addressed this issue by contrasting speech sounds with spectrally rotated speech (Scott, Blank, Rosen, & Wise, 2000). The latter is produced by inverting speech sounds in the frequency domain, thus maintaining their acoustic complexity but rendering the original phonemes mostly unintelligible (Blesser, 1972). The results

show what appears to be a further subdivision within the speech sound region. On the lateral STG, anterolateral to the primary auditory cortex, the responses were as strong for spectrally rotated speech as for normal speech, suggesting processing at an auditory level. Further ventrally, in the STS, the responses were stronger for speech than for spectrally rotated speech, suggesting neural activity related to phoneme recognition.

These findings indicate the existence of a hierarchical processing stream concerned with speech perception that is composed of at least three stages located within the STG and STS. In accord with anatomical and neurophysiological studies of the auditory cortex, the earliest stage involves sensory processors located in primary and belt auditory regions on the superior temporal plane, including the PT, which respond to relatively simple frequency and intensity information (Galaburda & Pandya, 1983; Mendelson & Cynader, 1985; Merzenich & Brugge, 1973; Morel et al., 1993; Phillips & Irvine, 1981; Rauschecker, Tian, Pons, & Mishkin, 1997). Further anterolaterally, on the lateral surface of the STG, are areas that respond to more complex and combinatorial acoustic phenomena, such as configurations of spectral peaks and dynamic spectral and intensity modulations (Rauschecker, 1998; Rauschecker et al., 1997; Tian, Reser, Durham, Kustov, & Rauschecker, 2001). Still further ventrally, within the STS, are cortical regions that appear to respond selectively in the presence of intelligible phonemes (Scott et al., 2000). The anterior and ventral course of this processing stream has been remarked on already.

What is perhaps most strikingly different about this model in comparison with the conventional view of Wernicke's area, however, is that none of these processing stages involve access to words or word meanings. That is, all of the processes so far discussed pertain specifically to recognition of speech sounds rather than comprehension of words. This model thus agrees well with neurolinguistic descriptions of patients with pure word deafness who have bilateral lesions in the STG and/or the STS. These patients have disturbed perception of speech phonemes, but do not have difficulty comprehending word meaning (when tested with visually presented words) or accessing words during speech production.

Processing Word Forms

According to the processing model described earlier and illustrated in schematic form in figure 9.2, comprehension of heard or seen words requires mapping from unimodal sensory representations, such as phonemes or graphemes, to semantic representations. As discussed at points throughout this chapter and illustrated in figure 9.3, the arbitrary and nonlinear nature of these mappings suggests the need for intermediate processing levels that represent combinations of phonemes or graphemes. Theories that envision these combinatorial representations as localized and equivalent to whole words describe them as the "phonological lexicon" and "orthographic lexicon."

In other theories, intermediate levels represent phoneme and letter combinations in a distributed manner with no one-to-one relationship between words and representational units. Common to both of these theoretical positions is the idea that the intermediate levels enable mapping from phoneme or grapheme information to semantics, and that the intermediate levels represent information pertaining to the (phonological or orthographic) structure of words. The neutral expression "word-form processing" captures these commonalities and so will be used to refer to intermediate levels of processing.

Many functional imaging studies have addressed word-form processing using either spoken or printed stimuli. The studies summarized here are those in which brain activation from word or wordlike stimuli was compared with activation from stimuli that were not wordlike. One issue complicating the interpretation of these data is that stimuli can have varying degrees of "wordlikeness" (reflecting, for example, such factors as the frequency of letter combinations, number of orthographic or phonological neighbors, frequency of neighbors, and pronounceability), and many imaging studies do not incorporate any clear metric for this crucial variable. For the most part, however, the contrasting conditions in these studies have involved extremely different stimuli in order to create clear distinctions between stimuli with or without word form.

Another issue complicating many of these experiments is that activation of word-form information may be accompanied by activation of semantic information, particularly when real words are used as stimuli and when subjects are encouraged to process the words for meaning. To avoid this confound, the following discussion focuses on studies in which either (1) stimuli used in the word-form condition were wordlike but were not real words (i.e., were pseudowords), or (2) semantic processing requirements were matched in the word-form and baseline tasks.

In phonological word-form studies, the usual contrast is between spoken words and reversed words (i.e., recordings of spoken words played backward). Although reversed playback of spoken words makes them unrecognizeable as meaningful words, this manipulation does not completely remove phonological structure since subjects reliably report phonemes on hearing such stimuli and there is even a degree of consistency across subjects in the particular phoneme sequences heard (Binder et al., 2000). Indeed, several studies have shown no differences in brain activation by words and reversed words (Binder et al., 2000; Hirano et al., 1997). Other investigators, however, have observed activation differences favoring words (Howard et al., 1992; Perani et al., 1996; Price et al., 1996b). The peak activation foci observed in these word versus reversed speech contrasts are distinctly separate from those in the STG and STS described earlier in association with speech versus nonspeech contrasts. As shown in figure 9.12, the word versus reversed speech peak activations lie in the middle temporal and posterior inferior temporal gyri, areas adjacent to but distinct from the superior temporal auditory cortex. Unlike the speech sound activations observed in the STG and STS, activation in these areas is strongly lateralized to the left hemisphere.

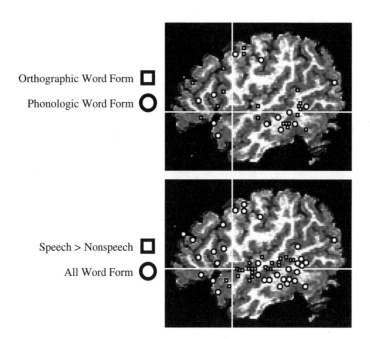

Orthographic Word Form ☐

Phonologic Word Form ◯

Speech > Nonspeech ☐

All Word Form ◯

Figure 9.12
Activation sites associated with word-form processing, almost all of which have been found in the left hemisphere. The top panel shows left hemisphere activation peaks from seven word form experiments (Perani, Dehaene, Grassi, Cohen, Cappa, Dupouz, Fazio, Mehler, 1996; Price, Wise, Warburton et al., 1996; Price et al., 1994; Price, Wise, & Frackowiak, 1996; Tagamets, Novick, Chalmers, & Friedman, 2000). The bottom panel illustrates segregation of these word-form activation foci (circles) from speech perception areas (squares); the latter are also found in the right hemisphere (see figure 9.11).

In orthographic word-form studies, the usual contrast is between words or pseudowords (pronounceable nonwords that look like words, e.g., tweal) and consonant letter strings (Bavelier et al., 1997; Herbster, Mintun, Nebes, & Becker, 1997; Howard et al., 1992; Indefrey et al., 1997; Petersen, Fox, Snyder, & Raichle, 1990; Price et al., 1994; Price, Wise, & Frackowiak, 1996c; Small et al., 1996; Tagamets, Novick, Chalmers, & Friedman, 2000). Consonant strings (e.g., mpfjc) differ from wordlike stimuli in two ways. First, they tend to contain letter combinations that do not occur or occur only infrequently in the language (e.g., mp at the initial position or jc at the final position of mpfjc). These stimuli thus do not have a familiar orthographic

structure and presumably produce only weak activation at the orthographic word-form level. Second, consonant strings in English are typically unpronounceable (except by an effortful insertion of schwa sounds between consonants) and should thus produce only weak activation of phonological word form and output phoneme representations. These two factors are, of course, inextricably linked to some degree. Because of the quasi-regular relationship between graphemes and phonemes, increasing the degree of orthographic structure tends to increase the degree of phonological structure, leading to increased pronounceability.

As shown in figure 9.12, the peak activation foci in studies contrasting orthographically wordlike stimuli with consonant strings have tended to cluster in the posterior MTG, the posterior STS, and the posterior ITG (Bavelier et al., 1997; Herbster et al., 1997; Howard et al., 1992; Indefrey et al., 1997; Price et al., 1994; Price et al., 1996c; Small et al., 1996; Tagamets et al., 2000). Similar activation peaks were observed in these studies whether the word-form stimuli used were real words or meaningless pseudowords, a finding that lends credence to the notion that the processing level or levels being identified are presemantic in nature. Like the activation sites observed in spoken word-form studies, these foci have almost all been in the left hemisphere.

One striking aspect of these results is the considerable overlap between regions identified in spoken and printed word-form studies (figure 9.12). This suggests that the phonological word-form system used to map input phonemes to semantics and the orthographic word-form system used to map input graphemes to semantics are at least partially overlapping in the posterior MTG and ITG. Another possible explanation for this overlap is that both the spoken and written word-form conditions activate representations of output phonemes. These representations are activated explicitly in tasks requiring the repetition of heard speech or reading aloud of orthographic stimuli, but are probably also engaged automatically whenever the brain is presented with stimuli that have a phonological structure (Macleod, 1991; Van Orden, 1987). Thus, some of the overlap in figure 9.12 could be due to activation of output phoneme representations or intermediate levels that lead to output phonemes.

Semantic Processing

Semantic processes are those concerned with storing, retrieving, and using knowledge about the world, and are a key component of such ubiquitous behaviors as naming, comprehending and formulating language, problem solving, planning, and thinking. Our focus here is on tasks involving comprehension of word meaning. As should be clear by now, understanding the meaning of words

is a complex process that engages multiple representational stages and nonlinear transformations. The following review summarizes functional imaging studies that attempted to isolate the final stage of this processing sequence, in which semantic representations are activated (Binder et al., 1999; Chee, O'Craven, Bergida, Rosen, & Savoy, 1999; Démonet et al., 1992; Mummery, Patterson, Hodges, & Price, 1998; Poldrack et al., 1999; Price, Moore, Humphreys, & Wise, 1997; Pugh et al., 1996). The semantic tasks used in these studies required that meaning-based judgments be made about words. These tasks included deciding if a word represented a concept from a particular category (e.g., living or nonliving, foreign or domestic, and abstract or concrete), deciding whether two words were related in meaning, or deciding which of two words was closer in meaning to a third word.

The identification of brain activation related to semantic access during such tasks requires the same sort of subtraction strategy employed in the speech perception and word-form experiments just reviewed. For tasks engaging semantic access, the appropriate control condition is one in which identical sensory, phoneme or grapheme, and word-form processing occurs, but without activation of (or with less activation of) semantic information.

Two types of experimental design have been used. In the first, control stimuli are pseudowords (either spoken or written), and the control task involves a judgment about the phonological structure (word form) of the pseudowords. These control tasks have included deciding whether pseudowords contain a target phoneme (Binder et al., 1999; Démonet et al., 1992), whether two written pseudowords rhyme (Pugh et al., 1996), and whether a written pseudoword has two syllables (Poldrack et al., 1999). Because the words and pseudowords are matched on low-level sensory and word-form characteristics, differences in the activation level between conditions are likely to be related to semantic processes. Activated areas in these studies (i.e., those in which activation was greater for the semantic condition than for the control condition) are shown, for those studies that reported activation peaks, in figure 9.13. These areas included the left angular gyrus, the left superior frontal gyrus, the left inferior frontal gyrus, the left fusiform gyrus and parahippocampus, and the left posterior cingulate cortex.

The second type of experiment is similar, except that the control task involves a judgment about the phonological structure of words rather than pseudowords. This design provides a tighter control for word-form processing because even carefully constructed pseudowords may not be as wordlike in structure as real words. For theorists who embrace the idea of localized whole-word representations that are accessed only in the presence of real words, using real words as control stimuli is necessary in order to "subtract" activation due to lexical (as opposed to semantic) processing. A potential disadvantage of this design is the possibility that using real words in the control condition may result in some degree of automatic activation of semantic information, even when the task being performed is not semantic (Binder & Price, 2001). In all of these studies, the control task required the subjects to judge whether the word contained a particular number of syllables (Chee et al., 1999; Mummery et al., 1998; Poldrack et al., 1999; Price et al., 1997).

As shown in figure 9.13, the activations in these studies were nearly identical to those observed in the experiments using pseudoword control stimuli, and included the angular gyrus, the superior frontal gyrus, the inferior frontal gyrus, the ventral temporal cortex, the MTG and ITG, and the posterior cingulate cortex in the left hemisphere. It should be noted that in two of these studies only the frontal lobe was imaged (Demb et al., 1995; Poldrack et al., 1999).

Although they are not perfectly consistent, these results indicate a distributed group of left hemisphere brain regions engaged specifically during activation and retrieval of semantic information. One of the more consistently identified areas (in four of the five studies in which it was imaged) is the angular gyrus (Brodmann area 39). Brodmann area 39 is a phylogenetically recent brain area that is greatly expanded in the human relative to the nonhuman primate brain (Geschwind, 1965). It is situated strategically between visual, auditory, and somatosensory centers, making it one of the more reasonable candidates for a multimodal convergence area involved in storing or processing very abstract representations of sensory experience and word meaning.

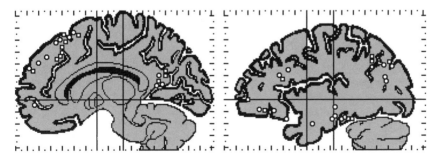

Figure 9.13
Activation peaks where a semantic task produced stronger activation than a phonological task in seven imaging studies of semantic processing (Binder, Frost, Hammeke, Bellgowan, Rao, Cox, 1999; Chee, O'Craven, Bergida, Rosen, & Savoy, 1999; Demonet et al., 1992; Mummery, Patterson, Hodges, & Price, 1998; Poldrack et al., 1999 (two studies); Price, Moore, Humphreys, & Wise, 1997). Squares indicate experiments using pseudowords in the phonological task; sites marked by circles are from experiments using words in the phonological task.

Other areas frequently identified in these semantic studies include the dorsal prefrontal cortex in the superior frontal gyrus and sulcus (seven of seven studies), the ventral temporal cortex in the fusiform and parahippocampal gyri (four of five studies), the inferior frontal gyrus (four of seven studies), and the posterior cingulate cortex and adjacent ventral precuneus (three of five studies). These regions are well outside the area damaged in Wernicke's aphasia and so are not discussed further here (see Binder and Price, 2001, for a discussion of these and related results).

In a few studies, activation foci were observed in the left MTG and ITG (Chee et al., 1999; Mummery et al., 1998; Price et al., 1997), suggesting that a subset of this ventrolateral temporal region may subserve semantic-level processes in addition to word-form processes. Several functional imaging studies have demonstrated enhanced activation of the posterior MTG when subjects identify objects in the tool category compared with objects from other categories, and when subjects generate verbs relative to generating nouns (Martin, 2001). The proximity of these activation sites to the visual motion-processing region (human "area MT") has led to speculation that the posterior MTG may store semantic representations related to visual motion, which are particularly salient semantic features for manipulable objects and verbs (Martin, 2001).

Phonological Production

The functional imaging studies discussed to this point have concerned transformations from spoken or visual word input to semantics, that is, the pathways engaged during comprehension of speech and written text. Speech production, another language process impaired in Wernicke's aphasia, has received some attention in functional imaging studies. As discussed earlier, deficits of ordered phoneme selection, which result in phonemic paraphasia, are the hallmark of posterior perisylvian lesions damaging the posterior STG and STS, the posterior insula, or the ventral supramarginal gyrus. On the basis of this correlation, a reasonable pre-

diction is that these regions should show activation under task conditions that engage output phoneme selection relative to conditions that do not activate output phonemes.

One source of information on this question has already been mentioned: studies contrasting pronounceable with unpronounceable letter strings. As shown in figure 9.12, activation peaks in these studies were found in the posterior left MTG and ITG, but also involved the posterior left STS. In fact, some studies have shown particularly strong effects in the posterior STS (Bavelier et al., 1997; Howard et al., 1992; Indefrey et al., 1997; Price et al., 1994; Small et al., 1996). As noted earlier, however, it is difficult to attribute the posterior STS activation specifically to processing of output phonemes because the pronounceable and unpronounceable items in these studies also differed along orthographic dimensions. Findings from the auditory word-form comparisons, however, provide indirect support for such an interpretation. These studies, in which spoken words were contrasted with reversed forms of the words, reveal activation of the left MTG and ITG, but do not generally show differential activation in the posterior STS. If we assume that both normal and reversed speech input produce some degree of activation of output phonemes (i.e., that isolated phonemes may be perceived in these stimuli even if they do not have word form), a contrast between these stimuli would not be expected to show activation of output phoneme systems.

Other evidence corroborating a specific role for the posterior left STS in processing output phonemes comes from a study by Wise et al. (2001). These authors reported common activation of the posterior left STS in three experiments. In the first of these, passive listening to words was contrasted with passive listening to signal-modulated noise (white noise that was amplitude modulated using the amplitude contours of speech sounds). Regions selectively activated by words included the anterior STS and the anterolateral STG bilaterally, which is consistent with other speech-nonspeech comparisons (see figure 9.11). In the left hemisphere, this activation spread posteriorly to involve the posterior STS. In the second experiment, posterior left STS activation was observed during a silent word-generation task ("think of as many words as possible that are related to a cue word") relative to a resting state. Other temporoparietal regions activated in this contrast included the adjacent posterior left STG, the posterior left MTG, and the left supramarginal gyrus. These results are consistent with several other studies that showed posterior STG and/or STS activation during word generation contrasted with rest (Fiez et al., 1996a; Hickok et al., 2000). In the final and most compelling experiment, the subjects generated words either aloud or silently at various rates that were controlled by varying the rate of presentation of cue words. The analysis searched for brain regions in which the activation level was correlated with the combined rate of hearing and internally generating words. Only the posterior left STS showed such a correlation.

The selection of output phonemes may lead to overt speech production by movement of the vocal tract, or to some form of "internal speech" without articulation or phonation. If output phonemes are represented in the posterior left STS, then overt speech production must involve an interface between this brain region and speech articulation mechanisms located in the inferior frontal lobe. The lesion literature on phonemic paraphasia suggests that this interface exists within the cortical and subcortical pathways lying between the posterior STS and the inferior frontal lobe, i.e., in the posterior STG, supramarginal gyrus, and posterior insula. It is likely that this interface also involves proprioceptive and other somatosensory input from the adjacent inferior parietal cortex, which provides dynamic feedback concerning position and movement of the vocal tract (Luria, 1966). For longer utterances, it may also be necessary to maintain a short-term record of the phoneme sequence to be uttered so that this information does not fade while articulation is in progress (Caplan & Waters, 1992). This "phonological buffer" is particularly implicated in internal speech and in tasks in which the phoneme sequence must be maintained in con-

sciousness for an extended period without overt articulation.

Although little convergent data regarding this phoneme-to-articulation pathway are yet available, a few imaging results are suggestive. Paus et al. (Paus, Perry, Zatorre, Worsley, & Evans, 1996) had subjects whisper two syllables repeatedly at varying rates. Auditory input was held constant across conditions by presenting continuous white noise that masked any perception of speech. The investigators searched for brain regions in which the activation level was correlated with the rate of speech articulation. One area showing this pattern was a small focus in the left planum temporale. Activation in the left precentral gyrus, a motor area associated with speech production, also varied with rate. The authors suggested that the left planum temporale and left premotor cortex function together during speech production, possibly as an interactive feed-forward and feedback system.

Wise et al. (2001) also searched for brain regions that are activated during speech production independent from auditory input. Their subjects were given a phrase ("buy Bobby a poppy") and asked to (1) say the phrase repeatedly aloud; (2) mouth the phrase with lip movement but no sound production; (3) sound out the phrase by substituting the syllable "uh" for the original syllables, thereby activating diaphragm, vocal cord, and glottal components of production without lip or tongue articulators; and (4) internally vocalize the phrase repeatedly without movement or sound. The authors contrasted the first three conditions, all of which involved overt motor production, with the internal vocalization condition. Similar to the study by Paus et al., activated regions included the left ventral motor cortex and a small focus in the posterior left sylvian fissure (coordinates −42, −40, +20). This focus is at the most posterior and medial aspect of the sylvian fissure, at the junction of the planum temporale, the supramarginal gyrus, and the posterior insula. It is worth noting that the posterior left STS, which we have suggested may be involved in representation of output phonemes, was not identified in this study, a result predicted by the fact that all four conditions in this experiment (including internal vocalization) would have activated output phoneme codes.

A third study on this topic was made by Hickok et al. (2000), who examined posterior STG activation during a silent picture-naming task. Many other studies of picture naming have not shown activation of this region, possibly because the task involved internal speech without articulation (Smith et al., 1996) or because a control task was used that also involved overt articulation (Murtha, Chertkow, Beauregard, & Evans, 1999; Price, Moore, Humphreys, Frackowiak, & Friston, 1996; Zelkowicz, Herbster, Nebes, Mintun, & Becker, 1998). In the study by Hickok et al. (2000), the subjects were asked to name pictures silently, but with overt articulation movements, while the baseline task—passive viewing of nonsense images—did not require covert or overt speech. Two activation foci were identified in the left planum temporale. Together, the studies by Paus et al. (1994), Wise et al. (2000), and Hickok et al. suggest that the left planum temporale and adjacent areas (SMG, posterior insula) are activated in concert with left premotor and ventral motor areas specifically during speech production (and not during internal speech without motor movements). Although the specific processes carried out by this region are not yet clear, the findings are consistent with a role in mapping output phonemes to motor programs.

Finally, there is some evidence that the ventral supramarginal gyrus plays a role in the short-term storage of phonological information. This region was activated bilaterally when subjects held a string of letters in memory compared with a task that did not require short-term memory (Paulesu, Frith, & Frackowiak, 1993). In another study, the ventral left supramarginal gyrus was more active during a phoneme detection task that involved multisyllabic nonwords (e.g., /redozabu/) than during a semantic decision task on words (Démonet, Price, Wise, & Frackowiak, 1994a). If the phoneme task makes a greater demand on short-term memory for phoneme sequences than does the semantic task, this finding is consistent with a short-term memory

role for the left supramarginal gyrus. Several other studies intended to test this hypothesis, however, have not shown activation of the ventral supramarginal cortex during short-term verbal maintenance tasks (Fiez et al., 1996b; Jonides et al., 1998).

Still other evidence suggests that the ventral supramarginal gyrus is activated as strongly by holding a tone series in memory as by holding a phoneme series (Binder et al., 1997; Démonet et al., 1992; Démonet, Price, Wise, & Frackowiak, 1994b). It may be that the supramarginal gyrus is sensitive to stimuli composed of smaller elements and to tasks that require a parsing of the stimulus into these elements. Such parsing might aid in the short-term storage of long utterances and unfamiliar utterances (e.g., nonwords or low-frequency words) during both comprehension and production tasks.

Conclusions and Future Directions

Wernicke aphasia is a multifaceted syndrome, the principal behavioral characteristics of which include impaired speech comprehension, impaired reading comprehension, impaired word retrieval, paraphasic speech with both phoneme and word selection errors, and paragraphia. The paraphasic and paragraphic errors are generally observed in all output tasks, including propositional speech, writing, reading, naming, repeating, and writing to dictation. Phoneme and grapheme perception are generally intact, as are speech articulation and speech prosody. Variations on this typical profile may occur. Comprehension and production deficits may differentially affect spoken or written language; paraphasic errors may be predominantly phonemic or verbal; and reading and writing deficits may primarily affect nonwords or exception words.

Wernicke aphasics retain the ability to discriminate between phonemes (i.e., to discern when two phonemes are identical or different), indicating that the sensory perceptual mechanism for speech sounds is, for the most part, intact (Blumstein, 1994). Functional imaging studies clearly place this speech perceptual mechanism in the middle and anterior STG and STS (figure 9.11), which would seem to present a paradox because this area is often damaged in Wernicke patients. The inescapable conclusion is that Wernicke aphasics retain the ability to distinguish phonemes because this perceptual system exists bilaterally, and the undamaged right STG and STS are sufficient to carry out the task. This model is consistent with both the functional imaging data, which show bilateral STG and STS responses to speech sounds, and with the lesion literature on pure word deafness. In this syndrome, which is characterized by a relatively isolated speech perceptual deficit, the causative lesion nearly always involves the STG or STS bilaterally. This model is also consistent with evidence from intracarotid amobarbital studies showing that during left hemisphere anesthesia, the isolated right hemisphere can still accurately perform phoneme discriminations (Boatman et al., 1998). Although these early speech perceptual mechanisms are represented bilaterally, this does not necessarily imply that they function identically in the two hemispheres. Functional imaging studies have shown varying degrees of asymmetry in STG activation during speech sound perception tasks (Binder et al., 2000; Démonet et al., 1992; Mazoyer et al., 1993; Mummery et al., 1999; Scott et al., 2000; Zatorre et al., 1992), but a full explanation of these asymmetries awaits further study.

In contrast to these sensory perceptual mechanisms, the speech comprehension deficit in Wernicke aphasia represents an inability to reliably access semantic representations associated with phonemes. For example, Wernicke aphasics are deficient in associating phonemes with their written letter equivalents and in associating spoken words with meanings. The processing loci where damage could induce such a deficit could include either intermediate phonological word-form representations in the mapping from input phonemes to semantics, damage to the semantic representations themselves, or both.

While some researchers have argued for intact semantic representations in Wernicke aphasia, other evidence points to a disturbance within semantics.

Functional imaging data suggest that the left MTG and posterior ITG are likely candidates for a phonological word-form processing region. This anatomical model is broadly consistent with the lesion data in two respects. First, unilateral lesions confined to the left STG, which commonly produce conduction aphasia, do not appear to cause word comprehension deficits. Second, lesions that spread beyond the left STG to involve the MTG do cause such deficits, and the severity and long-term recovery of word comprehension appear to depend on the degree of MTG damage. Functional imaging and lesion studies indicate that the left ventral temporal lobe (fusiform gyrus, parahippocampus, ITG, and posterior MTG) and the left angular gyrus are nodes in a distributed system involved in processing and storing semantic representations. Lesions in Wernicke's aphasia commonly involve the left angular gyrus and the posterior MTG, which could account for a disturbance at the semantic level in at least some patients.

Thus, the model proposed here accounts for the speech comprehension disturbance in Wernicke's aphasia by damage to a phonological word-form processor located in the left MTG and posterior ITG, which interrupts the processing stream connecting input phoneme representations in the anterior STS with semantic representations in the left angular gyrus and ventral temporal lobe (figure 9.11–9.13). Damage to the left angular gyrus undoubtedly contributes to the problem by partially damaging the distributed system of semantic representations on which comprehension ultimately depends.

The model accounts for reading comprehension deficits in a similar manner. Functional imaging studies suggest that the posterior left MTG and ITG also play a role in orthographic word-form processing, linking input grapheme codes (processed in the posterior ventral temporal lobe) with semantic representations in the left angular gyrus and more anterior ventral temporal regions. The reading comprehension disturbance in Wernicke's aphasia is thus due to combined damage to the orthographic word-form system in the posterior left MTG and to semantic representations in the left angular gyrus.

Isolated damage to the left angular gyrus may produce more severe deficits of reading comprehension than of speech comprehension ("alexia with agraphia"), a finding difficult to account for on the basis of currently available functional imaging data. One possible explanation is that the orthographic word-form system may project primarily to the angular gyrus, while the phonological word-form system projects more widely to the angular gyrus and ventral temporal semantic regions. The result is that reading comprehension is more dependent on the integrity of the angular gyrus than is speech comprehension. Conversely, isolated lesions of the middle and anterior left temporal lobe may produce more severe deficits of speech comprehension than of reading comprehension. This pattern suggests that the pathway from input phonemes to semantics is organized somewhat anteriorly in the MTG and ITG relative to the pathway from input graphemes to semantics. These conclusions are based on a relatively small body of lesion data and so must be regarded as tentative.

Further studies using functional imaging or lesion correlation methods combined with carefully matched phoneme-semantic and grapheme-semantic tasks are needed to clarify the extent of functional and anatomical overlap between these systems. An improved understanding of the intrinsic organization of the semantic system itself, currently an area of intense study by researchers using functional imaging, lesion correlation, and computational modeling techniques, will also aid in understanding the various patterns of comprehension deficit seen in patients with temporal and parietal lesions.

Paraphasia represents a disturbance in mapping from semantic codes to output phonemes. Wernicke aphasics make a mixture of word- and phoneme-level errors, and interactive neural network models of speech production suggest that such mixed error patterns are generally to be expected (Dell et al., 1997). However, there is evidence that isolated posterior perisylvian lesions may produce exclusively phonemic errors, whereas lesions in ventral temporal areas may cause a preponderance of semantic errors. This suggests that word and phoneme selection errors may have a somewhat distinct functional and anatomical basis. One proposal is that lesions confined to the output phoneme level cause relatively isolated phoneme errors (Hillis et al., 1999). Conversely, lesions confined to the semantic level may primarily disrupt word selection while sparing phoneme selection. This account, together with the lesion data just cited, is in good agreement with available functional imaging data, which suggest that output phoneme representations are processed in the posterior perisylvian cortex (the STS and STG), while semantic representations are localized in ventral temporal zones.

The early success in modeling such paraphasic syndromes as varying combinations of representational and transmission defects supports more widespread application of this approach. In particular, modeling error patterns using local rather than global lesions, which so far has been attempted in only a few patients, may offer functionally and biologically plausible accounts of paraphasia at a level of precision previously unknown.

The processes involved in spelling and writing have been less well studied with functional imaging, and proposals concerning their anatomical basis remain rather speculative. Isolated paragraphia without paraphasia has been linked to posterior and dorsal parietal injury, but writing disturbances have been observed with lesions in a variety of other parietal and temporal lobe locations. Writing impairments involving phoneme-to-grapheme translation (phonological dysgraphia) are closely associated with damage to the supramarginal gyrus. The actual motor production of graphemes, like the motor production of phonemes, is likely to be a complex process involving the coordination of output grapheme, motor sequencing, sensory feedback, and short-term memory systems. Some of these pathways may well involve the inferior parietal cortex and so might be damaged in Wernicke's aphasia, further contributing to the writing disturbance in many cases.

According to the account given here, Wernicke's aphasia is far from being a simple, unitary disturbance of the sound-word image or of the comprehension center. Rather, some components of the syndrome reflect a central deficit that disrupts the translational processes to and from semantics, whereas the phonemic paraphasia component reflects a more peripheral disturbance involving phoneme selection and phoneme-to-articulation mapping. This distinction is made clearer by considering the related posterior aphasia syndromes of transcortical sensory aphasia and conduction aphasia. The former, according to the current model, results from a lesion at the word-form or semantic level, disrupting processes involving word meaning, but sparing those involving phoneme selection and production. In contrast, conduction aphasia results from damage to the phoneme output pathway, with sparing of word-form and semantic processes. Wernicke's aphasia, simply put, consists of the combination of these syndromes and results from a larger lesion that encompasses both lexical-semantic and phoneme output systems.

Notes

1. "The uneducated man with little practice in reading understands the written word only when he hears himself say it. The scholar, practiced since childhood, skims over a page and understands its meaning without becoming conscious of individual words. The former will show symptoms of alexia as well as aphasia, while the latter, in striking contrast to his inability to understand speech, will be able to understand all written material." (Wernicke, 1874/1968, pp. 53–54.)

2. Intermediate units, often referred to as *hidden units* in neural network parlance, are necessary whenever there are unpredictable relationships between adjacent representational levels. A simple example relevant to semantics and phonology are the four words mother, father, woman, and man (Dell et al., 1997). In attempting to map from semantics to phonology, there is no simple mapping that predicts whether the word in question should begin with the phoneme /m/ on the basis of the semantic features /female/ and /parent/. In this example, /m/ is the correct phoneme

choice if the concept includes both of these semantic features (mother) or neither (man), but not if it includes only one of the features, which makes the mapping formally equivalent to an exclusive-OR function. Exclusive-OR and other "linearly inseparable" mappings require an intermediate layer of hidden nodes between the levels to be mapped (Ackley et al., 1985; Hornik et al., 1989; Minsky & Papert, 1969). The intermediate units capture information about combinations of active nodes in the adjacent layers, allowing mappings to occur on the basis of conjunctions of features (for a review see Rumelhart, McClelland, & PDP Group, 1986).

Each node in the intermediate level can contain information about many feature conjunctions, and each possible conjunction can be represented across many intermediate nodes. Similarly, the intermediate nodes connecting phoneme and semantic layers in the model may simply carry distributed information about conjunctions of semantic and phonological features, and may thus bear little resemblance to the conventional notion of whole-word entries in a lexicon.

3. Although the nodes at the lemma level are represented in figure 9.6 by words, this was done for the sake of simplicity and is not meant to imply that there are necessarily discrete representations of words (or phonemes or phonetic features, for that matter) in the brain. On the contrary, as previously mentioned, some theorists have explicitly held that word representations are distributed across many nodes (Plaut et al., 1996; Seidenberg & McClelland, 1989). In this sense, the lemma level is simply an intermediate layer that permits the mapping between semantics and phonology to occur (see note 2).

4. Phonetic features are essentially the articulatory elements that define a given phoneme (Ladefoged & Maddieson, 1996). For example, the set of features defining the phoneme /b/ include bilabial (referring to the fact that it is produced at the lips), stop (produced by sudden opening of the vocal tract), and voiced (produced with the vocal cords vibrating).

5. "Now, under no circumstances can a direct path be available from the sense images that form the concept to the motor center, over which writing movements could be innervated while the sound images were circumvented." (Wernicke, 1874/1968, p. 57.)

6. "By clinical observation the existence of two forms of word-deafness, the word-sound-deafness and the word-comprehension-deafness, is proved. Consequently there exist two centres: (1) of word-sound, (2) of word-

comprehension. In consequence of this theory, we ought to accept three forms of word-deafness:

1. A *pseudo-word-deafness*, essentially only a form of deafness . . .

2. *Perceptive word-deafness*, a consequence of the destruction of the centre for word-sounds in T1 [STG] or of the conduction between Ttr [Heschl's gyrus] and T1 or of the conduction between T1 and the center for comprehension of words . . .

3. *Associative word-deafness* with troubles of the internal word, also of spontaneous speech, as a consequence of the destruction of the centre of word-comprehension, which is probably situated in T2 and T3.

The confusion about this matter—the real nature of word-deafness—is very remarkable, and difficult to understand. This confusion is, after my opinion, a consequence of an erroneous localisation and limitation of the hearing centre in relation to the word-centre, the authors localizing those to the same surface in the temporal lobe." (Henschen, 1918–1919, pp. 440–441).

References

Ackley, D. H., Hinton, G. E., & Sejnowski, T. J. (1985). A learning algorithm for Boltzmann machines. *Cognitive Science*, 9, 147–169.

Alajouanine, T. (1956). Verbal realization in aphasia. *Brain*, 79, 1–28.

Alexander, M. P., & Benson, D. F. (1993). The aphasias and related disturbances. In R. J. Joynt (Ed.), *Clinical neurology* (pp. 1–58). Philadelphia: J. B. Lipincott.

Alexander, M. P., Friedman, R. B., Loverso, F., & Fischer, R. S. (1992). Lesion localization of phonological agraphia. *Brain and Language*, 43, 83–95.

Alexander, M. P., Hiltbrunner, B., & Fischer, R. S. (1989). Distributed anatomy of transcortical sensory aphasia. *Archives of Neurology 46*, 885–892.

Allport, A., MacKay, D. G., & Prinz, W. (1987). *Language perception and production: Relationships between listening, speaking, reading and writing*. London: Academic Press.

Allport, D. A. (1984). Speech production and comprehension: One lexicon or two. In W. Prinz & A. F. Sanders (Eds.), *Cognition and motor processes* (pp. 209–228). Berlin: Springer-Verlag.

Allport, D. A., & Funnell, E. (1981). Components of the mental lexicon. *Philosophical Transactions of the Royal Society of London, Ser. B*, 295, 379–410.

Anderson, J. M., Gilmore, R., Roper, S., Crosson, B., Bauer, R. M., Nadeau, S., et al. (1999). Conduction aphasia and the arcuate fasciculus: A reexamination of the Wernicke-Geschwind model. *Brain and Language*, 70, 1–12.

Baars, B. J., Motley, M. T., & MacKay, D. G. (1975). Output editing for lexical status from artificially elicited slips of the tongue. *Journal of Verbal Learning and Verbal Behavior*, 14, 382–391.

Barrett, A. M. (1910). A case of pure word-deafness with autopsy. *Journal of Nervous and Mental Disease*, 37(2), 73–92.

Basso, A., Casati, G., & Vignolo, L. A. (1977). Phonemic identification defect in aphasia. *Cortex*, 13, 85–95.

Basso, A., Lecours, A. R., Moraschini, S., & Vanier, M. (1985). Anatomoclinical correlations of the aphasia as defined through computerized tomography: Exceptions. *Brain and Language*, 26, 201–229.

Basso, A., Taborelli, A., & Vignolo, L. A. (1978). Dissociated disorders of speaking and writing in aphasia. *Journal of Neurology, Neurosurgery, and Psychiatry*, 41, 556–563.

Bavelier, D., Corina, D., Jezzard, P., Padmanabhan, S., Clark, V. P., Karni, A., Prinster, A., Braun, A., Lalwani, A., Rauschecker, J. P., Turner, R., & Neville, H. (1997). Sentence reading: A functional MRI study at 4 tesla. *Journal of Cognitive Neuroscience*, 9, 664–686.

Baylis, G. C., Rolls, E. T., & Leonard, C. M. (1987). Functional subdivisions of the temporal lobe neocortex. *Journal of Neuroscience*, 7, 330–342.

Becker, S., Moscovitch, M., Behrmann, M., & Joordens, S. (1997). Long-term semantic priming: A computational account and empirical evidence. *Journal of Experimental Psychology: Learning, Memory, and Cognition*, 23, 1059–1082.

Belin, P., Zatorre, R. J., Lafaille, P., Ahad, P., & Pike, B. (2000). Voice-selective areas in human auditory cortex. *Nature*, 403, 309–312.

Benson, D. F. (1979). *Aphasia, alexia and agraphia*. New York: Churchill Livingstone.

Benson, D. F., & Geschwind, N. (1969). The alexias. In P. J. Vinken & G. W. Bruyn (Eds.), *Handbook of clinical neurology* (pp. 112–140). Amsterdam: North-Holland.

Benson, D. F., Sheremata, W. A., Bouchard, R., Segarra, J. M., Price, D., & Geschwind, N. (1973). Conduction aphasia. A clinicopathological study. *Archives of Neurology, 28,* 339–346.

Besner, D., Twilley, L., McCann, R. S., & Seergobin, K. (1990). On the association between connectionism and data: Are a few words necessary? *Psychological Review, 97,* 432–446.

Best, W. (1996). When racquets are baskets but baskets are biscuits, where do the words come from? A single-case study of formal paraphasic errors in aphasia. *Cognitive Neuropsychology, 13,* 443–480.

Binder, J. R., Frost, J. A., Hammeke, T. A., Bellgowan, P. S. F., Rao, S. M., & Cox, R. W. (1999). Conceptual processing during the conscious resting state: A functional MRI study. *Journal of Cognitive Neuroscience, 11*(1), 80–93.

Binder, J. R., Frost, J. A., Hammeke, T. A., Rao, S. M., & Cox, R. W. (1996). Function of the left planum temporale in auditory and linguistic processing. *Brain, 119,* 1239–1247.

Binder, J. R., Frost, J. A., Hammeke, T. A., Cox, R. W., Rao, S. M., & Prieto, T. (1997). Human brain language areas identified by functional MRI. *Journal of Neuroscience, 17*(1), 353–362.

Binder, J. R., Frost, J. A., Hammeke, T. A., Bellgowan, P. S. F., Springer, J. A., Kaufman, J. N., & Possing, E. T. (2000). Human temporal lobe activation by speech and nonspeech sounds. *Cerebral Cortex, 10,* 512–528.

Binder, J. R., & Price, C. J. (2001). Functional imaging of language. In R. Cabeza & A. Kingstone (Eds.), *Handbook of functional neuroimaging of cognition* (pp. 187–251). Cambridge, MA: MIT Press.

Binder, J. R., Rao, S. M., Hammeke, T. A., Frost, J. A., Bandettini, P. A., & Hyde, J. S. (1994a). Effects of stimulus rate on signal response during functional magnetic resonance imaging of auditory cortex. *Cognitive Brain Research, 2,* 31–38.

Binder, J. R., Rao, S. M., Hammeke, T. A., Yetkin, Y. Z., Jesmanowicz, A., Bandettini, P. A., Wong, E. C., Estkowski, L. D., Goldstein, M. D., Haughton, V. M., & Hyde, J. S. (1994b). Functional magnetic resonance imaging of human auditory cortex. *Annals of Neurology, 35,* 662–672.

Blanken, G. (1990). Formal paraphasias: A single case study. *Brain and Language, 38,* 534–554.

Blesser, B. (1972). Speech perception under conditions of spectral transformation: I. Phonetic characteristics. *Journal of Speech and Hearing Research, 15,* 5–41.

Blumstein, S. E. (1973). *A phonological investigation of aphasic speech.* The Hague: Mouton.

Blumstein, S. E. (1994). Impairments of speech production and perception in aphasia. *Philosophical Transactions of the Royal Society of London, Ser. B, 346,* 29–36.

Blumstein, S. E., Baker, E., & Goodglass, H. (1977). Phonological factors in auditory comprehension in aphasia. *Neuropsychologia, 15,* 19–30.

Blumstein, S. E., Burton, M., Baum, S., Waldstein, R., & Katz, D. (1994). The role of lexical status on the phonetic categorization of speech in aphasia. *Brain and Language, 46,* 181–197.

Blumstein, S. E., Cooper, W. E., Zurif, E., & Caramazza, A. (1977). The perception and production of voice-onset time in aphasia. *Neuropsychologia, 15,* 371–383.

Blumstein, S. E., Milberg, W., & Shrier, R. (1982). Semantic processing in aphasia: Evidence from an auditory lexical decision task. *Brain and Language, 17,* 301–315.

Blumstein, S. E., Tartter, V. C., Nigro, G., & Statlender, S. (1984). Acoustic cues for the perception of place of articulation in aphasia. *Brain and Language; 22,* 128–149.

Boatman, D., Hart, J., Lesser, R. P., Honeycutt, N., Anderson, N. B., Miglioretti, D., & Gordon, B. (1998). Right hemisphere speech perception revealed by amobarbital injection and electrical interference. *Neurology, 51,* 458–464.

Bogen, J. E., & Bogen, G. M. (1976). Wernicke's region— where is it? *Annals of the New York Academy of Science, 290,* 834–843.

Boller, F. (1973). Destruction of Wernicke's area without language disturbance. A fresh look at crossed aphasia. *Neuropsychologia, 11,* 243–246.

Brookshire, R. H. (1972). Visual and auditory sequencing by aphasic subjects. *Journal of Communication Disorders, 5,* 259–269.

Buchman, A. S., Garron, D. C., Trost-Cardamone, J. E., Wichter, M. D., & Schwartz, D. (1986). Word deafness: One hundred years later. *Journal of Neurology, Neurosurgery, and Psychiatry, 49,* 489–499.

Buckingham, H. W. (1980). On correlating aphasic errors with slips-of-the-tongue. *Applied Psycholinguistics, 1,* 199–220.

Buckingham, H. W., & Kertesz, A. (1976). *Neologistic jargon aphasia.* Amsterdam: Swets & Zeitlinger.

Buckingham, H. W., & Rekart, D. M. (1979). Semantic paraphasia. *Journal of Communication Disorders*, *12*, 197–209.

Butterworth, B. (1979). Hesitation and the production of verbal paraphasias and neologisms in jargon aphasia. *Brain and Language*, *8*, 133–161.

Caplan, D., Gow, D., & Makris, N. (1995). Analysis of lesions by MRI in stroke patients with acoustic-phonetic processing deficits. *Neurology*, *45*, 293–298.

Caplan, D., & Waters, G. (1992). Issues arising regarding the nature and consequences of reproduction conduction aphasia. In S. E. Kohn (Ed.), *Conduction aphasia* (pp. 117–149). Hillsdale, NJ: Lawrence Erlbaum Associates.

Cappa, S., Cavallotti, G., & Vignolo, L. A. (1981). Phonemic and lexical errors in fluent aphasia: Correlation with lesion site. *Neuropsychologia*, *19*, 171–177.

Caramazza, A. (1988). Some aspects of language processing revealed through the analysis of acquired aphasia: The lexical system. *Annual Review of Neuroscience*, *11*, 395–421.

Caramazza, A., Berndt, R. S., & Basili, A. G. (1983). The selective impairment of phonological processing: A case study. *Brain and Language*, *18*, 128–174.

Caramazza, A., & Hillis, A. E. (1990). Where do semantic errors come from? *Cortex*, *26*, 95–122.

Chee, M. W. L., O'Craven, K. M., Bergida, R., Rosen, B. R., & Savoy, R. L. (1999). Auditory and visual word processing with fMRI. *Human Brain Mapping*, *7*, 15–28.

Chenery, H. J., Ingram, J. C. L., & Murdoch, B. E. (1990). Automatic and volitional semantic processing in aphasia. *Brain and Language*, *38*, 215–232.

Chertkow, H., Bub, D., Deaudon, C., & Whitehead, V. (1997). On the status of object concepts in aphasia. *Brain and Language*, *58*, 203–232.

Collins, A. M., & Loftus, E. (1975). A spreading-activation theory of semantic processing. *Psychological Review*, *82*, 407–428.

Coltheart, M., Curtis, B., Atkins, P., & Haller, M. (1993). Models of reading aloud: Dual-route and parallel-distributed-processing approaches. *Psychological Review*, *100*, 589–608.

Creutzfeld, O., Ojemann, G., & Lettich, E. (1989). Neuronal activity in the human lateral temporal lobe. I. Responses to speech. *Experimental Brain Research*, *77*, 451–475.

Damasio, H. (1981). Cerebral localization of the aphasias. In M. T. Sarno (Ed.), *Acquired aphasia* (pp. 27–50). Orlando, FL: Academic Press.

Damasio, H. (1989). Neuroimaging contributions to the understanding of aphasia. In F. Boller & J. Grafman (Eds.), *Handbook of neuropsychology* (pp. 3–46). Amsterdam: Elsevier.

Damasio, H., & Damasio, A. R. (1980). The anatomical basis of conduction aphasia. *Brain*, *103*, 337–350.

Damasio, H., & Damasio, A. R. (1989). *Lesion analysis in neuropsychology*. New York: Oxford University Press.

Dehaene, S., Dupoux, E., Mehler, J., Cohen, L., Paulesu, E., Perani, D., van de Moortele, P.-F., Lehéricy, S., & Le Bihan, D. (1997). Anatomical variability in the cortical representation of first and second language. *Neuroreport*, *8*, 3809–3815.

Déjerine, J. (1891). Sur un cas de cécité verbal avec agraphie, suivi d'autopsie. *Comptes Rendus des Séances de la Société de Biologie*, *3*, 197–201.

Déjerine, J. (1892). Contribution à l'étude anatomo-pathologique et clinique des différentes variétés de cécité verbale. *Comptes Rendus des Séances de la Société de Biologie*, *44*, 61–90.

Dell, G. S. (1986). A spreading-activation theory of retrieval in sentence production. *Psychological Review*, *93*(3), 283–321.

Dell, G. S., & O'Seaghdha, P. G. (1992). Stages of lexical access in language production. *Cognition*, *42*, 287–314.

Dell, G. S., & Reich, P. A. (1981). Stages in sentence production: An analysis of speech error data. *Journal of Verbal Learning and Verbal Behavior*, *20*, 611–629.

Dell, G. S., Schwartz, M. F., Martin, N., Saffran, E. M., & Gagnon, D. A. (1997). Lexical access in aphasic and non-aphasic speakers. *Psychological Review*, *104*(4), 801–838.

Demb, J. B., Desmond, J. E., Wagner, A. D., Vaidya, C. J., Glover, G. H., & Gabrieli, J. D. E. (1995). Semantic encoding and retrieval in the left inferior prefrontal cortex: A functional MRI study of task difficulty and process specificity. *Journal of Neuroscience*, *15*, 5870–5878.

Démonet, J.-F., Chollet, F., Ramsay, S., Cardebat, D., Nespoulous, J.-L., Wise, R., Rascol, A., & Frackowiak, R. (1992). The anatomy of phonological and semantic processing in normal subjects. *Brain*, *115*, 1753–1768.

Démonet, J.-F., Price, C., Wise, R., & Frackowiak, R. S. J. (1994a). Differential activation of right and left posterior sylvian regions by semantic and phonological tasks: A positron emission tomography study in normal human subjects. *Neuroscience Letters*, *182*, 25–28.

Démonet, J.-F., Price, C. J., Wise, R., & Frackowiak, R. S. J. (1994b). A PET study of cognitive strategies in normal subjects during language tasks: Influence of phonetic ambiguity and sequence processing on phoneme monitoring. *Brain, 117,* 671–682.

Desimone, R., & Gross, C. G. (1979). Visual areas in the temporal cortex of the macaque. *Brain Research, 178,* 363–380.

Dhankhar, A., Wexler, B. E., Fulbright, R. K., Halwes, T., Blamire, A. M., & Shulman, R. G. (1997). Functional magnetic resonance imaging assessment of the human brain auditory cortex response to increasing word presentation rates. *Journal of Neurophysiology, 77,* 476–483.

Dronkers, N. F., Redfern, B. B., & Ludy, C. A. (1995). Lesion localization in chronic Wernicke's aphasia. *Brain and Language, 51,* 62–65.

Duvernoy, H. (1991). *The human brain. Surface, three-dimensional sectional anatomy, and MRI.* Vienna/New York: Springer-Verlag.

Efron, R. (1963). Temporal perception, aphasia, and déjà vu. *Brain, 86,* 403–424.

Ellis, A. W., Miller, D., & Sin, G. (1983). Wernicke's aphasia and normal language processing: A case study in cognitive neuropsychology. *Cognition, 15,* 111–144.

Faglia, L., Rottoli, M. R., & Vignolo, L. A. (1990). Aphasia due to lesions confined to the right hemisphere in right-handed patients: A review of the literature including the Italian cases. *Italian Journal of Neurological Sciences, 11,* 131–144.

Faglioni, P., Spinnler, H., & Vignolo, L. A. (1969). Contrasting behavior of right and left hemisphere-damaged patients on a discriminative and a semantic task of auditory recognition. *Cortex, 5,* 366–389.

Farah, M. J., & McClelland, J. L. (1991). A computational model of semantic memory impairment: Modality specificity and emergent category specificity. *Journal of Experimental Psychology: General, 120,* 339–357.

Fay, D., & Cutler, A. (1977). Malapropisms and the structure of the mental lexicon. *Linguistic Inquiry, 8,* 505–520.

Fiez, J. A., Raichle, M. E., Balota, D. A., Tallal, P., & Petersen, S. E. (1996a). PET activation of posterior temporal regions during auditory word presentation and verb generation. *Cerebral Cortex, 6,* 1–10.

Fiez, J. A., Raichle, M. E., Miezin, F. M., Petersen, S. E., Tallal, P., & Katz, W. F. (1995). PET studies of auditory and phonological processing: Effects of stimulus characteristics and task demands. *Journal of Cognitive Neuroscience, 7,* 357–375.

Fiez, J. A., Raife, E. A., Balota, D. A., Schwarz, J. P., Raichle, M. E., & Petersen, S. E. (1996b). A positron emission tomography study of short-term maintenance of verbal information. *Journal of Neuroscience, 16,* 808–822.

Flechsig, P. (1908). Bemerkungen über die hörsphäre des menschlichen gehirns. *Neurologische Zentralblatte, 27,* 2–7.

Foix, C. (1928). Aphasies. In G. H. Roger, F. Widal, & P. J. Teissier (Eds.), *Nouveau triète de medecine.* Paris: Masson.

Forde, E. M. E., & Humphreys, G. W. (1999). Category-specific recognition impairments: A review of important case studies and influential theories. *Aphasiology, 13,* 169–193.

Foundas, A. L., Leonard, C. M., Gilmore, R., Fennell, E., & Heilman, K. M. (1994). Planum temporale asymmetry and language dominance. *Neuropsychologia, 32,* 1225–1231.

Freud, S. (1891/1953). *On aphasia: A critical study* (E. Stengel, Trans.). Madison, CT: International Universities Press.

Fromkin, V. A. (1971). The nonanomolous nature of anomolous utterances. *Language, 47,* 27–52.

Gagnon, D. A., Schwartz, M. F., Martin, N., Dell, G. S., & Saffran, E. M. (1997). The origins of formal paraphasias in aphasics' picture naming. *Brain and Language, 59,* 450–472.

Gainotti, G., Silveri, M. C., & Villa, G. (1986). Anomia with and without lexical comprehension disorders. *Brain and Language, 29,* 18–33.

Galaburda, A., & Sanides, F. (1980). Cytoarchitectonic organization of the human auditory cortex. *Journal of Comparative Neurology, 190,* 597–610.

Galaburda, A. M., LeMay, M., Kemper, T., & Geschwind, N. (1978). Right-left asymmetries in the brain. Structural differences between the hemispheres may underlie cerebral dominance. *Science, 199,* 852–856.

Galaburda, A. M., & Pandya, D. N. (1983). The intrinsic architectonic and connectional organization of the superior temporal region of the rhesus monkey. *Journal of Comparative Neurology, 221,* 169–184.

Gandour, J., Ponglorpisit, S., Khunadorn, F., Dechongkit, S., Boongird, P., & Boonklam, R. (1992). Timing characteristics of speech after brain damage: Vowel length in Thai. *Brain and Language, 42,* 337–345.

Garrett, M. F. (1975). The analysis of sentence production. In G. H. Bower (Ed.), *The psychology of learning and motivation* (pp. 133–177). New York: Academic Press.

Garrett, M. F. (1984). The organization of processing structure of language production: Application to aphasic speech. In D. Caplan, A. Lecours, & A. Smith (Eds.), *Biological perspectives on language*. Cambridge, MA: MIT Press.

Garrett, M. F. (1992). Disorders of lexical selection. *Cognition, 42*, 143–180.

Geschwind, N. (1965). Disconnection syndromes in animals and man. *Brain, 88*, 237–294, 585–644.

Geschwind, N. (1971). Aphasia. *New England Journal of Medicine, 284*, 654–656.

Geschwind, N., & Levitsky, W. (1968). Human brain: Left-right asymmetries in temporal speech region. *Science, 161*, 186–187.

Gloning, I., Gloning, K., Haub, G., & Quatember, R. (1969). Comparison of verbal behavior in right-handed and non right-handed patients with anatomically verified lesion of one hemisphere. *Cortex, 5*, 41–52.

Goldblum, M. C., & Albert, M. (1972). Phonemic discrimination in sensory aphasia. *International Journal of Mental Health, 1*, 25–29.

Goldstein, K. (1948). *Language and language disturbances*. New York: Grune & Stratton.

Goldstein, M. (1974). Auditory agnosia for speech ("pure word deafness"): A historical review with current implications. *Brain and Language, 1*, 195–204.

Goodglass, H., & Baker, E. (1976). Semantic field, naming, and auditory comprehension in aphasia. *Brain and Language, 3*, 359–374.

Goodglass, H., & Kaplan, E. (1972). *The assessment of aphasia and related disorders*. Philadelphia: Lea and Febiger.

Grady, C. L., Van Meter, J. W., Maisog, J. M., Pietrini, P., Krasuski, J., & Rauschecker, J. P. (1997). Attention-related modulation of activity in primary and secondary auditory cortex. *Neuroreport, 8*, 2511–2516.

Grober, E., Perecman, E., Kellar, L., & Brown, J. (1980). Lexical knowledge in anterior and posterior aphasia. *Brain and Language, 10*, 318–330.

Grossman, M. (1980). The aphasics' identification of a superordinate's referents with basic object level and subordinate level terms. *Cortex, 16*, 459–469.

Grossman, M. (1981). A bird is a bird is a bird: Making reference within and without superordinate categories. *Brain and Language, 12*, 313–331.

Hagoort, P. (1993). Impairments of lexical-semantic processing in aphasia: Evidence from the processing of lexical ambiguities. *Brain and Language, 45*, 189–232.

Hammond, W. (1900). *Medical Record, 58*, 1011–1015.

Harley, T. A. (1984). A critique of top-down independent level models of speech production: Evidence from non-plan-internal speech errors. *Cognitive Science, 8*, 191–219.

Hart, J., & Gordon, B. (1990). Delineation of single-word semantic comprehension deficits in aphasia, with anatomic correlation. *Annals of Neurology, 27*, 226–231.

Head, H. (1926). *Aphasia and kindred disorders of speech*. New York: Macmillan.

Hécaen, H., & Albert, M. L. (1978). *Human neuropsychology*. New York: Wiley.

Heilman, K. M., Rothi, L., Campanella, D., & Wolfson, S. (1979). Wernicke's and global aphasia without alexia. *Archives of Neurology, 36*, 129–133.

Henschen, S. E. (1918–1919). On the hearing sphere. *Acta Oto-laryngologica, 1*, 423–486.

Henschen, S. E. (1920–1922). *Klinische und anatomische Beitrage zur Pathologie des Gehirns* (Vols. V–VII). Stockholm: Nordiska Bokhandeln.

Herbster, A. N., Mintun, M. A., Nebes, R. D., & Becker, J. T. (1997). Regional cerebral blood flow during word and nonword reading. *Human Brain Mapping, 5*, 84–92.

Hickok, G., Erhard, P., Kassubek, J., Helms-Tillery, A. K., Naeve-Velguth, S., Strupp, J. P., Strick, P. L., & Ugurbil, K. (2000). A functional magnetic resonance imaging study of the role of left posterior superior temporal gyrus in speech production: Implications for the explanation of conduction aphasia. *Neuroscience Letters, 287*, 156–160.

Hickok, G., & Poeppel, D. (2000). Towards a functional neuroanatomy of speech perception. *Trends in Cognitive Sciences, 4*, 131–138.

Hier, D. B., & Mohr, J. P. (1977). Incongruous oral and written naming. *Brain and Language, 4*, 115–126.

Hikosawa, K., Iwai, E., Saito, H.-A., & Tanaka, K. (1988). Polysensory properties of neurons in the anterior bank of the caudal superior temporal sulcus of the macaque monkey. *Journal of Neurophysiology, 60*, 1615–1637.

Hillis, A. E., Boatman, D. B., Hart, J., & Gordon, B. (1999). Making sense out of jargon. A neurolinguistic and computational account of jargon aphasia. *Neurology, 53*, 1813–1824.

Hillis, A. E., & Caramazza, A. (1991). Category-specific naming and comprehension impairment: A double dissociation. *Brain*, *114*, 2081–2094.

Hillis, A. E., & Caramazza, A. (1995). Representation of grammatical categories of words in the brain. *Journal of Cognitive Neuroscience*, *7*, 396–407.

Hinton, G. E., McClelland, J. L., & Rumelhart, D. E. (1986). Distributed representations. In D. E. Rumelhart & J. L. McClelland (Eds.), *Parallel distributed processing: Explorations in the microstructure of cognition* (pp. 77–109). Cambridge, MA: MIT Press.

Hinton, G. E., & Shallice, T. (1991). Lesioning an attractor network: Investigations of acquired dyslexia. *Psychological Review*, *98*(1), 74–95.

Hirano, S., Naito, Y., Okazawa, H., Kojima, H., Honjo, I., Ishizu, K., Yenokura, Y., Nagahama, Y., Fukuyama, H., & Konishi, J. (1997). Cortical activation by monaural speech sound stimulation demonstrated by positron emission tomography. *Experimental Brain Research*, *113*, 75–80.

Hoeft, H. (1957). Klinisch-anatomischer Beitrag zur Kenntnis der Nachsprechaphasie (Leitungsaphasie). *Deutsche Zeitschrift Nervenheilk*, *175*, 560–594.

Hornik, S., Stinchcombe, M., & White, H. (1989). Multilayer feedforward networks are universal approximators. *Neural Networks*, *2*, 359–366.

Howard, D., & Franklin, S. (1987). Three ways for understanding written words, and their use in two contrasting cases of surface dyslexia. In D. G. MacKay, A. Allport, W. Prinz, & E. Scheerer (Eds.), *Language perception and production* (chap. 16). Orlando, FL: Academic Press.

Howard, D., Patterson, K., Wise, R., Brown, W. D., Friston, K., Weiller, C., & Frackowiak, R. (1992). The cortical localization of the lexicons. *Brain*, *115*, 1769–1782.

Indefrey, P., Kleinschmidt, A., Merboldt, K.-D., Krüger, G., Brown, C., Hagoort, P., & Frahm, J. (1997). Equivalent responses to lexical and nonlexical visual stimuli in occipital cortex: A functional magnetic resonance imaging study. *Neuroimage*, *5*, 78–81.

Ingles, J. L., Mate-Kole, C. C., & Connolly, J. F. (1996). Evidence for multiple routes of speech production in a case of fluent aphasia. *Cortex*, *32*, 199–219.

Jäncke, L., Shah, N. J., Posse, S., Grosse-Ryuken, M., & Müller-Gärtner, H.-W. (1998). Intensity coding of auditory stimuli: An fMRI study. *Neuropsychologia*, *36*(9), 875–883.

Jauhiainen, T., & Nuutila, A. (1977). Auditory perception of speech and speech sounds in recent and recovered aphasia. *Brain and Language*, *4*, 572–579.

Jones, E. G., & Burton, H. (1976). Areal differences in the laminar distribution of thalamic afferents in cortical fields of the insular, parietal and temporal regions of primates. *Journal of Comparative Neurology*, *168*, 197–247.

Jones, E. G., & Powell, T. S. P. (1970). An anatomical study of converging sensory pathways within the cerebral cortex of the monkey. *Brain*, *93*, 793–820.

Jonides, J., Schumacher, E., Smith, E., Koeppe, R., Awh, E., Reuter-Lorenz, P. A., Marshuetz, C., & Willis, C. R. (1998). The role of the parietal cortex in verbal working memory. *Journal of Neuroscience*, *18*, 5026–5034.

Kaas, J. H., & Hackett, T. A. (1998). Subdivisions of auditory cortex and levels of processing in primates. *Audiology Neuro-Otology*, *3*, 73–85.

Kempen, G., & Huijbers, P. (1983). The lexicalization process in sentence production and naming: Indirect election of words. *Cognition*, *14*, 185–209.

Kertesz, A., & Benson, D. F. (1970). Neologistic jargon: A clinicopathological study. *Cortex*, *6*, 362–386.

Kertesz, A., Harlock, W., & Coates, R. (1979). Computer tomographic localization, lesion size, and prognosis in aphasia and nonverbal impairment. *Brain and Language*, *8*, 34–50.

Kertesz, A., Lau, W. K., & Polk, M. (1993). The structural determinants of recovery in Wernicke's aphasia. *Brain and Language*, *44*, 153–164.

Kertesz, A., Sheppard, A., & MacKenzie, R. (1982). Localization in transcortical sensory aphasia. *Archives of Neurology*, *39*, 475–478.

Kinsbourne, M., & Warrington, E. K. (1963). Jargon aphasia. *Neuropsychologia*, *1*, 27–37.

Kirschner, H. S., & Webb, W. G. (1982). Alexia and agraphia in Wernicke's aphasia. *Journal of Neurology, Neurosurgery, and Psychiatry*, *45*, 719–724.

Kirschner, H. S., Webb, W. G., & Duncan, G. W. (1981). Word deafness in Wernicke's aphasia. *Journal of Neurology, Neurosurgery, and Psychiatry*, *44*, 197–201.

Klatt, D. H. (1989). Review of selected models of speech perception. In W. D. Marslen-Wilson (Eds.), *Lexical representation and process* (pp. 169–226). Cambridge, MA: MIT Press.

Kleist, K. (1962). *Sensory aphasia and amusia*. London: Pergamon Press.

Kohn, S. E., & Smith, K. L. (1994). Evolution of impaired access to the phonological lexicon. *Journal of Neurolinguistics*, *8*, 267–288.

Kudo, T. (1987). Aphasics' appreciation of hierarchical semantic categories. *Brain and Language*, *30*, 33–51.

Ladefoged, P., & Maddieson, I. (1996). *The sounds of the world's languages*. Oxford: Blackwell.

Laiacona, M., Capitani, E., & Barbarotto, R. (1997). Semantic category dissociations: A longitudinal study of two cases. *Cortex*, *33*, 441–461.

Lebrun, Y. (1987). Anosognosia in aphasics. *Cortex*, *23*, 251–263.

Lecour, A. R., & Rouillon, F. (1976). Neurolinguistic analysis of jargonaphasia and jargonagraphia. In H. Whitaker & H. Whitaker (Eds.), *Studies in neurolinguistics*. New York: Academic Press.

Leinonen, L., Hyvärinen, J., & Sovijärvi, A. R. A. (1980). Functional properties of neurons in the temporo-parietal association cortex of awake monkey. *Experimental Brain Research*, *39*, 203–215.

Levelt, W. J. M., Schriefers, H., Vorberg, D., Meyer, A. S., Pechmann, T., & Havinga, J. (1991). The time course of lexical access in speech production: A study of picture naming. *Psychological Review*, *98*, 122–142.

Liberman, A. M., Cooper, F. S., Shankweiler, D. P., & Studdert-Kennedy, M. (1967). Perception of the speech code. *Psychological Review*, *74*, 431–461.

Lichtheim, L. (1885). On aphasia. *Brain*, *7*, 433–484.

Liègeois-Chauvel, C., Musolino, A., & Chauvel, P. (1991). Localization of the primary auditory area in man. *Brain*, *114*, 139–153.

Liepmann, H., & Pappenheim, M. (1914). Über einem FALL von sogenannter LEITUNGSAPHASIE mit anatomischer BEFUND. *Zeitschrift für Gesamtes des Neurologie und Psychiatrie*, *27*, 1–41.

Luria, A. R. (1966). *Higher cortical functions in man* (B. Haigh, trans.). New York: Basic Books and Plenum.

Luria, A. R., & Hutton, A. (1977). A modern assessment of the basic forms of aphasia. *Brain and Language*, *4*, 129–151.

MacKay, D. G. (1970). Spoonerisms: The structure of errors in the serial order of speech. *Neuropsychologia*, *8*, 323–350.

Macleod, C. M. (1991). Half a century of research on the Stroop effect: An integrative review. *Psychological Bulletin*, *109*, 163–203.

Maher, L. M., Gonzalez Rothi, L. J., & Heilman, K. M. (1994). Lack of error awareness in an aphasic patient with relatively preserved auditory comprehension. *Brain and Language*, *46*, 402–418.

Margolin, D. (1991). Cognitive neuropsychology: Resolving enigmas about Wernicke's aphasia and other higher cortical disorders. *Archives of Neurology*, *48*, 751–765.

Marie, P. (1888/1971). On aphasia in general and agraphia in particular according to the teaching of Professor Charcot. Reprinted from Le Progres Medical, Series 2, 1888, 7: 81–84. In *Pierre Marie's Papers on Speech Disorders*. New York: Hafner.

Marie, P., & Foix, C. (1917). Les aphasies de guerre. *Revue Neurologique*, *24*, 53–87.

Marshall, R. C., Rappaport, B. Z., & Garcia-Bunuel, L. (1985). Self-monitoring behavior in a case of severe auditory agnosia with aphasia. *Brain and Language*, *24*(297–313).

Martin, A. (2001). Functional imaging of semantic memory. In R. Cabeza & A. Kingstone (Eds.), *Handbook of functional neuroimaging of cognition* (pp. 153–186). Cambridge, MA: MIT Press.

Martin, N., Dell, G. S., Saffran, E. M., & Schwartz, M. F. (1994). Origins of paraphasias in deep dysphasia: Testing the consequences of a decay impairment to an interactive spreading activation model of lexical retrieval. *Brain and Language*, *47*, 609–660.

Martin, N., Gagnon, D. A., Schwartz, M. F., Dell, G. S., & Saffran, E. M. (1996). Phonological facilitation of semantic errors in normal and aphasic speakers. *Language and Cognitive Processes*, *11*, 257–282.

Masson, M. E. J. (1995). A distributed model of semantic priming. *Journal of Experimental Psychology: Learning, Memory, and Cognition*, *21*, 3–23.

Mayeux, R., & Kandel, E. R. (1985). Natural language, disorders of language, and other localizable disorders of cognitive function. In E. R. Kandel & J. Schwartz (Eds.), *Principles of neural science* (pp. 688–703). New York: Elsevier.

Mazoyer, B. M., Tzourio, N., Frak, V., Syrota, A., Murayama, N., Levrier, O., Salamon, G., Dehaene, S., Cohen, L., & Mehler, J. (1993). The cortical representation of speech. *Journal of Cognitive Neuroscience*, *5*, 467–479.

McCleary, C. (1988). The semantic organization and classification of fourteen words by aphasic patients. *Brain and Language*, *34*, 183–202.

McCleary, C., & Hirst, W. (1986). Semantic classification in aphasia: A study of basic, superordinate, and function relations. *Brain and Language*, *27*, 199–209.

McClelland, J. L., & Rumelhart, D. E. (1986). A distributed model of human learning and memory. In J. L.

McClelland & D. E. Rumelhart (Eds.), *Parallel distributed processing: Vol. 2: Psychological and biological models* (pp. 170–215). Cambridge, MA: MIT Press.

McRae, K., de Sa, V. R., & Seidenberg, M. S. (1997). On the nature and scope of featural representations of word meaning. *Journal of Experimental Psychology: General, 126*, 99–130.

Mendelson, J. R., & Cynader, M. S. (1985). Sensitivity of cat primary auditory cortex (AI) to the direction and rate of frequency modulation. *Brain Research, 327*, 331–335.

Merzenich, M. M., & Brugge, J. F. (1973). Representation of the cochlear partition on the superior temporal plane of the macaque monkey. *Brain Research, 60*, 315–333.

Mesulam, M. M. (1990). Large-scale neurocognitive networks and distributed processing for attention, language, and memory. *Annals of Neurology, 28*, 597–613.

Mesulam, M.-M., & Pandya, D. N. (1973). The projections of the medial geniculate complex within the Sylvian fissure of the rhesus monkey. *Brain Research, 60*, 315–333.

Metz-Lutz, M.-N., & Dahl, E. (1984). Analysis of word comprehension in a case of pure word deafness. *Brain and Language, 23*, 13–25.

Meyer, D. E., & Schvaneveldt, R. W. (1971). Facilitation in recognizing pairs of words: Evidence of a dependence between retrieval operations. *Journal of Experimental Psychology, 90*, 227–234.

Miceli, G., Gainotti, G., Caltagirone, C., & Masullo, C. (1980). Some aspects of phonological impairment in aphasia. *Brain and Language, 11*, 159–169.

Milberg, W., & Blumstein, S. E. (1981). Lexical decision and aphasia: Evidence for semantic processing. *Brain and Language, 14*, 371–385.

Milberg, W., Blumstein, S. E., & Dworetzky, B. (1987). Processing of lexical ambiguities in aphasia. *Brain and Language, 31*, 138–150.

Milberg, W., Blumstein, S. E., & Dworetzky, B. (1988a). Phonological factors in lexical access: Evidence from an auditory lexical decision task. *Bulletin of the Psychonomic Society, 26*, 305–308.

Milberg, W., Blumstein, S. E., & Dworetzky, B. (1988b). Phonological processing and lexical access in aphasia. *Brain and Language, 34*, 279–293.

Milberg, W., Blumstein, S. E., Saffran, J., Hourihan, J., & Brown, T. (1995). Semantic facilitation in aphasia: Effects of time and expectancy. *Journal of Cognitive Neuroscience, 7*, 33–50.

Minsky, M., & Papert, S. A. (1969). *Perceptrons: An introduction to computational geometry.* Cambridge, MA: MIT Press.

Mitchum, C. C., Ritgert, B. A., Sandson, J., & Berndt, R. (1990). The use of response analysis in confrontation naming. *Aphasiology, 4*, 261–280.

Moerman, C., Corluy, R., & Meersman, W. (1983). Exploring the aphasiac's naming disturbances: A new approach using the neighbourhood limited classification method. *Cortex, 19*, 529–543.

Mohr, J. P., Gautier, J. C., & Hier, D. B. (1992). Middle cerebral artery disease. In H. J. M. Barnett, J. P. Mohr, B. M. Stein, & F. M. Yatsu (Eds.), *Stroke. Pathophysiology, diagnosis, and management* (pp. 361–417). New York: Churchill Livingstone.

Monsell, S. (1987). On the relation between lexical input and output pathways for speech. In A. Allport, D. G. MacKay, & W. Prinz (Eds.), *Language perception and production: Relationships between listening, speaking, reading, and writing* (pp. 273–311). London: Academic Press.

Morel, A., Garraghty, P. E., & Kaas, J. H. (1993). Tonotopic organization, architectonic fields, and connections of auditory cortex in macaque monkeys. *Journal of Comparative Neurology, 335*, 437–459.

Morton, J., & Patterson, K. (1980). A new attempt at an interpretation, or, an attempt at a new interpretation. In M. Coltheart, K. Patterson, & J. C. Marshall (Eds.), *Deep dyslexia* (pp. 91–118). London: Routledge & Kegan Paul.

Moss, H. E., Hare, M. L., Day, P., & Tyler, L. K. (1994). A distributed memory model of the associative boost in semantic priming. *Connection Science, 6*, 413–427.

Mummery, C. J., Ashburner, J., Scott, S. K., & Wise, R. J. S. (1999). Functional neuroimaging of speech perception in six normal and two aphasic subjects. *Journal of the Acoustical Society of America, 106*, 449–457.

Mummery, C. J., Patterson, K., Hodges, J. R., & Price, C. J. (1998). Functional neuroanatomy of the semantic system: Divisible by what? *Journal of Cognitive Neuroscience, 10*, 766–777.

Murtha, S., Chertkow, H., Beauregard, M., & Evans, A. (1999). The neural substrate of picture naming. *Journal of Cognitive Neuroscience, 11*, 399–423.

Naeser, M., Hayward, R. W., Laughlin, S. A., & Zatz, L. M. (1981). Quantitative CT scan studies of aphasia. I. Infarct size and CT numbers. *Brain and Language, 12*, 140–164.

Naeser, M. A., Gaddie, A., Palumbo, C. L., & Stiassny-Eder, D. (1990). Late recovery of auditory comprehension in global aphasia. Improved recovery observed with subcortical temporal isthmus lesion vs Wernicke's cortical area lesion. *Archives of Neurology*, *47*, 425–432.

Naeser, M. A., Helm-Estabrooks, N., Haas, G., Auerbach, S., & Srinivasan, M. (1987). Relationship between lesion extent in 'Wernicke's area' on computed tomographic scan and predicting recovery of comprehension in Wernicke's aphasia. *Archives of Neurology*, *44*, 73–82.

Neely, J. H. (1977). Semantic priming over retrieval from lexical memory: Roles of inhibitionless spreading activation and limited-capacity attention. *Journal of Experimental Psychology: General*, *106*, 226–254.

Nickels, L., & Howard, D. (1995). Phonological errors in aphasic naming: Comprehension, monitoring and lexicality. *Cortex*, *31*, 209–237.

Nielsen, J. M. (1938). The unsolved problems in aphasia. II. Alexia resulting from a temporal lesion. *Bulletin of the Los Angeles Neurological Society*, *4*, 168–175.

Nielsen, J. M. (1946). *Agnosia, apraxia, aphasia. Their value in cerebral localization.* New York: Paul B. Hoeber.

Nooteboom, S. G. (1969). The tongue slips into patterns. In A. G. Sciarone, A. J. van Essen, & A. A. Van Raad (Eds.), *Leyden studies in linguistics and phonetics* (pp. 114–132). The Hague: Mouton.

Oden, G. C., & Massaro, D. W. (1978). Integration of featural information in speech perception. *Psychological Review*, *85*, 172–191.

Ojemann, G. A. (1983). Brain organization for language from the perspective of electrical stimulation mapping. *Behavioral and Brain Sciences*, *2*, 189–230.

O'Leary, D. S., Andreasen, N. C., Hurtig, R. R., Hichwa, R. D., Watkins, G. L., Boles-Ponto, L. L., Rogers, M., & Kirchner, P. T. (1996). A positron emission tomography study of binaurally and dichotically presented stimuli: Effects of level of language and directed attention. *Brain and Language*, *53*, 20–39.

Ono, M., Kubik, S., & Abernathey, C. D. (1990). *Atlas of the cerebral sulci.* Stuttgart: Georg Thieme Verlag.

Palumbo, C. L., Alexander, M. P., & Naeser, M. A. (1992). CT scan lesion sites associated with conduction aphasia. In S. E. Kohn (Ed.), *Conduction aphasia* (pp. 51–75). Hillsdale, NJ: Lawrence Erlbaum Associates.

Paulesu, E., Frith, C. D., & Frackowiak, R. S. J. (1993). The neural correlates of the verbal component of working memory. *Nature*, *362*, 342–345.

Paus, T., Perry, D. W., Zatorre, R. J., Worsley, K. J., & Evans, A. C. (1996). Modulation of cerebral blood flow in the human auditory cortex during speech: Role of motor-to-sensory discharges. *European Journal of Neuroscience*, *8*, 2236–2246.

Perani, D., Dehaene, S., Grassi, F., Cohen, L., Cappa, S. F., Dupoux, E., Fazio, F., & Mehler, J. (1996). Brain processing of native and foreign languages. *Neuroreport*, *7*, 2439–2444.

Petersen, S. E., Fox, P. T., Posner, M. I., Mintun, M., & Raichle, M. E. (1988). Positron emission tomographic studies of the cortical anatomy of single-word processing. *Nature*, *331*, 585–589.

Petersen, S. E., Fox, P. T., Snyder, A. Z., & Raichle, M. E. (1990). Activation of extrastriate and frontal cortical areas by visual words and word-like stimuli. *Science*, *249*, 1041–1044.

Phillips, D. P., & Irvine, D. R. F. (1981). Responses of single neurons in physiologically defined primary auditory cortex (AI) of the cat: Frequency tuning and responses to intensity. *Journal of Neurophysiology*, *45*, 48–58.

Pick, A. (1909). *Über das Sprachverständnis.* Leipzig: Barth.

Pick, A. (1913). *Die agrammatischen Sprachstörungen.* Berlin: Springer.

Pick, A. (1931). *Aphasia.* Berlin: Springer.

Plaut, D. C., McClelland, J. L., Seidenberg, M. S., & Patterson, K. (1996). Understanding normal and impaired word reading: Computational principles in quasi-regular domains. *Psychological Review*, *103*, 45–115.

Plaut, D. C., & Shallice, T. (1993). Deep dyslexia: A case study of connectionist neuropsychology. *Cognitive Neuropsychology*, *10*, 377–500.

Poldrack, R. A., Wagner, A. D., Prull, M. W., Desmond, J. E., Glover, G. H., & Gabrieli, J. D. E. (1999). Functional specialization for semantic and phonological processing in the left inferior prefrontal cortex. *Neuroimage*, *10*, 15–35.

Price, C. J., Moore, C. J., Humphreys, G. W., Frackowiak, R. S. J., & Friston, K. J. (1996a). The neural regions sustaining object recognition and naming. *Proceedings of the Royal Society of London, Ser. B*, *263*, 1501–1507.

Price, C. J., Moore, C. J., Humphreys, G. W., & Wise, R. J. S. (1997). Segregating semantic from phonological processes during reading. *Journal of Cognitive Neuroscience*, *9*, 727–733.

Price, C. J., Wise, R. S. J., & Frackowiak, R. S. J. (1996c). Demonstrating the implicit processing of visually presented words and pseudowords. *Cerebral Cortex, 6,* 62–70.

Price, C., Wise, R., Ramsay, S., Friston, K., Howard, D., Patterson, K., & Frackowiak, R. (1992). Regional response differences within the human auditory cortex when listening to words. *Neuroscience Letters, 146,* 179–182.

Price, C. J., Wise, R. J. S., Warburton, E. A., Moore, C. J., Howard, D., Patterson, K., Frackowiak, R. S. J., & Friston, K. J. (1996b). Hearing and saying. The functional neuro-anatomy of auditory word processing. *Brain, 119,* 919–931.

Price, C. J., Wise, R. J. S., Watson, J. D. G., Patterson, K., Howard, D., & Frackowiak, R. S. J. (1994). Brain activity during reading. The effects of exposure duration and task. *Brain, 117,* 1255–1269.

Pugh, K. R., Shaywitz, B. A., Shaywitz, S. E., Constable, R. T., Skudlarski, P., Fulbright, R. K., Bronen, R. A., Shankweiler, D. P., Katz, L., Fletcher, J. M., & Gore, J. C. (1996). Cerebral organization of component processes in reading. *Brain, 119,* 1221–1238.

Pujol, J., Deus, J., Losilla, J. M., & Capdevila, A. (1999). Cerebral lateralization of language in normal left-handed people studied by functional MRI. *Neurology, 52,* 1038–1043.

Quigg, M., & Fountain, N. B. (1999). Conduction aphasia elicited by stimulation of the left posterior superior temporal gyrus. *Journal of Neurology, Neurosurgery and Psychiatry, 66,* 393–396.

Rademacher, J., Caviness, V. S., Steinmetz, H., & Galaburda, A. M. (1993). Topographical variation of the human primary cortices: Implications for neuroimaging, brain mapping and neurobiology. *Cerebral Cortex, 3,* 313–329.

Rapcsak, S. Z., & Rubens, A. B. (1994). Localization of lesions in transcortical aphasia. In A. Kertesz (Eds.), *Localization and neuroimaging in neuropsychology* (pp. 297–329). San Diego: Academic Press.

Rauschecker, J. P. (1998). Parallel processing in the auditory cortex of primates. *Audiology and Neuro-Otology, 3,* 86–103.

Rauschecker, J. P., Tian, B., Pons, T., & Mishkin, M. (1997). Serial and parallel processing in rhesus monkey auditory cortex. *Journal of Comparative Neurology, 382,* 89–103.

Reidl, K., & Studdert-Kennedy, M. (1985). Extending formant transitions may not improve aphasics' perception of stop consonant place of articulation. *Brain and Language, 24,* 223–232.

Roelofs, A. (1992). A spreading-activation theory of lemma retrieval in speaking. *Cognition, 42,* 107–142.

Roeltgen, D. P., Sevush, S., & Heilman, K. M. (1983). Phonological agraphia: Writing by the lexical-semantic route. *Neurology, 33,* 755–765.

Romanski, L. M., Tian, B., Fritz, J., Mishkin, M., Goldman-Rakic, P. S., & Rauschecker, J. P. (1999). Dual streams of auditory afferents target multiple domains in the primate prefrontal cortex. *Nature Neuroscience, 2,* 1131–1136.

Rosch, E., Mervis, C. B., Gray, W. D., Johnson, D. M., & Boyes-Braem, D. (1976). Basic objects in natural categories. *Cognitive Psychology, 8,* 382–439.

Rubens, A. B., Mahowald, M. W., & Hutton, J. T. (1976). Asymmetry of the lateral (sylvian) fissures in man. *Neurology, 26,* 620–624.

Rumelhart, D. E., McClelland, J. L., & The PDP Research Group (1986). *Parallel distributed processing, Vol 1: Foundations.* Cambridge, MA: MIT Press.

Rumsey, J. M., Horwitz, B., Donohue, B. C., Nace, K., Maisog, J. M., & Andreason, P. (1997). Phonological and orthographic components of word recognition. A PET-rCBF study. *Brain, 120,* 739–759.

Ryalls, J. (1986). An acoustic study of vowel production in aphasia. *Brain and Language, 29,* 48–67.

Schwartz, M. F., Saffran, E. M., Bloch, D. E., & Dell, G. S. (1994). Disordered speech production in aphasic and normal speakers. *Brain and Language, 47,* 52–88.

Scott, S. K., Blank, C., Rosen, S., & Wise, R. J. S. (2000). Identification of a pathway for intelligible speech in the left temporal lobe. *Brain, 123,* 2400–2406.

Seidenberg, M. S., & McClelland, J. L. (1989). A distributed, developmental model of word recognition and naming. *Psychological Review, 96,* 523–568.

Seidenberg, M. S., & McClelland, J. L. (1990). More words but still no lexicon: Reply to Besner et al. (1990). *Psychological Review, 97,* 447–452.

Selnes, O. A., Knopman, D. S., Niccum, N., Rubens, A. B., & Larson, D. (1983). Computed tomographic scan correlates of auditory comprehension deficits in aphasia: A prospective recovery study. *Annals of Neurology, 13,* 558–566.

Selnes, O. A., & Niccum, N. (1983). Alexia and agraphia in Wernicke's aphasia. *Journal of Neurology, Neurosurgery and Psychiatry, 46,* 462–463.

Selnes, O. A., Niccum, N., Knopman, D. S., & Rubens, A. B. (1984). Recovery of single word comprehension: CT-scan correlates. *Brain and Language*, *21*, 72–84.

Seltzer, B., & Pandya, D. N. (1978). Afferent cortical connections and architectonics of the superior temporal sulcus and surrounding cortex in the rhesus monkey. *Brain Research*, *149*, 1–24.

Seltzer, B., & Pandya, D. N. (1994). Parietal, temporal, and occipital projections to cortex of the superior temporal sulcus in the rhesus monkey: A retrograde tracer study. *Journal of Comparative Neurology*, *343*, 445–463.

Semenza, C., Cipolotti, L., & Denes, G. (1992). Reading aloud in jargon aphasia: An unusual dissociation in speech input. *Journal of Neurology, Neurosurgery and Psychiatry*, *55*, 205–208.

Sevush, S., Roeltgen, D. P., Campanella, D. J., & Heilman, K. M. (1983). Preserved oral reading in Wernicke's aphasia. *Neurology*, *33*, 916–920.

Shapiro, L. P., Gordon, B., Hack, N., & Killackey, J. (1993). Verb-argument structure processing in complex sentences in Broca's and Wernicke's aphasia. *Brain and Language*, *45*, 423–447.

Shattuck-Hufnagel, S., & Klatt, D. (1979). The limited use of distinctive features and markedness in speech production: Evidence from speech error data. *Journal of Verbal Learning and Verbal Behavior*, *18*, 41–55.

Silveri, C. M., & Gainotti, G. (1988). Interaction between vision and language in category-specific semantic impairment. *Cognitive Neuropsychology*, *5*, 677–709.

Sirigu, A., Duhamel, J.-R., & Poncet, M. (1991). The role of sensorimotor experience in object recognition. *Brain*, *114*, 2555–2573.

Small, S. L., Noll, D. C., Perfetti, C. A., Hlustik, P., Wellington, R., & Schneider, W. (1996). Localizing the lexicon for reading aloud: Replication of a PET study using fMRI. *Neuroreport*, *7*, 961–965.

Smith, C. D., Andersen, A. H., Chen, Q., Blonder, L. X., Kirsch, J. E., & Avison, M. J. (1996). Cortical activation in confrontation naming. *Neuroreport*, *7*, 781–785.

Springer, J. A., Binder, J. R., Hammeke, T. A., Swanson, S. J., Frost, J. A., Bellgowan, P. S. F., Brewer, C. C., Perry, H. M., Morris, G. L., & Mueller, W. M. (1999). Language dominance in neurologically normal and epilepsy subjects: A functional MRI study. *Brain*, *122*, 2033–2045.

Starr, M. A. (1889). The pathology of sensory aphasia, with an analysis of fifty cases in which Broca's centre was not diseased. *Brain*, *12*, 82–101.

Steinmetz, H., Rademacher, J., Jäncke, L., Huang, Y., Thron, A., & Zilles, K. (1990). Total surface of temporoparietal intrasylvian cortex: Diverging left-right asymmetries. *Brain and Language*, *39*, 357–372.

Steinmetz, H., Volkmann, J., Jäncke, L., & Freund, H.-J. (1991). Anatomical left-right asymmetry of language-related temporal cortex is different in left- and right-handers. *Annals of Neurology*, *29*, 315–319.

Stemberger, J. P. (1982). The nature of segments in the lexicon: Evidence from speech errors. *Lingua*, *56*, 235–259.

Stemberger, J. P. (1985). An interactive activation model of language production. In A. W. Ellis (Ed.), *Progress in the psychology of language* (pp. 143–186). Hillsdale, NJ: Lawrence Erlbaum Associates.

Stengel, E. (1933). Zur LEHRE von der LEITUNGSAPHASIE. *Zeitschrift für Gesamte des Neurologie und Psychiatrie*, *149*, 266–291.

Stevens, K. N., & Blumstein, S. E. (1981). The search for invariant acoustic correlates of phonetic features. In P. D. Eimas & J. L. Miller (Eds.), *Perspectives on the study of speech* (pp. 1–38). Hillsdale, NJ: Lawrence Erlbaum Associates.

Tagamets, M.-A., Novick, J. M., Chalmers, M. L., & Friedman, R. B. (2000). A parametric approach to orthographic processing in the brain: An fMRI study. *Journal of Cognitive Neuroscience*, *12*, 281–297.

Tallal, P., & Newcombe, F. (1978). Impairment of auditory perception and language comprehension in dysphasia. *Brain and Language*, *5*, 13–24.

Tallal, P., & Piercy, M. (1973). Defects of non-verbal auditory perception in children with developmental aphasia. *Nature*, *241*, 468–469.

Tanaka, Y., Yamadori, A., & Mori, E. (1987). Pure word deafness following bilateral lesions: a psychophysical analysis. *Brain*, *110*, 381–403.

Tian, B., Reser, D., Durham, A., Kustov, A., & Rauschecker, J. P. (2001). Functional specialization in the rhesus monkey auditory cortex. *Science*, *292*, 290–293.

Van Orden, G. C. (1987). A ROWS is a ROSE: Spelling, sound, and reading. *Memory and Cognition*, *15*, 181–198.

von Economo, C., & Horn, L. (1930). Über Windungsrelief, Maße und Rindenarchitektonik der Supratemporalfläche, ihre individuellen und ihre seitenunterscheide. *Zeitschrift für Neurologie und Psychiatrie*, *130*, 678–757.

Wada, J. A., Clarke, R., & Hamm, A. (1975). Cerebral hemispheric asymmetry in humans. *Archives of Neurology*, *32*, 239–246.

Warburton, E., Wise, R. J. S., Price, C. J., Weiller, C., Hadar, U., Ramsay, S., & Frackowiak, R. S. J. (1996). Noun and verb retrieval by normal subjects. Studies with PET. *Brain*, *119*, 159–179.

Warrington, E. K., & Shallice, T. (1984). Category specific semantic impairments. *Brain*, *107*, 829–854.

Wernicke, C. (1874/1968). *Der aphasische SYMPTO-MENKOMPLEX*. Breslau: Cohn & Weigert. Reprinted in English in *Boston Studies in the Philosophy of Science* (Vol. IV, pp. 34–97). Dordrecht, Netherlands: Kluwer Academic Publishers.

Wernicke, C. (1881). *Lehrbuch der GEHIRNKRANK-HEITEN*. Kassel, Germany: Theodore Fischer.

Westbury, C. F., Zatorre, R. J., & Evans, A. C. (1999). Quantifying variability in the planum temporale: A probability map. *Cerebral Cortex*, *9*, 392–405.

Wise, R., Chollet, F., Hadar, U., Friston, K., Hoffner, E., & Frackowiak, R. (1991). Distribution of cortical neural networks involved in word comprehension and word retrieval. *Brain*, *114*, 1803–1817.

Wise, R. S. J., Scott, S. K., Blank, S. C., Mummery, C. J., Murphy, K., & Warburton, E. A. (2001). Separate neural subsystems within "Wernicke's area." *Brain*, *124*, 83–95.

Witelson, S. F., & Kigar, D. L. (1992). Sylvian fissure morphology and asymmetry in men and women: Bilateral differences in relation to handedness in men. *Journal of Comparative Neurology*, *323*, 326–340.

Zatorre, R. J., Evans, A. C., Meyer, E., & Gjedde, A. (1992). Lateralization of phonetic and pitch discrimination in speech processing. *Science*, *256*, 846–849.

Zelkowicz, B. J., Herbster, A. N., Nebes, R. D., Mintun, M. A., & Becker, J. T. (1998). An examination of regional cerebral blood flow during object naming tasks. *Journal of the International Neuropsychological Society*, *4*, 160–166.

Zurif, E., Caramazza, A., Myerson, R., & Galvin, J. (1974). Semantic feature representations for normal and aphasic language. *Brain and Language*, *1*, 167–187.

Zurif, E., Swinney, D., Prather, P., Solomon, J., & Bushell, C. (1993). An on-line analysis of syntactic processing in Broca's and Wernicke's aphasia. *Brain and Language*, *45*, 448–464.

10 Apraxia: A Disorder of Motor Control

Scott Grafton

Apraxia is a disturbance of goal-directed motor behavior characterized by an inability to perform previously learned movements in the absence of weakness or sensory defects (Leiguarda & Marsden, 2000). There is a striking preservation of perception, attention, coordination, motivation, and comprehension. Thus it represents a high-level disorder of movement representation. There is significant variation in the clinical manifestations. Patients may have selective deficits in their ability to generate actions performed by the limb or the mouth and face. Apraxic patients may be unable to move with respect to imitation, verbal command, or both. Apraxia is often associated with deficits of more complex movements such as gestures, pantomime, and sequential movement. There may be failure to perform a movement in response to an object or failure to handle an object correctly. Motor errors vary in severity, ranging from an inability to generate any appropriate movement to mild clumsiness in generating a complex movement. Inaccuracy of arm movements, particularly reaching, pointing, and grasping, can be observed and form an important link to optic ataxia and related disorders of visually guided movement.

The unusual clinical features of apraxia have generated numerous fundamental theories of how movements are represented within the nervous system. In this chapter these historically important ideas are examined within a broader perspective of contemporary anatomy, motor physiology, lesion studies, and brain imaging.

Case Report

Mr. T., a 48-year-old government official presented with an acute onset of confusion and a mixed pattern of aphasia with inconsistent impairments in language comprehension and reduced verbal output (Rothi & Heilman, 1996). The cranial nerves were intact and there was no evidence of hemiplegia, sensory loss, ataxia, or gait disturbance. The patient would only use the right hand to follow commands, but invariably failed in following almost all instructions involving actions with the right arm. Attempts to use the right arm typically produced bizarre and distorted movements. He was unable to use his right arm to point at a ringing bell, to respond to written instructions, to imitate gestures performed by the examiner, to scratch when tickled on the right ear, or to point at named objects. Surprisingly, commands such as "stand up and walk to the window" were performed without difficulty. Moreover, when forced to use the left arm, he could perform all of the limb tasks, suggesting a preservation of comprehension. There was preservation of reading and writing (when forced to use the left hand).

In examining the deficit of the right hand more closely, it was found that the patient made systematic errors when reaching for and grasping objects. When multiple objects were displayed, the patient would consistently grasp an object adjacent to the target. Reach and grasp improved when there were no distracters. The patient also displayed signs consistent with bimanual discoordination. When asked to pour from a jug held with the left hand into a glass held in the right hand, the right hand and glass would move to the mouth before the left had time to fill the glass. The patient displayed little dismay when making errors with the right hand, unless they were pointed out to him. In this case, he would become exceedingly embarrassed.

This case report is particularly relevant because it is a synopsis of the patient described by Liepmann in 1900 (Liepmann, 1977). In his interpretation of the case, Liepmann proposed novel concepts that continue to be relevant to our understanding of apraxia today. First, he was able to exclude the presence of "asymbolia" or agnosia, i.e., deficits of comprehension, which he called "sensory apraxia." He proposed instead a disturbance in the control of motor communication, which he called "motor apraxia." The patient's lack of concern for his right-hand errors led Liepmann to propose a relationship between movement planning and mechanising for online detection and correction of errors. Liepmann's detection of systematic errors in reaching when distracted provided early evidence for a connection between representational motor disorders and motor attentional defects.

Bedside Tests for Apraxia

The first challenge in testing a patient with a deficit of complex movement is to establish that there is no loss of comprehension (Rothi, Ochipa, and Heilman, 1997). For a patient without aphasia, this can be determined by asking them to repeat and explain a verbal command. In the aphasic patient with non-fluent aphasia, it is often possible to confirm intact comprehension by means of simple "yes" or "no" questions.

Clinical tests for apraxia begin with simple verbal commands such as "look upward" or "close the eyes." Commands for whole-body movements such as "stand up" or "turn around" are also useful in delineating the severity of coexistent comprehension impairment as well as defects of axial motor control. Deficits may be segmental in distribution, so it is useful to examine limb, buccofacial, and axial body movements separately. Imitation of familiar movements or gestures across these same body segments is then tested. Imitation of meaningless gestures can also be tested. Patients with concomitant aphasia and normal praxis may be able to imitate an examiner despite difficulty following detailed verbal instruction.

Next, the patient is asked to generate transitive movements, i.e., the manipulation of objects. Instructions include "show me how you brush your hair," "how you blow out a candle," and "pretend to throw a ball." Intransitive movements such as "wave hello" are also tested. Patients are examined for irregular movements, use of inappropriate body parts, perseveration, and verbal repetition rather than movement. Patients may form the hand into the shape of the tool rather than pantomime holding a tool. Spatial errors in limb movement are probably common, but are often difficult to observe without the assistance of video-kinematic analysis (Poizner et al., 1995).

If patients show deficits in pantomiming or gesturing, attempting to induce the movement with another stimulus can be a useful technique to rule out coexistent weakness, uncoordination, or akinesia. For transitive movements, the most powerful stimulus is the tool itself. For example, patients may not be able to show how to comb their hair unless they are holding a comb. Another interesting test of transitive representation is tool selection. Some patients will be impaired in selecting the appropriate tool to complete a task (e.g., a hammer to pound a nail). In relation to this, it is useful to establish if the apraxic deficit is specific to cues provided via a single sensory modality. For example, optic ataxia, a disorder of visually guided reaching and grasping, can be considered as a form of apraxia limited to one sensory modality (vision) (Perenin & Vighetto, 1988; Pisella et al., 2000). On closer examination these patients manifest the impairment only when movements are directed at visually presented objects; when items are specified through another sensory modality (e.g., haptically), their performance improves considerably.

Categorization of the Clinical Findings of Apraxia

Apraxia has been categorized with many different schemes. Early approaches by Liepmann as well as Geschwind emphasized the involved body segment as a starting point (Geschwind & Damasio, 1985; Liepmann, 1920). The heuristic value of this categorization with respect to limb or buccofacial involvement remains unclear with respect to motor representation and response selection. This approach has been deemphasized over the past decade. An alternative categorization relies on an approach based on the ideas of DeRenzi (1988) and Rothi, Ochipa, and Heilman (1997). As a starting point, clinical findings associated with apraxia are divided into two large domains, production and conceptualization. As shown in the following sections, this approach turns out to be particularly useful for linking apraxia to human behavioral, functional imaging and nonhuman primate experiments.

Production Domain

The "production domain" refers to the ability of patients to produce simple forms of movement. This domain can be further divided into different types of movement. Intransitive movements consist of nonrepresentational, body-centered actions ("look up," "show me your teeth") and representational movements ("wave hello"). Transitive movements are linked to the use of objects ("use a knife," "use a paintbrush"). These can be tested using real objects under verbal, visual, or tactile conditions. Movement imitation including both meaningful and meaningless movements, sequences, and postures are included in this domain.

Conceptual Domain

The conceptual domain refers to higher cognitive deficits associated with action and tool use. Deficits can be observed on sequential tasks ("mount a picture on the wall using a hammer and nail"), *tool selection tasks* (selecting the appropriate tool for a half-finished job or picking another tool to finish a task if the best is not available) and gesture recognition tasks (naming meaningful gestures performed by the examiner). For aphasics, naming can be tested nonverbally using picture cards or tools that match the object that is involved in a gesture.

Clinical Classification of Apraxia

Ideational and Conceptual Apraxia

It is generally agreed that impairment of the conceptual system leads to errors in the performance of transitive movements (Heilman, Maher, Greenwald, & Rothi, 1997). A patient told to pantomime brushing their hair might make movements resembling shaving or tooth brushing. In other words, the wrong tool is associated with the corresponding action. There can also be incorrect selection of a tool for a given object or verbal instruction. In such a case, a patient will not have a deficit of tool

naming per se. There can be loss of general mechanical knowledge so that the next best tool is not chosen if the primary one is not available. In addition to selection errors, there are sequencing errors in the performance of the actions between tools and objects. Sequencing errors are particularly disruptive for the performance of the activities of daily living.

Whether or not there is a form of ideational apraxia that is distinct from conceptual apraxia is debated. Pick, Liepmann, and others used the expression "ideational apraxia" to refer to an inability to carry out a series of actions with more than one object (Leiguarda & Starkstein, 1998). A good example is the inability of Liepmann's patient, Mr. T., to pour a glass of water. Others have argued that it is a disruption of using a single tool appropriately or is the inappropriate selection of a single tool. These could both result from an inability to remember the correct action associated with a tool, obscuring the distinction with conceptual apraxia.

Ochipa has argued that ideational apraxia is a failure of sequencing actions that lead to a goal whereas conceptual apraxia is the loss of tool-action knowledge (Ochipa, Rothi, & Heilman, 1989). Thus, a patient with pure "ideational" apraxia would be able to recognize and name objects, but would not be able to identify inappropriate sequences of actions in photographs or movies. The main problem with this refined distinction between conceptual and ideational apraxia is that many patients with sequencing errors, if tested carefully, will also display errors of tool-action or single-object use (Leiguarda & Marsden, 2000).

Ideomotor Apraxia

Ideomotor apraxia is a disturbance in programming the timing, sequencing, and spatial organization of gestural movements (Rothi, Ochipa, & Heilman, 1997). The errors tend to be temporal and spatial in nature, with irregular speed, sequencing, amplitude, and orienting with respect to objects (Clark et al., 1994; Poizner, Mack, Verfaellie, Rothi, Heilman, 1990b). It is common to observe inappropriate limb posture and the use of a body part as an object (Poizner et al., 1995). Although the movements are wrong, the goal of the intended action can usually be recognized. Actions tend to be worse with transitive gestures, although they can be improved if a real object is provided or if the patient is allowed to imitate the examiner (Rothi & Heilman, 1996).

Kinematic analysis of patients with ideomotor apraxia who are performing simple aiming movements demonstrates that they are particularly impaired in response implementation, with decoupling of the spatial and temporal features of movement (Haaland, Harrington, & Knight, 1999). The aiming error can be subtle and is magnified by occluding the patient's view of the moving limb or the target, suggesting a disruption of the neural representation linking egocentric and allocentric information.

Callosal Apraxia

Sectioning of the genu and body of the corpus callosum can lead to a variety of apraxic signs (Graff-Radford, Welsh, & Godersky, 1987; Watson & Heilman, 1983). The classic test is to give patients spoken commands to be pantomimed with the left hand. The basic finding of a deficit associated with spoken words is consistent with Geschwind's formulation that a spoken command, once interpreted in the left hemisphere, is transformed into a motor plan within the left hemisphere (Goldenberg, Wimmer, Holzner, & Wessely, 1985). In the callosal patient, this information is not accessible to the right hemisphere. Praxis is preserved if instructions are provided with modalities such as vision or tactile cues that are accessible to the right hemisphere. Depending on the case series, some but not all patients have been able to perform normally when given an object in the left hand or during imitation.

Studies of commissurotomized (i.e., split-brain) patients suggest that the distal control needed for grasping is primarily exercised within the hemisphere contralateral to the response hand (Gazzaniga, Bogen, & Sperry, 1967; Milner & Kolb, 1985). However, these human studies also indicate an asymmetry in motor control that favors the left hemisphere. Gazzaniga et al. (1967), for example, reported that patients accurately mimicked postures of visually presented hands when stimuli were presented to the hemisphere contralateral to the response hand. The most accurate responses occurred when stimuli were presented to the left hemisphere and responses were executed with the dominant right hand. When stimuli were presented to the left hemisphere, performance with the ipsilateral left hand was moderately impaired; yet substantial dyspraxia was evident when stimuli were presented to the right hemisphere and responses were made with the ipsilateral right hand.

A very different pattern emerged when commissurotomized patients were required to point toward a visually presented target—a task primarily involving control of proximal limb segments of the upper arm and shoulder. Under these conditions, patients performed well with the hand ipsilateral to the stimulated hemisphere. When the target was presented to the left hemisphere, reaching with the left hand was highly accurate; when the target was presented to the right hemisphere, reaching with the right arm was moderately accurate. However, it was also apparent that right hemisphere control of the right arm was not exclusive, because contradictory information presented simultaneously to the left and right hemispheres interfered significantly with reach accuracy.

It is also worth noting that right-handed patients with right frontal lesions sometimes exhibit apraxic behaviors normally associated with left frontal damage. The impairments of these so-called "crossed apraxics" suggest that there may be individual variability in the cerebral organization of the systems involved in hand dominance and skilled movements of the hands (Haaland & Flaherty, 1984; Marchetti & Della Sala, 1997; Raymer et al., 1999) and face (Mani & Levine, 1988).

For reasons that are not entirely clear, patients with lesions of the corpus callosum secondary to stroke or other pathologies are much more likely to present with apraxic symptoms than those who have had surgical resections of this structure for intractable epilepsy (Hines, Chiu, McAdams, Bentler, & Lipcamon, 1992; Leiguarda, Starkstein, & Berthier, 1989). Although they are present soon after surgery, persistent apraxic behaviors following complete or anterior callosotomy are rare, and may only be apparent when patients are tested under conditions where cues are presented exclusively to one hemisphere at a time, as discussed earlier. Additional work is needed to determine whether this difference is attributable to the effects of nonsurgical lesions on adjacent gray matter, or whether partial sparing of the fiber tracts after a stroke is somehow responsible for destabilizing the system in a way not experienced with complete disconnection.

Modality-Specific or Disassociation Apraxia

Modality-specific deficits are isolated forms of apraxia in which the patient will commit errors when the movement instruction is provided in one but not all modalities (DeRenzi, Faglioni, & Sorgato, 1982; Rothi, Ochipa, & Heilman, 1997). Thus, the callosal apraxia syndrome with isolated verbal-praxis errors could be considered one form of modality-specific apraxia. The disturbance of visually guided movement in optic ataxia is another example of modality-specific apraxia (Perenin & Vighetto, 1988). Other forms are also described. For example, there are patients with ideational apraxia to seen objects who can still pantomime gestures in response to a spoken command (Rothi, Heilman, & Watson, 1985). Presumably this pattern is most likely to occur with lesions of visual-motor pathways. There are apraxics with deficits limited to the tactile modality (DeRenzi et al., 1982). Finally there are occasional patients with impaired imitation or pantomiming who could perform under other conditions (Rothi, Mack, & Heilman, 1986). For some, the deficit is particularly severe if the gestures are meaningless.

Limb-Kinetic Apraxia

The hallmark of limb-kinetic apraxia as originally defined by Kleist is an inability to perform tasks requiring individual finger movements (Kleist, 1907). He called it "innervatory apraxia" to stress the loss of finger dexterity. The clinical signs emerge with tasks such as tying a knot or using scissors. This has always been a controversial category of apraxia because the loss of hand deftness is common with many brain lesions, including pyramidal tract or premotor cortex lesions.

When limb apraxia is suspected to exist, there will often also be ideomotor apraxia. A useful approach is to consider this form of apraxia in relationship to the deftness that comes with hand dominance (Denes, Mantovan, Gallana, & Cappelletti, 1998). In patients with normal motor function who undergo (WADA) testing, there is evidence that the left hemisphere facilitates finger deftness in either hand, whereas the right hemisphere only facilitates the left hand (Heilman, Meador, & Loring, 2000).

Pathophysiological Substrates of Apraxia

Theoretical Context

Finkelnburg and Asymbolia

In the late 1800s Finkelnburg presented an influential viewpoint on the functional basis of apraxia (cited by Liepmann, 1908b). Finkelnburg considered apraxia, to be a particular form of asymbolia, the inability to convey a learned sign. In the case of apraxia, it was a sign denoted by hand movement rather than a spoken word that stood symbolically for another event or object. In the 1920s, Henry Head also emphasized that an act, when executed in isolation, requires a symbolic formulation that is not required with familiar usage (Head, 1926). A fundamental weakness of this asymbolia interpretation of apraxia is that patients with difficulty in producing the required manual acts on command usually also have difficulty in simple imitation. Imitation, particularly of meaningless gestures, does not necessarily require symbolic content.

Liepmann

One of the more remarkable intellectual developments in behavioral neurology was Liepmann's precise redefinition of the apraxia syndrome in his papers spanning 1900 through 1908 (Liepmann, 1900/1977, 1908a,b, 1905/1980, 1920; 1988; Liepmann & Maas, 1907). Although Steinthal had already proposed a classification of limb praxic disorders in 1871 and Finkelnburg had theorized the connection of asymbolia to apraxia, it was Liepmann who first proposed a coherent functional model that could incorporate all of the clinical variations of apraxia.

Liepmann proposed that actions be organized by formulae of movements. The formulae provide a description of movement through time and space. He identified the greater frequency of apraxia with left-brain injury and deduced that these space-time formulae must be represented within the left hemisphere. Furthermore, he made the bold deduction that the corpus callosum is essential for transmitting these formulae to the right motor cortex for movements performed by the left hand. He partitioned apraxia into three categories. Ideational apraxia was defined as a disruption of the retrieval or appropriate activation of the correct space-time formulae for a movement. The essential feature was that the patient could not generate the "idea" of the movement. The second category was ideomotor apraxia. In this case the formulae for generating actions are intact, but are disconnected from the centers in which they are implemented. Thus the patient knows what to do, but not how do it. Limb-kinetic apraxia was considered to be disruption within brain areas that generate the actual movements. The action is executed with disorganized coordination between appropriate muscle groups. Liepmann also defined the first patient with apraxia in the setting of a corpus callosum lesion. He distinguished functional deficits resulting from a focal cortical lesion from a white matter lesion that disconnected two cortical areas, i.e., the disconnection syndrome.

Liepmann's categorization for apraxia remains in widespread use. A potential drawback of his approach is the difficulty of distinguishing pure limb-kinetic apraxia from the pure motor deficits associated with corticospinal tract lesions. Both may lead to clumsy limb movements.

Geschwind

Liepmann's studies were largely ignored outside of Germany after World War I. Geschwind is credited for rediscovering Liepmann's work and promoting apraxia as a unique clinical syndrome. Influenced by Wernicke and convinced of the logic for disconnection syndromes, Geschwind argued that limb praxis should be categorized in relation to language processing (Geschwind, 1965; Geschwind & Damasio, 1985). The spoken command for a movement or gesture must first be decoded in receptive language areas, particularly left posterior temporal speech areas. Once comprehended, the command would then be transmitted to ipsilateral left premotor areas. Disconnection at this level would lead to impaired retrieval of actions, but preserved control of movements initiated internally via alternative pathways to motor command areas or movements triggered by external stimuli. For left-hand movements, the command would first have to pass into right motor association areas, then the right motor cortex. Geschwind provided additional evidence that apraxia was most common with left hemisphere cortical lesions. He also suggested that the anterior (frontal) portions of the corpus callosum were most important for transmitting movement representations between the hemispheres.

Geschwind emphasized the categorization of apraxia based on the body segments involved (limb, axial, or buccofacial). In some respects his work is a recapitulation of the asymbolia theory proposed by Finckelnburg and has the same limitation of not accounting for apraxic symptoms that were not clearly symbolic in form. Also undermining his theoretical approach was the clinical series by Kimura and Archibald (1974) that showed a strong correlation between traditional tests of apraxia based on spoken commands and tests requiring the imitation of meaningless gestures. Stated differently, Geschwind's definition of apraxia was overly restrictive relative to the remarkable clinical diversity of the disorder, and it did not adequately address the idea that motor programs and their execution could exist irrespective of conscious verbal operations.

Heilman and Rothi

Working as collaborators and also independently, Heilman and Rothi have presented numerous clinical series that define the scope of apraxia syndromes and their clinical variation (Rothi, Ochipa & Heilman, 1997). They have added anatomical clarity to Geschwind's model by showing that the left inferior parietal cortex is essential for representational motor planning, "upstream" of motor planning areas such as the supplementary motor area and the lateral premotor cortex. They confirmed the dissociation between ideomotor and ideational apraxias and the predominance of apraxia with left hemisphere lesions. More recently, Heilman and colleagues have clarified the clinical features of limb-kinetic apraxia (Heilman et al., 2000). They provide strong evidence that a subset of apraxia patients can be divided into disassociation (or modality-specific) syndromes. With modality-specific apraxia, the patient is unable to perform a movement described in one modality of instruction, but can respond to another form. This generalizes on Geschwind's approach in allowing logical alternatives other than deficits in following verbal instructions. Rothi also proposed a cognitive neuropsychological model of limb apraxia that distinguished verbal, object-based, and gestural pathways that provide input to motor areas (Rothi, Ochipa, & Heilman, 1991).

Roy and Square Model

How much do we need to know about a tool or object to use it? In 1985 Roy and Square proposed a cognitive neuropsychological model for action formation based on conceptual and production systems (Roy & Square, 1985). Within the conceptual system, they proposed the existence of three types of knowledge related to praxis: knowledge of actions independent of tools or objects, knowledge of objects and tools in relation to their action or functions, and knowledge of sequences of actions. In contrast, the production system represents the sensory-motor loops required for producing action and for online control of movement. Disruption of the conceptual system would lead to one of several forms of ideational apraxia, whereas disruption of the production system would lead to ideomotor apraxia.

Lesion Localization

Cortical Lesions

Apraxia is more common and severe with left hemisphere lesions. There is also a greater likelihood of defects in imitating gestures than with right hemisphere pathology (DeRenzi, Motti, & Nichelli, 1980). Left hemisphere lesions often cause many other motor deficits besides apraxia, such as deficits in the scheduling or timing of motor programs for simple or repetitive gestures. When apraxia is also present, there is usually an additional problem in preprogramming heterogeneous sequences, particularly when they contain three or more sequential hand positions (Harrington & Haaland, 1992).

Within the left hemisphere, approximate associations can be made between lesion location and type of apraxia, although these generalizations are subject to frequent exceptions. In general, posterior parietal lesions in the region of the intraparietal sulcus are linked to disturbances of visually guided movement, i.e., optic ataxia (Perenin & Vighetto, 1988). Parietal lesions are also closely associated with ideomotor and ideational apraxia. Lesions tend to be more frequent within the inferior rather than the superior parietal lobule. The parietal lobe is particularly critical for recognition of gestures. However, impairment of gesture recognition is often associated with a lesion extending into many other structures. Frontal lobe lesions within the premotor cortex near the primary motor cortex are associated with limb-akinetic apraxia. Injury or resection of the frontal lobe is also associated with impairments in learning long manual sequences and in the organization of spontaneous gestures (Canavan et al., 1989; Jason, 1985a). Imitation of simple or sequential movements is also impaired with frontal lesions, albeit to a milder degree than with parietal lesions (Jason, 1985b; Kolb & Milner, 1981).

By definition, apraxics are not hemiparetic or hemiplegic. Conversely, there is evidence that hemiparesis secondary to a cortical or subcortical stroke can occur without ideomotor apraxia. Recent behavioral studies suggest that not all hemiparetics are incapable of accurately representing at a conceptual level movements that they are incapable of executing. When tested soon after the onset of hemiparesis induced by a cerebrovascular accident, patients with focal lesions in a variety of motor structures (frontal, internal capsule, and basal ganglia) retain the ability to represent accurately the biomechanical constraints of the paralyzed limb when selecting how they would grasp objects appearing in various orientations (Johnson, 2000). Follow-up work indicates that these internal somatomotor representations are maintained even years after the onset of paralysis. Like ideomotor praxics, hemiparetic patients with parietal lobe damage have considerable difficulty with these tasks.

Subcortical Lesions

It is not uncommon for large hemispheric lesions in apraxic patients to extend into the basal ganglia, thalamus, or deep white matter (see the review by Leiguarda, and Marsden 2000). On the other hand, apraxia without aphasia is extremely uncommon in association with lesions restricted to the basal ganglia or thalamus. Thus the exact contribution of the basal ganglia function to apraxia remains poorly understood.

Experimental Research on Apraxia

Behavioral Studies

Apraxia results from an intrinsic, elemental defect of motor representation. An expanding repertoire of behavioral experiments is being applied to patients with parietal lobe lesions to better characterize the nature of a motor representation. For example, it is evident that parietal cortex damage leads to a profound difficulty in the mental rehearsal of movement, owing to either an inability to generate an appropriate kinesthetic reference for the intended or ongoing movement, or an inability to monitor motor outflow. Without an accurate efference copy it is difficult to subsequently compare kinesthetic information and motor goals (Sirigu et al., 1996). Different approaches for understanding motor representation that explain some of the clinical features of apraxia are discussed next.

Distorted Frame of Reference

It is now widely agreed that the parietal lobe is critical for merging information represented by different reference frames (Goodale & Haffenden, 1998). These reference frames can be described as coordinate frames oriented with respect to the retina, head, limb, or other body location. There are many instances where single neurons in the parietal cortex fire with respect to one or more of these reference frames. Or they can simply be distinguished by body-centered (egocentric) or extrapersonal space (allocentric). Here, also, neurons in the nonhuman primate motor cortex can be classified with respect to body- or world-referenced representations of space (Snyder, Grieve, Brotchie, & Andersen, 1998).

Disruption of a system that merges different frames of reference could lead to many different clinical defects (Goodale & Haffenden, 1998). The prototypical example is optic ataxia, in which visual information cannot be used to guide limb movement. More subtle defects can also be observed. Binkofski and colleagues describe a series of patients with an inability to point toward objects that are observed with a mirror (Binkofski, Buccino, Dohle, Seitz, & Freund, 1999a). In the severe form, called "mirror agnosia," the patients will repeatedly reach into the mirror, even if they are shown the actual location of the target. In the milder form, called "mirror ataxia," patients will reach in the direction of the object, but with increased errors of reach and grasp, suggesting that the visual information is not adequately transformed to a body-centered frame of reference.

Online Error Correction

In addition to merging different reference frames, the parietal lobe may be critical for maintaining a continuous internal representation of the current state of the body with respect to the external world (Wolpert, Goodbody, & Husain, 1998a). This information would be used for generating dynamic motor error signals based on a motor efference copy and evolving sensory feedback (Desmurget & Grafton, 2000). Patients with bilateral parietal lesions may show an inability to make online corrections of errors in reaching toward targets that are moved (Pisella et al., 2000). Similarly, transcranial magnetic stimulation of the parietal cortex in normal subjects at the onset of a reaching movement will block their ability to update a reaching movement toward a target that has shifted location (Desmurget et al., 1999). It is striking that reaches toward stationary targets are normal. These errors are subtler than the gross errors of reach and/or grasp observed with optic ataxia (Jeannerod, Decety, & Michel, 1994).

Disordered Body Schema

Successful goal-directed behavior, including the formation of gestures, is predicated on an accurate representation of the self and the body schema. In an intriguing study of three apraxic patients with parietal lobe lesions, Sirigu and colleagues identified an unusual disturbance of the body schema (Sirigu, Daprati, Pradat-Diehl, Franck, & Jeannerod, 1999). The patients observed gloved hand movements on a video monitor. The hand could be their own or that of an examiner in another room who was performing movements at the same time. The subjects were readily capable of distinguishing their own hand on the screen when the movement they performed was different than that generated by the examiner. However, when the movement was the same, they could not distinguish their own hand from that of the examiner, a task easily performed by normal subjects. This finding shows a complex, subtle disruption of body identification and the inability to compare internal with external feedback during movement in apraxic patients.

Motor Attention

Rushworth and colleagues propose a model of ideomotor apraxia that extends the well-known role of the right parietal cortex for covert attentional orientation (Rushworth, 2001). They argue that a complementary motor attentional system exists in the left hemisphere and that patients with ideomotor apraxia are unable to shift the focus of a motor-related attention from one movement in a sequence to the next (Rushworth, Nixon, Renowden, Wade, & Passingham, 1997c). Their patients with left parietal lesions were equal to control subjects in their attention to a movement, provided they were given advance warning with a precue. However, they were impaired in disengaging the focus of motor attention from one movement to another when the precue was incorrect.

Other clinical studies are consistent with this motor attention model. A striking example is the syndrome of magnetic misreaching described by Carey et al. (Carey, Coleman, & Sala, 1997). A patient with bilateral posterior parietal degeneration, when asked to reach to a target in her peripheral vision, would "slavishly" reach straight to a fovial fixation point. The reaches were determined by the place where she was looking, independent of the desired peripheral target. This problem can be thought of as an inability to disengage motor attention from a fixation point.

Short-Lived Motor Representation

A confounding problem in understanding how actions are organized is the observation that a motor representation can evolve along two fundamentally different levels, one semantic and conscious, the other implicit and highly automatic (Rossetti, 1998). Rossetti has proposed that control of eye and hand movements exhibits automatic features that are not always compatible with conscious control. Conscious intervention can contaminate or override short-lived motor representation, but the reciprocal influence does not occur. Immediate action is not mediated by the same neural system as delayed action. Patients may show an inability to consciously perceive or describe sensory information used to generate a motor behavior, but will perform the behavior well under natural conditions.

Patient D.F. described by Goodale and colleagues is a striking example (Goodale, Milner, Jakobson, & Carey, 1991). This patient had a severe form of visual agnosia secondary to bilateral lesions in the occipitoparietal cortex. She could not perceive shape or orientation when tested with an explicit perceptual test. However, she could readily insert an envelope through a slot with the proper hand orientation, a skill that required similar knowledge of orientation and target location. Apraxia patients can show a similar impairment of function when they are tested under explicit instruction, and they show dramatic improvement when stimuli such as tools are provided.

Animal Studies of Limb-Action Planning

There is no definitive behavioral correlate of apraxia in nonhuman primates. Research has focused instead on the role of the cortical and subcortical systems involved in various aspects of prehensile movements, including selection of movement, pointing, reaching, and grasping (Wise & Desimone, 1988). These studies detail the anatomical cortico-cortical connections between parietal and frontal areas and identify the electrophysiologically defined functional properties of neurons in localized areas of the cortex. In general, nonhuman primate studies show that the sensory-to-motor transformations involved in reaching and grasping visual objects are accomplished by two specialized subsystems that interconnect distinct regions of the parietal and frontal cortices (Jeannerod, Arbib, Rizzolatti, & Sakata, 1995).

Reaching toward a target in extrapersonal space involves a dorsal pathway that traverses the dorsal parietal cortex, the intraparietal sulcus, and the premotor cortex (Mountcastle, Lynch, Georgopoulos, Sakata, & Acuna, 1975). These areas are directly connected (Cavada & Goldman-Rakic, 1989) and appear to be critical for generating motor commands that can move the limb toward targets located with respect to proprioceptive or visual information. A second pathway traverses the inferior parietal, anterior intraparietal, and ventral premotor cortices (Luppino, Murata, Govini, & Matelli, 1999). Function in this ventral pathway is more closely associated with determining the properties of objects that are subsequently used to plan a grasp. These two pathways must share information to allow the close coordination and control of reach and grasp observed with normal prehension.

The dorsal pathway can be further segregated into functionally distinct domains. Lesions of the lateral intraparietal cortex and the adjacent inferior parietal lobule or in the white matter connecting the occipital and parietal cortices lead to inaccuracies in reaching toward visual targets (Haaxma & Kuypers, 1974; Rushworth, Nixon, & Passingham, 1997a). More dorsal lesions involving the medial intraparietal sulcus and the adjacent superior parietal lobule lead to errors in reaching toward targets in the dark. These areas appear to represent the limb in terms of spatial position and link motor output (copy efference) and proprioceptive information (Rushworth, Nixon, & Passingham, 1997b). Single-unit recording studies obtained during movement show that neurons in the medial intraparietal area are modulated by the direction of the hand movement, whereas cells in the lateral intraparietal area encode a predictive representation of the movement that is independent of the visual or motor output (Eskandar & Assad, 1999). Such a predictive signal would be a critical component of visuomotor transformations.

Parietal lesions do not disrupt the selection of a reaching movement based on instructional cues. In contrast, dorsal premotor cortex lesions lead to an impairment of learning new associations between instructional cues and reaching movements, i.e., the mapping of sensory-motor associations (Wise & Kurata, 1989). Cells within the dorsal premotor cortex show complex properties that are consistent with the capacity to transform target information into a motor command (Shen & Alexander, 1997).

Because the posterior parietal cortex can be divided into planning regions for different types of actions, it has been argued that each area should code the required movement in relation to a coordinate reference frame that is most appropriate for the respective movement (Colby, 1998). For example, within the more posterior parietal cortex of the dorsal pathway, there is growing electrophysiological evidence for a "parietal reach region" where sensorimotor transformations for reaching toward a target are generated with respect to an eye-centered reference (Batista, Buneo, Snyder, & Andersen, 1999). Additional areas showing both eye- and body-centered reference frames are found within the lateral intraparietal cortex. Within the inferior parietal lobule, there is evidence for an environment-centered frame of reference (Snyder et al., 1998).

Turning to the ventral pathway, a key area for action-oriented processing of an object appears to be the anterior intraparietal sulcus (AIP). There are other areas within the inferior temporal lobe that are essential for identifying objects. Unlike the inferior temporal cortex, which appears to be critical for object identification, the AIP appears to be critical for linking the properties of an object with the appropriate grasp attributes (Sakata, Taira, Kusunoki, Murata, & Tanaka, 1997). The AIP receives the binocular three-dimensional features of objects. Grasp planning in the AIP occurs in concert with the ventral premotor cortex, to which the AIP is reciprocally connected. The AIP contains several subpopulations of "manipulation" cells that code the specific hand configurations necessary for grasping objects (Taira et al., 1990), or a target object's three-dimensional characteristics (Murata, Gallese, Luppino, Kaseda, & Sakata, 2000).

Cells within the anatomically connected ventral premotor area appear to be involved in the prepara-tion and execution of visually and haptically guided grasping movements (Rizzolatti et al., 1990). Typical cells in this area show coordinate frames that are anchored to the eye, head, or body part (Graziano, Hu, & Gross, 1997b). Many cells in this area respond to objects viewed in close proximity to the face or arm of the animal. The neurons continue to fire in the dark, demonstrating object permanence (Graziano, Hu, & Gross, 1997a). Thus, the area appears to support sensorimotor transformations linking the body with an object.

Functional Neuroimaging Studies of Limb-Action Planning

Recent functional neuroimaging studies contribute to our understanding of the structures involved in various apraxic conditions. At present, there are few studies that use these techniques to directly explore the mechanisms responsible for apraxic behavior. Instead, work has concentrated primarily on mapping the systems involved in the production and conceptualization of movements in healthy adults. These findings yield insights into the distributed networks of the regions involved in these functions, and therefore provide a broader context in which the effects of focal brain injury and the associated behavioral impairments exhibited by the apraxic individual can be interpreted. There are two constraints that limit neuroimaging studies of human motor behavior: the requirement to maintain a constant head position during data acquisition, and the restrictive physical confines of current imaging systems. For these reasons, researchers have focused on a relatively small range of movements.

Production Domain

Simple Movements As noted earlier, a key element in the diagnosis of apraxia is ruling out impairments attributable to an explicit weakness that can arise from damage to a variety of peripheral and/or central structures. Having satisfied this criterion, however, apraxic patients may exhibit global difficulties in the production of simple movements. The past two decades have seen a large number of functional imaging studies of simple unilateral and bilateral movements involving the upper limbs. These studies support the existence of multiple somatotopically organized representations in a variety of structures within the cortical motor system including the M1, supplementary motor area (SMA), and premotor area (PMA) (Grafton, Woods, & Mazziotta, 1993). A typical result in these studies is that simple finger movements activate the contralateral M1 and the ipsilateral cerebellum, SMA, and S1 (Grafton, Mazziotta, Woods, & Phelps, 1992). An important variable in these studies is whether movements are generated in response to an external sensory stimulus (e.g., an auditory or visual pacing cue) or are generated internally by the subject (Jahanshahi et al., 1995). This distinction may underlie the common clinical observation that some apraxic patients have difficulty initiating movements spontaneously, yet may exhibit no difficulty in performing stimulus-driven responses such as covering the mouth when coughing.

Intransitive Actions   Double dissociation between intransitive and transitive movements suggests that these two classes of actions should be represented in relatively independent subsystems within the human brain. To date there have been no attempts to directly compare these two classes of actions in a single functional neuroimaging experiment. However, considerable attention has been devoted to the representation of meaningless and meaningful intransitive movements or gestures. One of the earliest gestures to develop, and the most ubiquitous, is pointing to locations in the environment. Studies of pointing to visual targets indicate the involvement of a widely distributed system of cortical and subcortical structures that include the contralateral motor, premotor, and ventral supplementary motor areas and the cingulate, superior parietal, and dorsal occipital cortices (Grafton, Fagg, Woods, & Arbib, 1996b). Several of these areas also contribute to gestures made in response to symbolic cues or imitated.

Iacoboni and colleagues recently identified a network of areas that were activated regardless of whether a finger movement was made in response to a visual cue or after observation of another's hand modeling the action (Iacoboni et al., 1999). Furthermore, two specific areas—the opercular region of the frontal cortex and the rostral, right, superior parietal lobe—showed increased activity when movements were initiated in response to an observed model. These findings were interpreted as supporting a view of gestural behavior in which perceiving an action automatically activates brain mechanisms that would be involved in producing the same behavior. This direct mapping or common coding hypothesis (CCH) originated with single-unit recordings in monkeys showing that some cells within the ventral premotor cortex respond to both observation and production of the same manual movements (Gallese, Fadiga, Fogassi, & Rizzolatti, 1996; Rizzolatti & Fadiga, 1998; Rizzolatti, Fadiga, Gallese, & Fogassi, 1996a).

There are now reasons to believe that the CCH may hold for several areas in the human brain. It has been known for some time that observation of movement induces electromyographical (EMG) changes in the muscles that would be involved in carrying out comparable actions (Berger & Hadley, 1975). This phenomenon appears to result from activity changes in the primary motor cortex associated with perception of movement. Indeed, observation of gestures selectively lowers the threshold for the stimulation of the motor cortex that is needed to induce motor-evoked potentials recorded from subjects' hand muscles (Fadiga, Fogassi, Pavesi, & Rizzolatti, 1995).

Transitive Actions   Recent positron emission tomography (PET) studies (Binkofski et al., 1999b; Binkofski et al., 1998; Grafton et al., 1996b) and investigations of the effects of localized brain lesions (Sirigu et al., 1996) suggest that sensory-to-motor transformations are accomplished by homologous parietofrontal circuits in humans.

Conceptual Domain

Intransitive Actions   To the extent that the CCH is valid, it should be possible to investigate many structures in the gesture production subsystem through paradigms that involve observation of gestures. The vast majority of functional neuroimaging studies have taken this approach because it allows one to study gestures while avoiding the difficulties associated with having subjects move during data acquisition. Because these studies do not involve explicit production of movement, they fall within the conceptual domain. The results of this work have revealed a network of areas in the frontal and parietal cortices that are activated by the perception of manual actions (Grafton, Arbib, Fadiga, & Rizzolatti, 1996a; Rizzolatti et al., 1996b) and meaning less gestures (Decety & Grezes, 1999; Grezes, Costes, & Decety, 1999). Many of these dorsal brain structures, including the primary motor and somatosensory cortices, are also involved in the production of comparable actions by the observer (Rizzolatti et al., 1996b). Furthermore, task demands appear to play an important role in determining which structures are activated during observation of gestures. More precisely, prefrontal structures associated with encoding of memory are engaged when subjects are instructed to observe gestures with the intention of performing an upcoming recognition task, whereas the intention to imitate gestures activates areas involved in motor planning and production (Grezes et al., 1999). Together, these results raise the interesting possibility that apraxics who have difficulties in producing intransitive gestures may also exhibit problems perceiving the same actions.

As initially novel gestures become recognizable, the gesture representation system exhibits considerable experience-dependent plasticity. Specifically, there is a decrease in parietal activation and an associated increase in regions of the frontal cortex, including the angular gyrus, with increasing familiarity (Decety et al., 1997; Grezes et al., 1999).

Meaningful Gestures   American Sign Language (ASL) is a gesture-based linguistic system that utilizes static hand postures, hand movements, and spatial locations to convey meaning (Bellugi, Poizner, & Klima, 1989; Poizner, Bellugi, & Klima, 1990a). While perception of meaningless gestures activates a network of areas on the dorsal surface of the brain, perception of ASL by expert signers involves more ventral areas located in and around the classic language centers of the left temporal lobe, as well as the primary motor cortex (Neville et al., 1998; Soderfeldt et al., 1997). Put differently, at some point during the acquisition of ASL, there appears to be a large-scale, experience-dependent reorganization in the neural representation of gestures that is related to their acquiring linguistic valence. At present, no single study has used neuroimaging to directly observe this shift in gesture representation related to expertise.

Transitive Actions   As noted earlier, apraxic patients often display the ability to produce action when they are provided with the appropriate tool or utensil, but fail to do so when they are required to mime (Sirigu et al., 1995). Although miming the use of tools has not been directly investigated, there are a number of neuroimaging studies that explored the representation of tools and their uses.

Representations of Tools   The question of whether different categories of objects (e.g., animals, faces, and buildings) are represented in separate cortical modules on the ventral surface of the temporal lobes has received copious attention in the neuroimaging literature (Farah & Aguirre, 1999). Of relevance to understanding apraxia is the observation that the left, premotor, dorsal (PMd) cortex is activated during either naming (Martin, Haxby, Lalonde, Wiggs, & Ungerleider, 1995; Martin, Wiggs, Ungerleider, & Haxby, 1996) or passive observation (Martin, et al., 1996) of familiar, graspable tools (e.g., a hammer) as opposed to other nontool objects. This has been interpreted as evidence that memory representations of objects belonging to the tool category are both visual and motor in nature.

As noted earlier, the PMd cortex is part of the parietofrontal network involved in visually guided reaching. This work suggests that damage to this circuit may disrupt not only object-oriented actions but also the perception of tools. Indeed, clinical observations indicate that ideomotor apraxics often have difficulty selecting the tools appropriate for solving a specific task.

Representations of Tool Use   In the earlier discussion of transitive actions, evidence was reviewed showing that the transformation of perceptual information into a motor plan—sensory-to-motor transformation—for reaching and grasping involves two dissociable frontoparietal networks (Jeannerod et al., 1995). Less well understood are the mechanisms involved in anticipating the consequences of potential actions on the body and the surrounding environment and using these predictions to select specific movements. In computational studies of motor control, these motor-to-sensory transformations are solved by systems that implement forward internal models and inverse internal models, respectively (Wolpert et al., 1998b).

One approach to investigating the mechanisms involved in motor-to-sensory transformations is through paradigms that involve mentally simulated actions, or motor imagery. Functional neuroimaging studies spanning two decades have shown that the imagining of movements activates many of the same brain structures as an actual action (Jeannerod, 1995; Johnson, 2000). Motor imagery tasks require subjects to plan actions in the absence of the sensory feedback that accompanies movements. To solve such tasks correctly, the subjects must instead construct accurate internal representations of the anticipated sensory consequences of would-be movements. A recent study by Johnson et al. (Jeannerod, 1995; Johnson, 2000) examined the areas of activation associated with deciding whether it would be natural to grasp a handle (appearing in a variety of different orientations) in an overhand grip. Their findings were consistent with the hypothesis that imagined grip selection involves parietal and frontal areas that contribute to sensory-to-motor transformations during manual prehension. Specifically, grip selection was accompanied by significant changes in the parietal and frontal areas believed to be homologous with the monkey "reach" circuit discussed earlier. Deciding how best to grasp the handle with either the left or right hand induced bilateral activation of the PMd cortex. These sites are consistent with those found in earlier studies of reaching (Grafton et al., 1996b) and movement selection (Grafton, Fagg, & Arbib, 1998) in humans and monkeys (Kalaska & Crammond, 1992, 1995; Kurata and Hoffman, 1994) and support the claim that the caudal PMd cortex is involved in the preparation and selection of conditional motor behavior (Grafton et al., 1998).

Grip selection also activated several areas within the superior (SPL) and inferior (IPL) parietal lobules. In contrast to the bilateral effects observed in the PMd cortex, activations within the parietal cortex were dependent in part on the hand on which grip decisions were based. Selection of a left-handed grip activated contralateral areas in the IPL located in anterior and medial regions along the intraparietal sulcus. These areas may be human homologs of the functional areas involved in grasping anterior intraparictal area (AIP) and reaching medial intraparetal area (MIP), respectively, in monkeys. Decisions based on the right hand also involved a region of the contralateral IPL, at a medial location along the bank of the intraparietal sulcus. This site may also correspond to the functional MIP. Consistent with this interpretation, the responses of cells within the monkey MIP are most pronounced when forthcoming actions will involve the contralateral hand (Colby & Duhamel, 1991). Together these findings suggest that the IPL may compute internal motor representations relative to the intended effector (Wise, Boussaoud, Johnson, & Caminiti, 1997).

Unexpectedly, grip decisions involving either hand also activated a common region of the right SPL. It is well known that the SPL is the major source of parietal input to the PMd cortex in monkeys and is involved in higher-level proprioception (Lacquaniti, Guigon, Bianchi, Ferraina, &

Caminiti, 1995; Mountcastle et al., 1975). Involvement in imagined grip selection is consistent with evidence that in humans the SPL participates in the representation of finger, hand, and arm movements (Grafton et al., 1992; Deiber et al., 1998), as well as in high-level spatial-cognitive processes such as mental rotation (Alivisatos & Petrides, 1997; Bonda, Petrides, Frey, & Evans, 1995) and the imitation of hand gestures (Iacoboni et al., 1999). As mentioned previously, patients with lesions in the SPL may show difficulties in visually guided reaching and eye movements, collectively known as optic ataxia (Perenin & Vighetto, 1988). Consistent with the right lateralization of SPL activations in grip selection, optic ataxics with right hemisphere damage have difficulty making visually guided reaches with either hand into the contralesional hemifield. By contrast, left hemisphere lesions affect only the contralateral right hand (DeRenzi, 1988; Goodale, 1990). Together, these findings suggest a specialization in the right SPL for processing the egocentric spatial information necessary for planning actions involving either limb.

Conclusions and Future Directions

There are many gaps in our understanding of apraxia in relation to the function of distinct cortical systems. Central to this issue is the need to define the relationship between apraxia and action-oriented perceptual processes. These processes include gesture recognition, tool representation, and the perception of intentionality. It remains unclear if behavioral testing of action-oriented processes with explicit measurements adequately captures operations that are normally performed implicitly (Rossetti, 1998).

Confounding experimental attempts to investigate movement, the experimental workspace of functional imaging has significant limitations on allowable actions. The artificial quality of allowable tasks can undermine the interpretation of brain mapping studies of action perception. For example, motor simulation is now commonly used to map the brain structures involved in motor planning by means of imagined movement or presentations of virtual reality. The connection between these simulated processes and real perceptions when planning natural actions remains unknown.

The development of praxis during infancy is understood in only the broadest terms. It will be critical to relate the overlearned, highly practiced movements of adulthood to the earliest emergence of primitive motor acts, such as reaching, grasping, and anticipating. As children, we have a profound capacity to learn by imitation. What is the connection between this childhood motor learning and acquisition of skills as adults?

In parallel, the importance of mirror systems as defined in nonhuman primates for human motor control and learning remains largely speculative. Although it is extremely attractive to think of mirror systems as fundamental substrates for imitative learning, this hypothesis remains untested in humans. Central to this problem is resolving the marked anatomical differences between the nonhuman primate cortex and that of humans, particularly in the parietal lobe. These anatomical differences limit our ability to generalize observations on neuron firing properties derived from the monkey. Similarly, functional brain imaging techniques can identify putative cortical areas involved in motor processes related to apraxia, but cannot ascribe functional causality with any certainty. Finally, the complex interaction between action and attention, which is profoundly distorted in apraxic patients, merits further study.

References

Alivisatos, B., & Petrides, M. (1997). Functional activation of the human brain during mental rotation. *Neuropsychologia, 35*, 111–118.

Batista, A. P., Buneo, C. A., Snyder, L. H., & Andersen, R. A. (1999). Reach plans in eye-centered coordinates. *Science, 285*, 257–260.

Bellugi, U., Poizner, H., & Klima, E. S. (1989). Language, modality and the brain. *Trends in Neuroscience, 12*, 380–388.

Berger, S. M., & Hadley, S. W. (1975). Some effects of a model's performance on an observer's electromyographic activity. *American Journal of Psychology, 88*, 263–276.

Binkofski, F., Buccino, G., Dohle, C., Seitz, R. J., & Freund, H.-J. (1999a). Mirror agnosia and mirror ataxia constitue different parietal lobe disorders. *Annals of Neurology, 46*, 51–61.

Binkofski, F., Buccino, G., Posse, S., Seitz, R. J., Rizzolatti, G., & Freund, H. (1999b). A frontoparietal circuit for object manipulation in man: Evidence from an fMRI study. *European Journal of Neuroscience, 11*, 3276–3286.

Binkofski, F., Dohle, C., Posse, S., Stephan, K. M., Hefter, H., Seitz, R. J., & Freund, H. J. (1998). Human anterior intraparietal area subserves prehension: A combined lesion and functional MRI activation study. *Neurology, 50*, 1253–1259.

Bonda, E., Petrides, M., Frey, S., & Evans, A. (1995). Neural correlates of mental transformations of the body-in-space. *Proceedings of the National Academy of Sciences, U.S.A., 92*, 11180–11184.

Canavan, A. G., Passingham, R. E., Marsden, C. D., Quinn, N., Wyke, M., & Polkey, C. E. (1989). Sequencing ability in parkinsonians, patients with frontal lobe lesions and patients who have undergone unilateral temporal lobectomies. *Neuropsychologia, 27*, 787–798.

Carey, D. P., Coleman, R. J., & Sala, S. D. (1997). Magnetic misreaching. *Cortex, 33*, 639–652.

Cavada, C., & Goldman-Rakic, P. S. (1989). Posterior parietal cortex in rhesus monkey: II Evidence for segregated corticocortical networks linking sensory and limbic areas with the frontal lobe. *Journal of Comparative Neurology, 287*, 422–445.

Clark, M. A., Merians, A. S., Kothari, A., Poizner, H., Macauley, B., Gonzalez Rothi, L. J., & Heilman, K. M. (1994). Spatial planning deficits in limb apraxia. *Brain, 117*, 1093–1106.

Colby, C. L. (1998). Action-oriented spatial reference frames in cortex. *Neuron, 20*, 15–30.

Colby, C. L., & Duhamel, J. R. (1991). Heterogeneity of extrastriate visual areas and multiple parietal areas in the macaque monkey. *Neuropsychologia, 29*, 517–537.

Decety, J., & Grezes, J. (1999). Neural mechanisms subserving the perception of human actions. *Trends in Cognition Science, 3*, 172–178.

Decety, J., Grezes, J., Costes, N., Perani, D., Jeannerod, M., Procyk, E., Grassi, F., & Fazio, F. (1997). Brain activity during observation of actions. Influence of action content and subject's strategy. *Brain, 120*, 1763–1777.

Deiber, M. P., Ibanez, V., Honda, M., Sadato, N., Raman, R., & Hallett, M. (1998). Cerebral processes related to visuomotor imagery and generation of simple finger movements studied with positron emission tomography. *Neuroimage, 7*, 73–85.

Denes, G., Mantovan, M. C., Gallana, A., & Cappelletti, J. Y. (1998). Limb-kinetic apraxia. *Movement Disorders, 13*, 468–476.

DeRenzi, E., Faglioni, P., & Sorgato, P. (1982). Modality-specific and supramodal mechanisms of apraxia. *Brain, 105*, 301–312.

DeRenzi, E., & Luchelli, F. (1998). Ideational apraxia. *Brain, 111*, 1173–1185.

DeRenzi, E., Motti, F., & Nichelli, P. (1980). Imitating gestures. A quantitative approach to ideomotor apraxia. *Archives of Neurology, 37*, 6–10.

Desmurget, M., Epstein, C. M., Turner, R. S., Prablanc, C., Alexander, G. E., & Grafton, S. T. (1999). Role of the posterior parietal cortex in updating reaching movements to a visual target. *Nature Neuroscience, 2*, 563–567.

Desmurget, M., & Grafton, S. T. (2000). Forward modeling allows feedback control for fast reaching movements. *Trends in Cognition Science, 4*, 423–431.

Eskandar, E. N., & Assad, J. A. (1999). Dissociation of visual, motor and predictive signals in parietal cortex during visual guidance. *Nature Neuroscience, 2*, 88–93.

Fadiga, L., Fogassi, L., Pavesi, G., & Rizzolatti, G. (1995). Motor facilitation during action observation: A magnetic stimulation study. *Journal of Neurophysiology, 73*, 2608–2611.

Farah, M. J., & Aguirre, G. K. (1999). Imaging visual recognition: PET and fMRI studies of the functional anatomy of human visual recognition. *Trends in Cognition Sciences, 3*, 179–186.

Gallese, V., Fadiga, L., Fogassi, L., & Rizzolatti, G. (1996). Action recognition in the premotor cortex. *Brain, 119*, 593–609.

Gazzaniga, M. S., Bogen, J. E., & Sperry, R. W. (1967). Dyspraxia following division of the cerebral commissures. *Archives of Neurology, 16*, 606–612.

Geschwind, N. (1965). Disconnexion syndromes in animals and man. I. *Brain, 88*, 237–294.

Geschwind, N., & Damasio, A. R. (1985). Apraxia. In V. J. Vinken, G. W. Brun & H. L. Klawans (Eds.), *Handbook of clinical neurology* Vol. 1. *Clinical neuropsychology* (pp. 423–432). Amsterdam: Elsevier. pp. 423–432.

Goldenberg, G., Wimmer, A., Holzner, F., & Wessely, P. (1985). Apraxia of the left limbs in a case of callosal disconnection: The contribution of medial frontal lobe damage. *Cortex, 21*, 135–148.

Goodale, M. A., & Haffenden, A. (1998). Frames of reference for perception and action in the human viisual system. *Neuroscience & Behavioral Reviews, 22*, 161–172.

Goodale, M. A., Milner, A. D., Jakobson, L. S., & Carey, D. P. (1991). A neurological dissociation between perceiving objects and grasping them. *Nature, 349*, 154–156.

Graff-Radford, N. R., Welsh, K., & Godersky, J. (1987). Callosal apraxia. *Neurology, 37*, 100–105.

Grafton, S. T., Arbib, M. A., Fadiga, L., & Rizzolatti, G. (1996a). Localization of grasp representations in humans by positron emission tomography. 2. Observation compared with imagination. *Experimental Brain Research, 112*, 103–111.

Grafton, S. T., Fagg, A. H., & Arbib, M. A. (1998). Dorsal premotor cortex and conditional movement selection: A PET functional mapping study. *Journal of Neurophysiology, 79*, 1092–1097.

Grafton, S. T., Fagg, A. H., Woods, R. P., & Arbib, M. A. (1996b). Functional anatomy of pointing and grasping in humans. *Cerebral Cortex, 6*, 226–237.

Grafton, S. T., Mazziotta, J. C., Woods, R. P., & Phelps, M. E. (1992). Human functional anatomy of visually guided finger movements. *Brain, 115*, 565–587.

Grafton, S. T., Woods, R. P., & Mazziotta, J. C. (1993). Within-arm somatotopy in human motor areas determined by positron emission tomography imaging of cerebral blood flow. *Experimental Brain Research, 95*, 172–176.

Graziano, M. S., Hu, X. T., & Gross, C. G. (1997a). Coding the locations of objects in the dark. *Science, 277*, 239–241.

Graziano, M. S., Hu, X. T., & Gross, C. G. (1997b). Visuospatial properties of ventral premotor cortex. *Journal of Neurophysiology, 77*, 2268–2292.

Grezes, J., Costes, N., & Decety, J. (1999). The effects of learning and intention on the neural network involved in the perception of meaningless actions. *Brain, 122*, 1875–1887.

Haaland, K. Y., & Flaherty, D. (1984). The different types of limb apraxia errors made by patients with left vs. right hemisphere damage. *Brain Cognition, 3*, 370–384.

Haaland, K. Y., Harrington, D. L., & Knight, R. T. (1999). Spatial deficits in ideomotor limb apraxia. A kinematic analysis of aiming movements. *Brain, 122*, 1169–1182.

Haaxma, R., & Kuypers, H. (1974). Role of occipito-frontal cortico-cortical connections in visual guidance of relatively independent hand and finger movements in rhesus monkeys. *Brain Research, 71*, 361–366.

Harrington, D. L., & Haaland, K. Y. (1992). Motor sequencing with left hemisphere damage. Are some cognitive deficits specific to limb apraxia? *Brain, 115*, 857–874.

Head, H. (1926). *Aphasia and kindred disorders of speech.* Cambridge: Cambridge University Press.

Heilman, K. M., Maher, L. M., Greenwald, M. L., & Rothi, L. J. (1997). Conceptual apraxia from lateralized lesions. *Neurology, 49*, 457–464.

Heilman, K. M., Meador, K. J., & Loring, D. W. (2000). Hemispheric asymmetries of limb-kinetic apraxia. *Neurology, 55*, 523–526.

Hines, M., Chiu, L., McAdams, L. A., Bentler, P. M., & Lipcamon, J. (1992). Cognition and the corpus callosum: Verbal fluency, visuospatial ability, and language lateralization related to midsagittal surface areas of callosal subregions. *Behavioral Neuroscience, 106(1)*, 3–14.

Iacoboni, M., Woods, R. P., Brass, M., Bekkering, H., Mazziotta, J. C., & Rizzolatti, G. (1999). Cortical mechanisms of human imitation. *Science, 286*, 2526–2528.

Jahanshahi, M., Jenkins, I. H., Brown, R. G., Marsden, C. D., Passingham, R. E., & Brooks, D. J. (1995). Self-initiated versus externally triggered movements. I. An investigation using measurement of regional cerebral blood flow with PET and movement-related potentials in normal and Parkinson's disease subjects. *Brain, 118*, 913–933.

Jason, G. W. (1985a). Gesture fluency after focal cortical lesions. *Neuropsychologia, 23*, 463–481.

Jason, G. W. (1985b). Manual sequence learning after focal cortical lesions. *Neuropsychologia, 23*, 483–496.

Jeannerod, M. (1995). Mental imagery in the motor context. *Neuropsychologia, 33*, 1419–1432.

Jeannerod, M., Arbib, M. A., Rizzolatti, G., & Sakata, H. (1995). Grasping objects: The cortical mechanisms of visuomotor transformation. *Trends in Neuroscience, 18*, 314–320.

Jeannerod, M., Decety, J., & Michel, F. (1994). Impairment of grasping movements following a bilateral posterior parietal lesion. *Neuropsychologia, 32*, 369–380.

Johnson, S. H. (2000). Imagining the impossible: Intact motor representations in hemiplegics. *Neuroreport, 11,* 729–732.

Kalaska, J. F., & Crammond, D. J. (1992). Cerebral cortical mechanisms of reaching movements. *Science, 255,* 1517–1523.

Kalaska, J. F., & Crammond, D. J. (1995). Deciding not to GO: Neuronal correlates of response selection in a GO/NOGO task in primate premotor and parietal cortex. *Cerebral Cortex, 5,* 410–428.

Klmura, D., & Archibald, Y. (1974) Motor function of the left hemisphere *Brain, 97,* 337–350.

Kleist, K. (1907). Kortikale (innervatorische) apraxie. *Jahrbuch für Psychiatrie und Neurologie, 28,* 46–112.

Kolb, B., & Milner, B. (1981). Performance of complex arm and facial movements after focal brain lesions. *Neuropsychologia, 19,* 491–503.

Kurata, K., & Hoffman, D. S. (1994). Differential effects of muscimol microinjection into dorsal and ventral aspects of the premotor cortex of monkeys. *Journal of Neurophysiology, 71,* 1151–1164.

Lacquaniti, F., Guigon, E., Bianchi, L., Ferraina, S., & Caminiti, R. (1995). Representing spatial information for limb movement: Role of area 5 in the monkey. *Cerebral Cortex, 5,* 391–409.

Leiguarda, R. C., & Marsden, C. D. (2000). Limb apraxias. Higher-order disorders of sensorimotor integration. *Brain, 123,* 860–879.

Leiguarda, R., Starkstein, S., & Berthier, M. (1989). Anterior callosal haemorrhage. A partial interhemispheric disconnection syndrome. *Brain, 112,* 1019–1037.

Leiguarda, R. C., & Starkstein, S. E. (1998). Apraxia in the syndromes of Pick complex. In A. Kertesz & D. G. Munoz (Eds.), *Pick's disease and Pick complex* (pp. 129–143). New York: Wiley-Liss.

Liepmann, H. (1900/1977). The syndrome of apraxia (motor asymboly) based on a case of unilateral apraxia. (Translated by W. H. O. Bohne, K. Liepmann, & D. A. Rottenberg from *Monatschrift für Psychiatrie und Neurologie 1900, 8,* 15–44). In D. A. Rottenberg & F. H. Hochberg (Eds.), *Neurological classics in modern translation.* New York: Hafner.

Liepmann, H. (1905/1980). The left hemisphere and action. (Translation from *Münchener Medizinische Wochenschriff 1905,* 48–49. Translations from Liepmann's essays on apraxia. Research Bulletin 506, Department of

Psychology, University of Western Ontario, London, Ontario.

Liepmann, H. (1908a). *Die linke hemisphere und das handeln* (The left hemisphere and handedness). Berlin: Karger.

Liepmann, H. (1908b). *Drei aufsätze aus dem apraxiegebiet.* Berlin: Karger.

Liepmann, H. (1920). Apraxie. *Ergebnisse der Gesamtem Medizin 1,* 516–543.

Liepmann, H., & Maas, O. (1907). Eie fall von linksseitiiger agraphie und apraxie bie rechtsseitiger lahmung. *Mschr Psychiatry Neurology, 10,* 214–227.

Liepmann, H. (1988) Apraxia. In Brown, J. W. (Ed.), *Agnosia and Aproxia: Selected papers of Liepmann, Lunge and Potzl* (pp. 3–43). Hillsdale, NJ.: Lawrence Erlbaum Associates.

Luppino, G., Murata, A., Govoni, P., & Matelli, M. (1999). Largely segregated parietofrontal connections linking rostral intraparietal cortex (areas AIP and VIP) and the ventral premotor cortex (areas F5 and F4). *Experimental Brain Research, 128,* 181–187.

Mani, R. B., & Levine, D. N. (1988). Crossed buccofacial apraxia. *Archives of Neurology, 45,* 581–584.

Marchetti, C., & Della Sala, S. (1997). On crossed apraxia. Description of a right-handed apraxic patient with right supplementary motor area damage. *Cortex, 33,* 341–354.

Martin, A., Haxby, J. V., Lalonde, F. M., Wiggs, C. L., & Ungerleider, L. G. (1995). Discrete cortical regions associated with knowledge of color and knowledge of action. *Science, 270,* 102–105.

Martin, A., Wiggs, C. L., Ungerleider, L. G., & Haxby, J. V. (1996). Neural correlates of category-specific knowledge. *Nature, 379,* 649–652.

Milner, B., & Kolb, B. (1985). Performance of complex arm movements and facial-movement sequences after cerebral commissurotomy. *Neuropsychologia, 23,* 791–799.

Mountcastle, V. B., Lynch, J. C., Georgopoulos, A., Sakata, & H., Acuna, C. (1975). Posterior parietal association cortex of the monkey: Command functions for operations within extrapersonal space. *Journal of Neurophysiology, 38,* 871–908.

Murata, A., Gallese, V., Luppino, G., Kaseda, M., & Sakata, H. (2000). Selectivity for the shape, size, and orientation of objects for grasping in neurons of monkey parietal area AIP. *Journal of Neurophysiology, 83,* 2580–2601.

Neville, H. J., Bavelier, D., Corina, D., Rauschecker, J., Karni, A., Lalwani, A., Braun, A., Clark, V., Jezzard, P., & Turner, R. (1998). Cerebral organization for language in deaf and hearing subjects: Biological constraints and effects of experience. *Proceeding of the National Academy of Science, U.S.A., 95*, 922–929.

Ochipa, C., Rothi, L. J., & Heilman, K. M. (1989). Ideational apraxia: A deficit in tool selection and use. *Annals of Neurology, 25*, 190–193.

Perenin, M. T., & Vighetto, A. (1988b). Optic ataxia: A specific disruption in visuomotor mechanisms. I. Different aspects of the deficit in reaching for objects. *Brain, 111*, 643–674.

Pisella, L., Grea, H., Tilikete, C., Vighetto, A., Desmurget, M., Rode, G., Boisson, D., & Rossetti, Y. (2000). An 'automatic pilot' for the hand in human posterior parietal cortex: Toward reinterpreting optic ataxia. *Nature Neuroscience, 3*, 729–736.

Poizner, H., Bellugi, U., & Klima, E. S. (1990a). Biological foundations of language: Clues from sign language. *Annual Review of Neuroscience, 13*, 283–307.

Poizner, H., Clark, M. A., Merians, A. S., Macauley, B., Gonzalez Rothi, L. J., & Heilman, K. M. (1995). Joint coordination deficits in limb apraxia. *Brain, 118*, 227–242.

Poizner, H., Mack, L., Verfaellie, M., Rothi, L. J., & Heilman, K. M. (1990b). Three-dimensional computer-graphic analysis of apraxia. Neural representations of learned movement. *Brain, 113*, 85–101.

Raymer, A. M., Merians, A. S., Adair, J. C., Schwartz, R. L., Williamson, D. J., Rothi, L. J., Poizner, H., & Heilman, K. M. (1999). Crossed apraxia: Implications for handedness. *Cortex, 35*, 183–199.

Rizzolatti, G., & Fadiga, L. (1998). Grasping objects and grasping action meanings: The dual role of monkey rostroventral premotor cortex (area F5). *Novartis Foundation Symposia, 218*, 81–95.

Rizzolatti, G., Fadiga, L., Gallese, V., & Fogassi, L. (1996a). Premotor cortex and recognition of motor actions. *Cognitive Brain Research, 3*, 131–141.

Rizzolatti, G., Fadiga, L., Matelli, M., Bettinardi, V., Paulesu, E., Perani, D., & Fazio, F. (1996b). Localization of grasp representations in humans by PET: 1. Observation versus execution. *Experimental Brain Research, 111*, 246–252.

Rizzolatti, G., Gentilucci, M., Camarda, R. M., Gallese, V., Luppino, G., Matelli, M., & Fogassi, L. (1990). Neurons related to reaching-grasping arm movements in the rostral part of area 6 (area 6a beta). *Experimental Brain Research, 82*, 337–350.

Rossetti, Y. (1998). Implicit short-lived motor representations of space in brain damaged and healthy subjects. *Consciousness and Cognition, 7*, 520–558.

Rothi, L. J. G., & Heilman, K. M. (1996). Liepmann (1900 and 1905): A definition of apraxia and a model of praxis. In C. Code, C.-W. Wallesch, Y. Joanett, & A. R. Lecours (Eds.), *Classic cases in neuropsychology* (pp. 111–122). East Sussex, UK: Psychology Press.

Rothi, L. J. G., Heilman, K. M., & Watson, R. T. (1985). Pantomime comprehension and ideomotor apraxia. *Journal of Neurology, Neurosurgery and Psychiatry, 48*, 207–210.

Rothi, L. J. G., Mack, L., & Heilman, K. M. (1986). Pantomime agnosia. *Journal of Neurology Neurosurgery and Psychiatry, 49*, 451–454.

Rothi, L. J. G., Ochipa, C., & Heilman, K. M. (1991). A cognitive neuropsychological model of limb praxis. *Cognitive Neuropsychology, 8*, 443–458.

Roy, E. A., & Square, P. A. (1985). Common considerations in the study of limb, verbal, and oral apraxia. In E. A. Roy (Ed.), *Neuropsychological studies of apraxia and related disorders* (pp. 111–161). Amsterdam: North-Holland.

Rushworth, M. F. (2001). The attentional role of the left parietal cortex: The distinct lateralization and localization of motor attention in the human brain. *Journal of Cognitive Neuroscience, 13*, 698–710.

Rushworth, M. F., Nixon, P. D., & Passingham, R. E. (1997a). Parietal cortex and movement. I. Movement selection and reaching. *Experimental Brain Research, 117*, 292–310.

Rushworth, M. F., Nixon, P. D., & Passingham, R. E. (1997b). Parietal cortex and movement. II. Spatial representation. *Experimental Brain Research, 117*, 311–323.

Rushworth, M. F., Nixon, P. D., Renowden, S., Wade, D. T., & Passingham, R. E. (1997c). The left parietal cortex and motor attention. *Neuropsychologia, 35*, 1261–1273.

Sakata, H., Taira, M., Kusunoki, M., Murata, A., & Tanaka, Y. (1997). The TINS Lecture. The parietal association cortex in depth perception and visual control of hand action. *Trends in Neuroscience, 20*, 350–357.

Shen, L., & Alexander, G. E. (1997). Preferential representation of instructed target location versus limb trajectory in dorsal premotor area. *Journal Neurophysiology, 77*, 1195–1212.

Sirigu, A., Cohen, L., Duhamel, J. R., Pillon, B., Dubois, B., & Agid, Y. (1995). A selective impairment of hand posture for object utilization in apraxia. *Cortex, 31*, 41–55.

Sirigu, A., Daprati, E., Pradat-Diehl, P., Franck, N., & Jeannerod, M. (1999). Perception of self-generated movement following left parietal lesion. *Brain, 122*, 1867–1874.

Sirigu, A., Duhamel, J. R., Cohen, L., Pillon, B., Dubois, B., & Agid, Y. (1996). The mental representation of hand movements after parietal cortex damage. *Science, 273*, 1564–1568.

Snyder, L. H., Grieve, K. L., Brotchie, P., & Andersen, R. A. (1998). Separate body- and world-referenced representations of visual space in parietal cortex. *Nature, 394*, 887–891.

Soderfeldt, B., Ingvar, M., Ronnberg, J., Eriksson, L., Serrander, M., & Stone-Elander, S. (1997). Signed and spoken language perception studied by positron emission tomography. *Neurology, 49*, 82–87.

Taira, M., Mine, S., Georgopoulos, A. P., Murata, A., & Sakata, H. (1990). Parietal cortex neurons of the monkey related to the visual guidance of hand movement. *Experimental Brain Research, 83*, 29–36.

Watson, R. T., & Heilman, K. M. (1983). Callosal apraxia. *Brain, 106*, 391–403.

Wise, S. P., Boussaoud, D., Johnson, P. B., & Caminiti, R. (1997). Premotor and parietal cortex: Corticocortical connectivity and combinatorial computations. *Annual Review of Neuroscience, 20*, 25–42.

Wise, S. P., & Desimone, R. (1988). Behavioral neurophysiology: Insights into seeing and grasping. *Science, 242*, 736–741.

Wise, S. P., & Kurata, K. (1989). Set-related activity in the premotor cortex of rhesus monkeys: Effect of triggering cues and relatively long delay intervals. *Somatosensorg Motor Research, 6*, 455–476.

Wolpert, D. M., Goodbody, S. J., & Husain, M. (1998a). Maintaining internal representations: The role of the human superior parietal lobe. *Nature Neuroscience, 1*, 529–533.

Wolpert, D. M., Miall, R. C., & Kawato, M. (1998b). Internal models in the cerebellum. *Trends in Cognitive Science, 2*, 338–347.

11 Lateral Prefrontal Syndrome: A Disorder of Executive Control

Robert T. Knight and Mark
D'Esposito

Evidence from neuropsychological, electrophysiological, and functional neuroimaging research supports a critical role for the lateral prefrontal cortex (PFC) in executive control of goal-directed behavior (Fuster, 1997). The extensive reciprocal PFC connections to virtually all cortical and subcortical structures place the PFC in a unique neuroanatomical position to monitor and manipulate diverse cognitive processes. For example, a meta-analysis of functional neuroimaging studies (Duncan & Owen, 2000) reveals the activation of common regions of the lateral PFC in a set of markedly diverse cognitive tasks. Activation in the PFC in these tasks centers in the posterior portions of the lateral PFC at the junction of the middle and inferior frontal gyri, including portions of the dorsal and ventral PFC (Brodmann areas 9, 44, 45, and 46) (Rajkowska & Goldman-Rakic, 1995a,b) (figure 11.1). Moreover, damage to the lateral PFC, excluding the language cortices in humans, results in a wide range of behavioral and cognitive deficits (Luria, 1966; Stuss & Benson, 1986; Damasio & Anderson, 1993; Mesulam, 1998). In short, patients with lateral PFC lesions have deficits in executive function, which is a term meant to capture a wide range of cognitive processes such as focused and sustained attention, fluency and flexibility of thought in the generation of solutions to novel problems, and planning and regulating adaptive and goal-directed behavior.

In contrast to lateral PFC damage, orbitofrontal damage spares many cognitive skills, but dramatically affects all spheres of social behavior (Stone, Baron-Cohen, & Knight, 1998; Bechera, Damasio, Tranel, & Anderson, 1998). The orbitofrontal patient is frequently impulsive, hyperactive, and lacking in proper social skills despite showing intact cognitive processing on a range of tasks that are typically impaired in patients with lateral PFC lesions. In some instances, the behavioral syndrome is so severe that the term *acquired sociopathy* has been used to describe the resultant personality profile of the orbitofrontal patient (Saver & Damasio, 1991). However, unlike true sociopaths, orbitofrontal patients typically feel remorse for their inappropriate behavior. Severe social and emotional dysfunction is typically observed only after bilateral orbitofrontal damage.

There has been a remarkable convergence of lesion, electrophysiological, and functional neuroimaging data from animals and humans on the role of the lateral PFC in cognition. The electrophysiological data provide important information on the timing of PFC modulation of cognitive processing. These data are complemented by functional neuroimaging findings defining the spatial characteristics of PFC involvement in a variety of cognitive processes, with evidence accruing for engagement of both inhibitory and excitatory processes. Finally, the neuropsychological data from studying patients with focal PFC lesions provide the crucial behavioral confirmation of electrophysiological and functional neuroimaging findings obtained in normal populations. In our view, the most complete picture will emerge from a fusion of classic neuropsychological approaches with powerful new techniques to measure the physiology of the human brain.

An exhaustive review and synthesis of the role of the PFC in cognition and behavior is beyond the scope of this chapter. Rather, we focus on the lateral PFC and specifically the role of this region in executive control. We begin by describing a typical patient with lateral PFC damage, followed by a clinical description of this syndrome, which has been gathered by observing other patients such as the one described in the case report. After a brief survey of the range of cognitive functions that have been attributed to the lateral PFC, we present experimental evidence derived from neuropsychological, electrophysiological, and functional neuroimaging research that supports a critical role for the lateral PFC in executive control of goal-directed behavior.

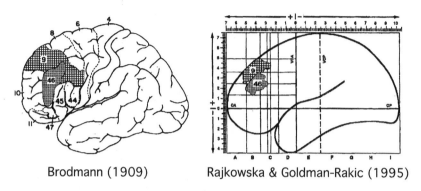

Brodmann (1909)   Rajkowska & Goldman-Rakic (1995)

Figure 11.1
The Brodmann classification and a more recent cytoarchitectonic postmortem definition of areas 9 and 46 of lateral pre-frontal cortex in humans. The cytoarchitectonic definitions of Rajkowska and Goldman-Rakic (1995a, b) are shown on the Talairach coordinate system and represent the overlap of these areas averaged from five subjects.

Case Report

Patient W.R., a 31-year-old lawyer, came to the neurology clinic because of family concern over his lack of interest in important life events. When queried as to why he was at the clinic, the patient stated that he had "lost his ego." His difficulties began 4 years previously when he had a tonic-clonic seizure after staying up all night and drinking large amounts of coffee while studying for midterm exams in his final year of law school. An extensive neurological evaluation conducted at that time, including an electro-encephalogram (EEG), a computed tomography (CT) scan, and a position emission tomography (PET) scan were all unremarkable. A diagnosis of generalized seizure disorder exacerbated by sleep deprivation was given and the patient was placed on dilantin.

W.R. graduated from law school, but did not enter a practice because he could not decide where to take the bar exam. Over the next year he worked as a tennis instructor in Florida. He then broke off a 2-year relationship with a woman and moved to California to live near his brother, who was also a lawyer. His brother reported that he was indecisive and procrastinated in carrying out planned activities, and that he was becoming progressively isolated from family and friends. The family attributed these problems to a "midlife crisis." Four months prior to neurological consultation, W.R.'s mother died. At the funeral and during the time surrounding his mother's death the family noted that he expressed no grief regarding his

mother's death. The family decided to have the patient reevaluated.

On examination, W.R. was pleasant but somewhat indifferent to the situation. A general neurological examination was unremarkable. A mild snout reflex was present. W.R. made both perseverative and random errors on the Luria hand-sequencing task and was easily distracted during the examination. His free recall was two out of three words at a 5-minute delay. He was able to recall the third word with a semantic cue. On being questioned about his mother's death, W.R. confirmed that he did not feel any strong emotions, either about his mother's death or about his current problem. The patient's brother mentioned that W.R. "had never lost it" emotionally during the week after his mother's death, at which point W.R. immediately interjected "and I'm not trying not to lose it." Regarding his mother's death, he stated "I don't feel grief, I don't know if that's bad or good." These statements were emphatic, but expressed in a somewhat jocular fashion (*witzelsucht*).

W.R. was asked about changes in his personality. He struggled for some minutes to describe changes he had noticed, but did not manage to identify any. He stated "Being inside, I can't see it as clear." He was distractible and perseverative, frequently reverting to a prior discussion of tennis, and repeating phrases such as "yellow comes to mind" in response to queries of his memory. When asked about either the past or the future, his responses were schematic and stereotyped. He lacked any plans for the future, initiated no future-oriented actions, and stated "It didn't matter that much, it never bothered me" that he never began to practice law.

A CT scan revealed a left lateral prefrontal glioblastoma that had grown through the corpus callosum into the lateral right frontal lobe. After discussion of the serious nature of the diagnosis, W.R. remained indifferent. The family were distressed by the gravity of the situation and showed appropriate anxiety and sadness. It is interesting that they noted that their sadness was alleviated in the presence of W.R.

In summary, W.R. remained a pleasant and articulate individual despite his extensive frontal tumor. However, he was unable to carry out the activities necessary to make him a fully functioning member of society. His behavior was completely constrained by his current circumstances. His jocularity was a reaction to the social situation of the moment, and was not influenced by the larger context of his recent diagnosis. He appeared to have difficulty with explicit memory and source monitoring; he had little confidence in his answers to memory queries, which were complicated by frequent intrusions from internal mental representations. He was distractible, and perseverative errors were common in both the motor and cognitive domain. A prominent aspect of his behavior was a complete absence of counterfactual expressions. In particular, W.R. expressed no counterfactual emotions, being completely unable to construe any explanation for his current behavioral state. He did not seem able to feel grief or regret, nor was he bothered by their absence even though he was aware of his brother's concern over his absence of emotion. The symptoms of this patient reveal the role of the lateral PFC in virtually all aspects of human cognition.

Clinical Description of Patients with Lateral PFC Damage

The development of human behavior is paralleled by a massive evolution of the PFC, which occupies up to 35% of the neocortical mantle in man. In contrast, in high-level nonhuman primates such as gorillas (Fuster, 1997), the PFC occupies only about 10–12% of the cortical mantle. Since the lateral PFC is involved in so many aspects of behavior and cognition, characterization of a "prefrontal" syndrome can be elusive. PFC damage from strokes, tumors, trauma, or degenerative disorders is notoriously difficult to diagnose since subtle behavioral

changes such as deficits in creativity and mental flexibility may be the only salient findings. The patient may complain that he is not able to pay attention as well and that his memory is not quite as sharp. In patients with degenerative disease, the symptoms related to PFC damage may become clinically obvious only if the patient has a job requiring some degree of mental flexibility and decision making. However, if the patient has a routinized job or lifestyle, PFC damage can be quite advanced before a diagnosis is made. Indeed, many PFC tumors are extensive at initial diagnosis.

As unilateral PFC lesions progress or become bilateral, pronounced behavioral and cognitive abnormalities invariably become evident. Advanced bilateral PFC damage leads to perseveration, which is manifested behaviorally as being fixed in the present and unable to effectively go forward or backward in time. In association with these deficits, confidence about many aspects of behavior deteriorates. Patients with PFC damage may be uncertain about the appropriateness of their behavior even when it is correct.

It is interesting that extensive frontal lobe damage may have little impact on the abilities measured by standardized intelligence tests or other neuropsychological tests, but these findings are in marked contrast to the way that these patients perform unintelligently in real life (Shallice & Burgess, 1991). Based on this observation, it is obvious that neuropsychological tests designed for the laboratory do not always capture the abilities that are necessary for success in real life. For example, real-life behavior requires heavy time processing demands (e.g., working memory) and a core system of values based on both inherited (e.g., drives, instincts) and acquired (e.g., education, socialization) information that is probably not necessary for most artificial problems posed by neuropsychological tasks (Damasio & Anderson, 1993). Tests of executive function, however, which are difficult to administer at the bedside, seem to capture the type of abilities that are typically impaired following lateral PFC damage. A brief review of these impairments is described next.

Inability to Modify Behavior in Response to Changing Circumstances

An impairment of this type is found when patients with frontal lobe injury perform the Wisconsin Card Sorting Test (WCST). In this test, a deck of cards is presented one at time to the patient, who must sort each one according to various stimulus dimensions (color, form, or number). Each card from the deck contains from one to four identical figures (stars, triangles, crosses, or circles) in one of four colors. The patient is told after each response whether the response is correct or not, and must infer from this information only (the sorting principle is not given by the examiner) what the next response should be. After ten correct sorts, the sorting principle is changed without warning.

During this test, frontal patients usually understand and can repeat the rules of the test, but are unable to follow them or use knowledge of incorrect performance to alter their behavior (Milner, 1963; Eslinger & Damasio, 1985). Recent findings in patients with lateral PFC damage indicate that these patients make both random errors and perseverative errors (Barcelo & Knight, 2002). Perseverative errors are traditionally viewed as a failure in inhibition of a previous response pattern, and on the WCST these errors are due to a failure to shift set to a new sorting criteria. A random error occurs when a patient is sorting correctly and switches to a new incorrect sorting category without any prompt from the examiner; this can be viewed as a transient failure in maintaining the goal at hand.

Inability to Handle Sequential Behavior Necessary for Organization, Planning, and Problem Solving

Patients with PFC lesions often have no difficulty with the basic operations of a given task, but nevertheless perform poorly. For example, when performing complex mathematical problems requiring multiple steps, the patient may initially respond impulsively to an early step and will be unable to string together and execute the component steps required for solving the problem (Stuss & Benson, 1984). However, the ability to perform in isolation each of the mathematical operations (i.e., addition and subtraction) required to complete the complex task might be intact. The problem, "The price of canned peas is two cans for 31 cents. What is the price of one dozen cans?" is almost impossible for patients with PFC lesions, even though these patients can perform the direct arithmetical task of multiplying 6 times 31 with ease (Stuss & Benson, 1984).

Inability to Inhibit Responses

The inability to inhibit responses can be detected with a measure called the "Stroop paradigm" (Stroop, 1935). It is based on the observation that it takes longer to name the color of a series of color words printed in conflicting colors (e.g., "red" printed in blue ink) than to name the color of a series of color blocks. This phenomenon is exaggerated in patients with frontal lesions (Perret, 1974). A related phenomenon is that patients with PFC lesions may display a remarkable tendency to imitate the examiner's gestures and behaviors even when no instruction has been given to do so, and even when this imitation entails considerable personal embarrassment. The mere sight of an object may also elicit the compulsion to use it, although the patient has not been asked to do so and the context is inappropriate—as in a patient who sees a pair of glasses and puts them on, even though he is already wearing his own pair. These symptoms have been called the "environmental dependency syndrome."

It has been postulated that the frontal lobes may promote distance from the environment and the parietal lobes foster approach toward one's environment. Therefore, the loss of frontal inhibition may result in overactivity of the parietal lobes. Without the PFC, our autonomy in our environment would not be possible. A given stimulus would automatically call up a predetermined response regardless of context (Lhermitte, 1986; Lhermitte, Pillon, & Sedarv, 1986).

Perseveration

Perseveration is defined as an abnormal repetition of a specific behavior. It can be present after frontal damage in a wide range of tasks, including motor acts, verbalizations, sorting tests, and drawing or writing.

Inability to Self-Monitor

Patients with lateral PFC damage are unable to monitor their own behavior. Two behaviors that capture self-monitoring, called "simulation behavior" and "reality checking," have been shown to be impaired after lateral PFC damage (Knight & Grabowecky, 2000). Simulation refers to the process of generating internal models of external reality. These models may represent an accurate past or an alternative past, present, or future and include models of the environment, of other people, and of the self. Simulation processes have been extensively studied in normal populations (Kahneman & Miller, 1986; Tversky & Kahneman, 1983). Judgments and decisions in any situation occur as a consequence of the evaluation of a set of internally generated alternatives.

One important type of simulation behavior is described as the ability to generate counterfactual scenarios. Counterfactual scenarios represent an alternative reality to the one experienced. Counterfactual expressions occur often in everyday life (for example, when one thinks "If I had ordered the pasta with white sauce instead of marinara this stain would be less obvious,"), and are very common in situations involving regret or grief. (For example, a distraught parent may say, "If only I had not given my son the keys to the car, the accident would not have occurred.")

According to Kahneman and Miller (1986), all events are compared with counterfactual alternatives. Counterfactuals are constructed to compare what happened with what could have happened. Without such simulations it is difficult to avoid making the same mistakes repetitively. Clinical observation suggests that patients with lateral PFC

damage may be impaired in their ability to generate and evaluate counterfactuals.

The expression "reality checking" refers to those aspects of monitoring the external world that have been called "reality testing" when they concern the present, and "reality monitoring" when they concern the past. Reality checking includes both an awareness of the difference between an internally generated alternative reality and a current reality, and the maintenance of a true past in the presence of counterfactual alternatives that one might construct. Memories are created for events experienced in the world and events experienced through internally constructed simulations. These two sources of memories must be treated differently in order for them to be used effectively during reality checking. Thus, what cues differentiate our internal models of reality from our internal simulations of reality?

Johnson and Raye (1981) studied normal subjects' abilities to discriminate between memories of external events and those of internally generated events. Memories of external events tend to be more detailed and have more spatial and temporal contextual information, whereas internally generated memories tend to be abstract and schematic, lacking in detail. Since these two memory representations form overlapping populations, similar internal and external events may become confused. Clinical observation suggests that such confusion may be more common in patients with PFC lesions, leading to impairments in the processes necessary for accurate reality checking and monitoring.

It is important to note that not all patients with lateral PFC lesions will exhibit all of the deficits described here. The clinical syndrome following lateral PFC lesions is heterogeneous, and the clinical signs that patients exhibit most likely reflect numerous factors such as the extent, location, and laterality of the lesions. Nevertheless, the myriad cognitive and behavioral disturbances observed in these patients have been well characterized, and such clinical descriptions have formed the foundation for understanding the role of the frontal lobes in cognition. In the next section, we review the experimental neuropsychological literature derived from studying patients with focal PFC lesions.

Neuropsychological Studies of Patients with Focal Frontal Lesions

Working Memory

Working memory is an evolving concept that refers to the short-term storage of information that is not accessible in the environment, and the set of processes that keep this information active for later use. It is a system that is critically important in cognition and seems to be necessary in the course of performing many other cognitive functions such as reasoning, language comprehension, planning, and spatial processing. Animal studies initially provided important evidence for the role of the lateral PFC in working memory (for a review see Fuster, 1997). For example, electrophysiological studies of awake, behaving monkeys have used delayed-response tasks to study working memory. In these tasks, the monkey must keep "in mind," or actively maintain a stimulus over a short delay. During such tasks, neurons within the lateral PFC persistently fire during the delay period of a delayed-response task when the monkey is maintaining information in memory prior to a making a motor response (Funahashi, Bruce, & Goldman-Rakic, 1989; Fuster & Alexander, 1971). The necessity of this region for active maintenance of information over short delays has been demonstrated in monkey studies that have shown that lesions of the lateral PFC impair performance on these tasks (Bauer & Fuster, 1976; Funahashi, Bruce, & Goldman-Rakic, 1993).

There are few studies in which human patients with focal lesions of the PFC performed delayed-response tasks (e.g., Chao & Knight, 1995, 1998; Muller, Machado, & Knight, 2002). In a recent review of such studies, we found that some groups of patients with PFC lesions can be impaired on delay tasks, and that these deficits tend to be more prominent when patients perform delay tasks that

include distraction during the delay period (D'Esposito & Postle, 1999). This finding might be understood as a reflection of the effects of this manipulation on information-processing demands. The rehearsal processes that suffice to support performance on a delay task without distraction may require the mediation of other PFC-supported processes when distraction during the delay interval presents a source of interference or attentional salience. These PFC-supported processes may include executive control processes, such as inhibition of prepotent responses (Diamond, 1988), or behaviorally irrelevant stimuli (Chao & Knight, 1995), shifting attention among stimuli and/or among different components of a task (Rogers & Monsell, 1995), maintaining or refreshing information in a noisy environment (Johnson, 1992), or selecting among competing responses (Thompson-Schill et al., 1997). These types of executive control processes have been linked to lateral PFC function in studies using both functional neuroimaging (e.g., D'Esposito et al., 1995; D'Esposito, Postle, Ballard, & Lease, 1999) and patients with focal lateral PFC lesions (Muller et al., 2002).

Episodic Long-Term Memory

Patients with damage to the PFC have episodic memory impairments. They differ from those with medial temporal damage in obvious ways. Hécaen and Albert (1978) summarized an enormous literature on frontal memory deficits and concluded that the impairments in memory were due to inefficiencies caused by poor attention or poor "executive" function. Patients with PFC lesions show consistent impairment in multiple-trial list learning tasks (Janowsky, Shimamura, Kritchevsky, & Squire, 1989a; Janowsky, Shimamura, & Squire, 1989b) in which they fail on recall measures, but have generally normal performance on recognition measures. This has been interpreted as defective retrieval—a function that requires strategy and effort—as opposed to normal storage—a function that is more passive (Shimamura, Janowsky, & Squire, 1991).

A major problem with this research is a failure to discriminate among lesions in different PFC regions. Comparisons are made between a group of patients with very specific and restricted lesions—medial temporal—and a group with very heterogeneous lesions—dorsolateral, orbital, polar, and superomedial—areas that may have greatly different roles in memory. There are substantially different effects on memory, depending on the specific frontal lesion site (Stuss et al., 1994). Patients with left dorsolateral PFC lesions are particularly impaired in list learning, and this deficit is highly correlated with deficits in lexicosemantic capacity measured by verbal fluency and naming tasks. Right PFC patients are particularly prone to perseverative errors in recall tasks. All frontal patients are defective in applying strategies to improve learning.

Patients with PFC lesions also have specific impairments in memory. They are defective in recall of temporal order, that is, recalling the context of learned items, even when they can remember these items (Shimamura, Janowsky, & Squire, 1990). Finally, they have defective metamemory, that is, they are very poor judges of knowing what they remember and how well their memory functions (Janowsky et al., 1989b). In summary, patients with damage to the PFC are impaired in the process involved in planning, organization and other strategic aspects of learning and memory that may facilitate encoding and retrieval of information (Shimamura et al., 1991). Some of these defective strategies may be specific to the frontal lesion site.

Inhibitory Control

There is long-standing evidence that distraction due to a failure in inhibitory control is a key element of the deficit observed in monkeys on delayed-response tasks (Malmo, 1942; Brutkowski, 1965; Bartus & Levere, 1977). For example, simple maneuvers such as turning off the lights in the laboratory or mildly sedating the animal, which would typically impair performance in intact animals, improved delay performance in animals with PFC lesions. Despite this evidence, remarkably little data

have been obtained in humans with PFC damage. The extant data center on failures in inhibition of early sensory input as well as problems in inhibition of higher-level cognitive processes.

In the sensory domain, it has been shown that the inability to suppress irrelevant information is associated with difficulties in sustained attention, target detection, and match-to-sample paradigms in both monkeys and humans (Woods & Knight, 1986; Richer et al., 1993; Chao & Knight, 1995, 1998). Delivery of task-irrelevant sensory information disproportionately reduces performance in patients with lateral PFC lesions. For example, presentation of brief high-frequency tone pips during a tone-matching delay task markedly reduces the performance of PFC patients. In essence, the patient with a lateral PFC lesion functions poorly in a noisy environment because of a failure in filtering out extraneous sensory information.

In the cognitive domain, inhibitory deficits in cognitive tasks that require suppression of prior learned material are also observed in patients with lateral PFC lesions (Shimamura, Jurica, Mangels, Gershberg, & Knight, 1995; Mangels, Gershberg, Shimamura, & Knight, 1996). Prior learned information irrelevant to the task at hand intrudes on performance. For example, words from a prior list of stimuli employed in a memory task may be inappropriately recalled during recall of a subsequent list of words. In essence, the PFC patient is unable to wipe the internal mental slate clean, resulting in the maintenance of an active neural representation of previously learned material. The inability to suppress previous incorrect responses may underlie the poor performance of PFC subjects in a wide range of neuropsychological tasks such as the Wisconsin Card Sorting Task and the Stroop Task (Shimamura, Gershberg, Jurica, Mangels, & Knight, 1992). It is interesting that there is some evidence that inhibitory failure extends to some aspects of motor control. For instance, lateral PFC damage results in a deficit in suppressing reflexive eye movements toward task-irrelevant spatial locations (Guitton, Buchtel, & Douglas, 1985).

Processing Novelty

The capacity to detect novelty in a stream of external sensory events or internal thoughts and the ability to produce novel behaviors is crucial for new learning, creativity, and flexible adjustments to perturbations in the environment. For example, behavioral and electrophysiological data have shown that novel events are better remembered than familiar ones (Von Restorff, 1933; Karis, Fabiani, & Donchin, 1984). Indeed, creative behavior in fields extending from science to the arts is commonly defined in direct relation to its degree of novelty.

Patients with lateral PFC lesions have difficulty solving novel problems and generating novel behaviors and have decreased interest in novel events. With significant PFC damage, deficits in orienting to novel stimuli emerge (Godfrey & Rousseaux, 1997; Dias, Robbins, & Roberts, 1997; Goldberg, Podell, & Lovell, 1994; Daffner et al., 2000a; Daffner et al., 2000b; Daffner et al., 2000c). Studies in normal subjects have shown that novel items generate a late-positive event-related potential (ERP) peaking in amplitude at about 300–500 ms that is maximal over the anterior scalp. This novelty ERP is proposed to be a central marker of the orienting response (Sokolov, 1963; Courchesne, Hillyard, & Galambos, 1975; Knight, 1984; Yamaguchi & Knight, 1991; Bahramali et al., 1997; Escera, Winkler, & Naatanen, 1998). In accord with clinical observations, PFC damage markedly reduces the scalp electrophysiological response to unexpected novel stimuli in the auditory (Knight, 1984; Knight & Scabini, 1998), visual (Knight, 1997), and somatosensory modalities (Yamaguchi & Knight, 1991, 1992). Also, single-unit data from monkeys have confirmed a prefrontal bias toward novelty (Rainer & Miller, 2000). Finally, functional neuroimaging findings in normal persons also support a critical role for the PFC in responding to novel events and solving new problems (see Duncan & Owen, 2000 for a review).

Novelty, of course, is an elusive concept that is dependent on both the sensory parameters of an event and the context in which it occurs. As an example, the unexpected occurrence of a visual fractal would typically engage the novelty system. Conversely, if one were presented with a stream of visual fractals and suddenly a picture of an apple occurred, this would also activate the novelty system. In the first case the visual complexity of the fractal initiates the novelty response whereas in the second situation the local context of repeated fractals would be violated by the insertion of a picture of an apple, engaging the novelty network.

Sensory parameters and local context have powerful effects on electrophysiological and behavioral responses to novelty (Comerchero & Polich, 1998, 1999; Katayama & Polich, 1998). Data from a series of probability learning experiments in patients with lateral PFC damage suggest that the appreciation of local context appears to be dependent on the lateral PFC. In one experiment, delivery of novel stimuli always predicted a subsequent target that required a behavioral response (100% condition). In another experiment, novel stimuli were randomly paired with targets so that novel stimuli occurred prior to targets on only 20% of trials (20% condition). The subjects were not informed about the novel stimuli–target pairing rules and had to extract this local context during the experiment. Control subjects learned the probability rules within two experimental blocks and altered their behavior as well as their electrophysiological response to the novel stimuli.

In the 100% novel stimuli–target condition, response times were faster and the brain ERP novelty response was attenuated. Conversely, in the 20% novel stimuli–target pairing condition, the response times were slower when a novel stimuli preceded a target, and a robust ERP novelty response was recorded for all novel events. This pattern of results fits with the notion that novel events are being used as alerting stimuli in the 100% condition and as distracters in the 20% condition. In contrast to normal subjects, PFC patients were unable to effectively use the local context of the experiments to extract and implement the probablity rules, even after twelve blocks of trials (Barcelo & Knight, 2000).

Experimental Studies of Executive Control

The diverse spectrum of deficits observed by clinicians and found in experimental neuropsychological studies in patients with lateral PFC damage may be considered to arise from difficulties with inhibitory and excitatory modulation of the distributed neural networks critical for cognitive processes. Evidence for this notion presented in this section is derived from electrophysiological and functional neuroimaging studies in normal subjects and patients with focal frontal lesions, as well as work in animals.

Inhibitory Control

PFC inhibitory control of subcortical (Edinger, Siegel, & Troiano, 1975) and cortical regions has been documented in a variety of mammalian preparations (Alexander, Newman, & Symmes, 1976; Skinner & Yingling, 1977; Yingling & Skinner, 1977). Galambos (1956) provided the first physiological evidence of an inhibitory auditory pathway in mammals with the description of the brainstem olivocochlear bundle. The olivocochlear bundle projects from the olivary nucleus in the brainstem to the cochlea in the inner ear. Stimulation of this bundle results in inhibition of transmission from the cochlea to the brainstem cochlear nucleus as measured by reductions in evoked responses in the auditory nerve. This pathway provides a system for early sensory suppression in the auditory system. The evidence for sensory filtering at the cochlear or brainstem level in humans is controversial, with most laboratories finding no evidence of attention-related manipulation of the brainstem auditory evoked response (Woods & Hillyard, 1978; Woldorff & Hillyard, 1991).

Research in the 1970s reported evidence of a multimodal prefrontal-thalamic inhibitory system in cats that regulates sensory flow to primary cortical regions. Reversible suppression of the cat PFC by cooling (cryogenic blockade) increased the amplitudes of evoked responses recorded in the primary cortex in all sensory modalities (Skinner & Yingling, 1977; Yingling & Skinner, 1977). Conversely, stimulation of the thalamic region (the nucleus reticularis thalami) surrounding the sensory relay nuclei resulted in modality-specific suppression of activity in the primary sensory cortex. This effect is also observed in all sensory modalities.

These data provided the first physiological evidence of a prefrontal inhibitory pathway regulating sensory transmission through thalamic relay nuclei. This prefrontal-thalamic inhibitory system provides a mechanism for modality-specific suppression of irrelevant inputs at an early stage of sensory processing. As noted, this system is modulated by an excitatory lateral PFC projection to the nucleus reticularis thalami, although the precise course of anatomical projections between these structures is not well understood. The nucleus reticularis thalami in turn sends inhibitory GABAergic projections to sensory relay nuclei, providing a neural substrate for selective sensory suppression (Guillery et al., 1998).

There is also evidence in humans that the PFC exerts control on other cortical and subcortical regions. For example, ERP studies in patients with focal PFC damage have shown that primary auditory- and somatosensory-evoked responses are enhanced (Knight, Scabini, & Woods, 1989; Yamaguchi & Knight, 1990; Chao & Knight, 1998), suggesting disinhibition of sensory flow to primary cortical regions. In a series of experiments, task-irrelevant auditory and somatosensory stimuli (monaural clicks or brief electric shocks to the median nerve) were presented to patients with comparably sized lesions in the lateral PFC, the temporal-parietal junction, or the lateral parietal cortex. Evoked responses from primary auditory (Kraus, Ozdamar, & Stein, 1982) and somatosensory (Leuders, Leser, Harn, Dinner, & Klem, 1983) cortices were recorded from these patients and age-matched controls (figure 11.2).

Damage to the primary auditory or somatosensory cortex in the temporal-parietal lesion group reduced the early latency (20–40 ms) evoked responses generated in these primary cortical regions.

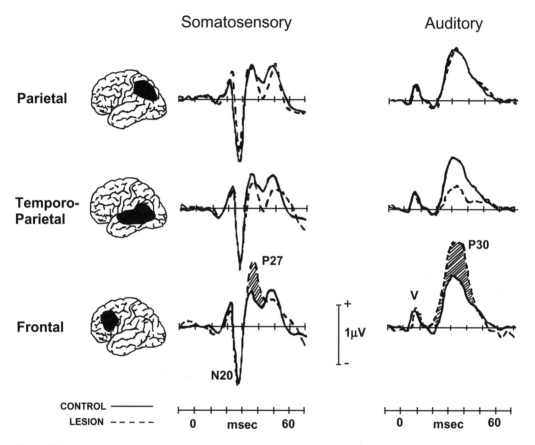

Figure 11.2
Inhibitory modulation. Primary cortical auditory and somatosensory evoked potentials are shown for controls (solid line) and patients (dashed line) with focal damage in the lateral parietal cortex (*top*, n = 8), temporal-parietal junction (*middle*, n = 13), or dorsolateral PFC (*bottom*, n = 13). Reconstructions of the center of damage in each patient group are shown on the left. For somatosensory stimuli, lateral parietal damage (sparing the primary somatosensory cortex) had no effect on the N20 or earlier spinal cord potentials. PFC damage, however, resulted in a selective increase in the amplitude of the P27 response (hatched area). For auditory stimuli, a temporal-parietal junction extending into the primary auditory cortex reduced P30 responses whereas lateral parietal damage (sparing the primary auditory cortex) had no effect on P30 responses. PFC damage resulted in normal brainstem potentials, but enhanced the P30 cortical response (hatched area).

Posterior association cortex lesions in the lateral parietal lobe that spared the primary sensory regions had no effect on early sensory potentials and served as a brain-lesioned control group. Lateral PFC damage resulted in enhanced amplitudes of both the primary auditory- and somatosensory-evoked responses (Knight et al., 1989; Yamaguchi & Knight, 1990; Chao & Knight, 1998). Spinal cord and brainstem potentials were not affected by lateral PFC damage, suggesting that the amplitude enhancements were due to abnormalities in either a prefrontal-thalamic or a prefrontal-sensory cortex mechanism. These results are in accord with the findings reported in the 1970s by Yingling and Skinner (1977) in their cat model of PFC-dependent sensory gating.

As mentioned previously, patients with lateral PFC lesions have deficits in tasks requiring inhibitory control. Moreover, several functional imaging studies have demonstrated a link between lateral PFC function and inhibitory control (e.g., Konishi, Nakajima, Uchida, Sekihara, & Miyashita, 1998; Garavan, Ross, & Stein, 1999; D'Esposito, Postle, Jonides, & Smith, 1999). However, this behavioral and imaging evidence of the involvement of the lateral PFC in inhibitory control does not provide direct support for the hypothesis that there are inhibitory signals from the PFC directed either toward early sensory cortices or excitatory PFC inputs to the GABAergic nucleus reticularis thalami that result in a net inhibitory control of sensory flow. In contrast, the combined ERP and patient studies described are able to measure the temporal dynamics of inhibitory control and provide powerful evidence that in humans the PFC provides a net inhibitory regulation of early sensory transmission.

Excitatory Control

Attention allows us to select from the myriad of closely spaced and timed environmental events. Attention is crucial for virtually all cognitive abilities. In addition to suppressing responses to irrelevant stimuli, as discussed in the previous section, humans must excite and sustain neural activity in distributed brain regions in order to perform most cognitive tasks.

Desimone (1998) has proposed a biased-competition model of visual attention in which neurons involved in processing different aspects of the visual world are mutually inhibitory. In this view, an excitatory signal (possibly from the PFC or the inferior parietal cortex) to selective visual neurons would result in the inhibition of nearby nontask-relevant visual neurons, resulting in a sharpening of the attentional focus. For example, visual attention increases V4 neuronal firing to an attended object, but suppresses firing to a nearby nonattended object (Luck, Chelazzi, Hillyard, & Desimone, 1997).

While this model may explain some aspects of sensory tuning, it does not fully explain such concepts as object-based attention since object representations (including form, color, and texture) would be stored in more distributed cortical representations. Full implementation of the model at a neural level would require extensive inhibition of many cortical regions. For example, if one were focusing on a baseball, the neural representation of every round object would need to be suppressed. This would entail a massive expenditure of energy as well as the engagement of a complex mechanism for parallel tagging and linking of all round objects. Nevertheless, the idea that the PFC may regulate top-down modulation of posterior association areas suggests that it is most likely an important mechanism for guiding goal-directed behavior.

Evidence for some aspects of this model exists in data from humans. Selective attention to an ear, a region of the visual field, or a digit increases the amplitude of sensory-evoked potentials for all stimuli delivered to that sensory channel (Hillyard, Hink, Schwent, & Picton, 1973). This provides evidence that attention reliably modulates neural activity at early sensory cortices (Woldorff et al., 1993; Grady et al., 1997; Somers, Dale, Seiffert, & Tootell, 1999; Steinmetz et al., 2000). Visual attention involves modulation in the excitability of extrastriate neurons through descending projections from hierarchically ordered brain structures

(Hillyard & Anllo-Vento, 1998). Single-cell recordings in monkeys (Fuster, Brodner, & Kroger, 2000; Funahashi et al., 1993; Rainer, Asaad, & Miller, 1998a,b), lesion studies in humans (Knight, 1997; Nielsen-Bohlman & Knight, 1999; Knight, Staines, Swick, & Chao, 1999; Barcelo, Suwazono, & Knight, 2000) and monkeys (Rossi, Rotter, Desimone, & Ungerleider, 1999), and blood flow data (McIntosh, Grady, Ungerleider, Haxby, Rapoport, & Horwitz, 1994; Büchel & Friston, 1997; Chawla, Rees, & Friston, 1999; Rees, Frackowiak, & Frith, 1997; Kastner, Pinsk, de Weerd, Desimone, & Ungerleider, 1999; Corbetta, 1998; Hopfinger, Buonocore, & Mangun, 2000) have linked the PFC to control of the extrastriate cortex during visual attention.

Functional imaging studies have reported activation of both the PFC and the parietal cortex during visual attention tasks. For example, Hopfinger and colleagues used event-related functional magnetic resonance imaging (fMRI) to study cued spatial attention (Hopfinger et al., 2000). These authors reported that the attention cue preceding presentation of a visual target activated the superior frontal, inferior parietal, and superior temporal cortices. However, owing to current constraints in temporal resolution, the fMRI studies of visual attention reported to date have not been able to demonstrate that a top-down signal originates in the PFC. In contrast, single-unit studies in monkeys and lesion and ERP studies in humans, which are discussed briefly later, provide evidence that the PFC activation seen in functional imaging studies most likely reflects top-down influences on visual processing.

Modulation of visual pathway activity has been extensively investigated in humans using ERPs. In normal human subjects, attended visual stimuli evoke distinct ERP signatures. For example, the most prominent extrastriate ERPs are a P1 component peaking at about 125 ms and an N1 component peaking at about 170–200 ms. Attention reliably enhances these early extrastriate ERP components for all stimuli in an attended channel (Heinze et al., 1994; Mangun, 1995; Martinez et al., 1999; Woldorff et al., 1997). These early human ERP

components have been linked to increased firing of extrastriate neurons in monkeys (Luck et al., 1997), providing a powerful parallel between the human and animal literature.

From ERP studies in patients with lateral PFC damage, evidence has accumulated that the human lateral PFC regulates attention-dependent extrastriate neural activity through three distinct mechanisms. These mechanisms include (1) an attention-dependent enhancement of the extrastriate cortex; (2) a tonic excitatory influence on ipsilateral posterior areas for all sensory information, including attended and nonattended sensory inputs; and (3) a phasic excitatory influence on ipsilateral posterior areas for all task-relevant stimuli. In these ERP studies, patients with unilateral PFC lesions (centered in Brodmann areas 9 and 46) performed a series of visual attention experiments. In the task, nontarget stimuli consisted of upright triangles that were presented rapidly to both visual fields (4 degrees from the fovea). Targets were rarely presented (10% of all stimuli) and consisted of inverted triangles presented randomly in each visual field. In one experiment, patients and age-matched controls were asked to press a button whenever a target appeared in either visual field (Barcelo et al., 2000). In another experiment, the subjects were required to allocate attention to only one visual field (Yago & Knight, 2000).

An interesting pattern of results emerged from these two experiments. First, both experiments revealed that the lateral PFC exerts a tonic excitatory influence on the ipsilateral extrastriate cortex. Specifically, the P1 component of the visual ERP is markedly reduced in amplitude for all stimuli presented to the contralesional field. It is important to note that this tonic influence is attention independent since a reduced P1 potential in the extrastriate cortex was found ipsilateral to PFC damage for *all* visual stimuli (attended and nonattended targets and nontargets) presented to the contralesional field. This tonic component may be viewed as a modulatory influence on extrastriate activity.

As noted previously, it is well known that attention increases the amplitude of extrastriate ERPs in normal persons, with the onset of effects about 100 ms after delivery of the stimulus. The second experiment (allocating attention to only one visual field) provided evidence of the temporal kinetics of prefrontal–extrastriate interactions. In essence, in PFC patients, attention effects on the extrastriate cortex were normal in the first 200 ms of processing, but were severely disrupted after 200 ms (Yago & Knight, 2000). This finding suggests that other cortical areas are responsible for attention-dependent regulation of the extrastriate cortex in the first 200 ms. A candidate structure for this influence, based on the neuroimaging and clinical literature, would be the inferior parietal cortex. It is conceivable that the inferior parietal cortex is responsible for the early reflexive component of attention whereas the PFC is responsible for the more controlled and sustained aspects of visual attention that begin after the parietal signal to the extrastriate cortices.

The third observation from these experiments is that the lateral PFC has been shown to send a top-down signal to the extrastriate cortex when a task-relevant event is detected during an attention task.

Two types of stimuli are typically presented in an attended channel, one task irrelevant and one requiring detection and a behavioral response. The amplitudes of both the irrelevant and relevant stimuli are enhanced in an attended channel. As discussed previously, the PFC is responsible for regulating this channel-specific attention enhancement. When a relevant target event is detected in an attended channel, another distinct electrophysiological event is generated in addition to the channel-specific enhancement. This top-down signal begins about 200 ms after a correct detection, extends throughout the ensuing 500 ms, and is superimposed on the channel-specific ERP attention enhancement (Suwazono, Machado, & Knight, 2000). Damage to the lateral PFC results in marked decreases in the top-down signal and is accompanied by behavioral evidence of impaired detection ability (Barcleo et al., 2000) (figure 11.3).

The temporal parameters of this human PFC-extrastriate top-down attention modulation are in accord with single-unit recordings in monkeys that reveal enhanced prefrontal activity related to stimulus detection 140 ms after presentation of the

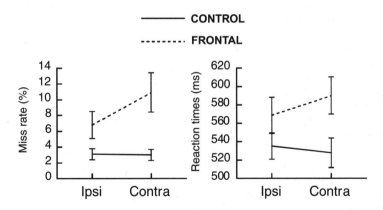

Figure 11.3
Visual attention deficits and PFC lesions. The miss rate (left) and reaction times (right) for patients and controls are given as a function of the visual field of target presentation. Contra, contralesional field for patients, right field for controls; Ipsi, ipsilesional field for patients, left field for controls (Barcelo, Suwazono, & Knight, 2000). A miss was defined as a failure to respond by 300–800 ms following presentation of a target. The interaction between group and visual field was significant for both measures. Vertical bars indicate the standard error of the mean.

stimulus (Rainer et al., 1998a,b) and other studies revealing top-down activation of inferior temporal neurons 180–300 ms after detection of the target (Tomita, Ohbayashi, Nakahara, Hasegawa, & Miyashita, 1999). For example, Rainer and colleagues (1998a,b) have provided evidence that visual detection of a target is associated with increased single-unit activity in the sulcus principalis, and Tomita and colleagues (1999) have provided additional evidence in monkeys that the sulcus principalis provides a top-down signal to the extrastriate cortex. These authors showed that in the absence of visual input, PFC single-unit activity was correlated with enhanced inferior temporal activity. Disruption of PFC–inferior temporal connections resulted in a severe performance deficit in the contralateral field.

The modulatory role of the PFC in intrahemispheric neural activity extends to other sensory modalities. For example, reductions of neural activity in the auditory association cortex have been observed after PFC damage in humans performing language, attention, and delay tasks (Knight Hillyard, Woods, & Neville, 1981; Swick & Knight, 1998; Swick, 1998; Chao & Knight, 1998). In one study PFC patients were tested in an auditory delayed match-to-sample task. The subjects reported whether a cue (S1) and a subsequent target (S2) sound were identical. Both the S1 and S2 stimuli generate a prominent N100 ERP response that measures neural activity in the auditory association cortex in the superior temporal plane (Woods, 1990). PFC lesions markedly reduced the N100 component generated to both the S1 and S2 stimuli throughout the hemisphere ipsilateral to the damage (Chao & Knight, 1998). A failure in excitatory modulation was readily observed in both the auditory and visual modalities (Knight 1997; Chao & Knight, 1998) (figure 11.4).

Anatomical studies in monkeys have supported this proposal of a PFC-posterior association area network. For example, projections from prefrontal areas 45 and 8 to inferior temporal areas TE and TEO have been demonstrated in monkeys (Webster, Bachevalier, & Ungerleider, 1994), providing a

possible glutamatergic pathway by which the lateral PFC could facilitate visual processing. Similarly, there are well-described PFC projections to the superior temporal plane that may subserve an excitatory PFC-auditory cortex circuit (Alexander et al., 1976).

While the mechanisms of interhemispheric coordination are not known, there is clear evidence of bilateral PFC recruitment during the performance of a wide range of cognitive tasks as determined by fMRI research (for a review see D'Esposito, Aguirre, Zarahn, & Ballard, 1998). There is also evidence in monkeys of bilateral engagement of the PFC in visual processing. For example, a PFC lesion results in impaired processing in the contralateral visual field in monkeys (Tomita et al., 1999; Rossi et al., 1999) and humans (Nielsen-Bohlman & Knight, 1999; Barcelo et al., 2000). However, transection of the corpus callosum in monkeys with PFC lesions dramatically worsens the visual processing deficit in the contralesional field (Rossi et al., 1999). This provides compelling evidence that these monkeys are transferring visual information to the intact hemisphere to solve the task at hand.

Our view is that virtually all tasks require parallel inhibitory and excitatory control of distributed neural activity which may be mediated by the PFC. However, the findings presented in the previous two sections address a critical conceptual issue. Why does the lateral PFC implement parallel inhibition and excitation to control distributed cognitive systems? The nervous system utilizes interleaved inhibition and excitation throughout the neuroaxis. Examples include spinal reflexes, cerebellar outputs, and the networks controlling basal ganglia movements. Thus it is not surprising that executive control would also utilize inhibition and excitation to control cognitive processing. It is likely that such parallel excitatory-inhibitory control entails large-scale neural control that might be involved in a PFC–thalamic gating network as well as direct excitatory PFC input to a specific cortical region. Local cortical tuning of attention through inhibition might entail long excitatory PFC projections that then

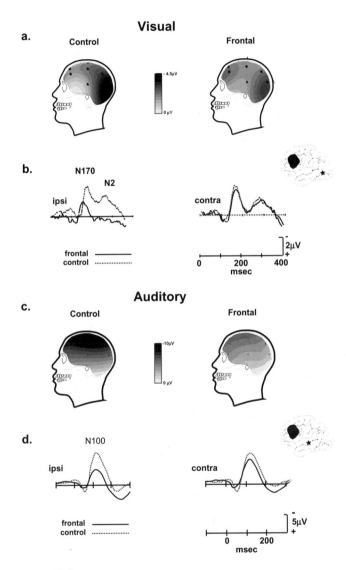

Figure 11.4

Excitatory modulation. Topographic maps in control subjects and PFC patients display the scalp voltage distribution of the N170 generated to visual targets and N100 to auditory targets. The shaded area on the brain shows the area of lesion overlap, while the star indicates a putative generator location for the N100 and N170. In the visual task, the extrastriate focus of the N170 is reduced ipsilaterally to PFC damage. Likewise, in the auditory task, the lateral temporal focus of the N100 is reduced ipsilaterally to PFC damage.

activate local inhibitory neurons, as proposed by Desimone and colleagues (1998). There is evidence in rodents that long-distance excitatory PFC projections terminate on GABA-immunoreactive neurons, providing a potential neuronal architecture for PFC-dependent inhibitory modulation (Carr & Sesack, 1998).

Conclusions and Future Directions

The role of the PFC in executive control has become a central issue in cognitive neuroscience. Indeed, given the vast expansion of the PFC in humans, explication of the function of this brain region appears to be a fundamental issue for understanding human cognition in both health and disease. Advances have been made in several domains. Cognitive psychology has provided a welcome addition to the classic neuropsychological approach, and several new areas of behavioral analysis have added to our understanding of PFC function. Newer approaches drawn from the discipline of social cognition and the study of behaviors such as decision making and reality monitoring are certain to provide a broader and ecologically valid approach to understanding PFC function.

One area likely to receive increasing attention is the contribution of the PFC to the evaluation and implementation of context in behavior (Barcelo & Knight, 2000). Context refers to the influence of the environment on current behavior. The notion of context is broadly used in the cognitive literature and has been applied to seemingly diverse areas, including probability learning, social regulation, and novelty detection. For instance, in the social domain, a behavior in one situation might be very appropriate while the same behavior could be quite counterproductive in another situation. Humans are able to draw on prior experience to set the appropriate context for the current situation. Research on the role of the PFC in the application of context-dependent parameters to behavior may prove critical for understanding the role of the PFC in mental flexibility. By mental flexibility we mean the ability

to rapidly alter behavior according to the requirements of the task at hand. The idea that the PFC may provide the substrate for supporting such flexibility in behavior is consistent with recent findings from single-unit electrophysiological studies in monkeys that suggest that PFC neurons are more plastic than traditional views might suggest (Rainer et al. 1998a,b; Rainer and Miller, 2000; Miller, 1999).

Determining how these executive processes are implemented at a neural level is perhaps the greatest challenge for a true understanding of PFC function. The notion that the engagement of parallel inhibition and excitation can be a useful construct for understanding PFC function is receiving support from single-unit, lesion, ERP, and functional neuroimaging research. Advances in the fusion of these experimental approaches may provide new insights into both the temporal and the spatial aspects of PFC-dependent executive control. Consideration of the neuropharmacology of PFC function will also be necessary for a complete understanding of prefrontal function.

Finally, knowledge of the nature of the neural code at both the local single-unit level and at the systems interaction level is central to a complete picture of PFC function. How do single units in a subregion of the PFC interact to produce the necessary signal to other brain regions? Are neurons concerned with inhibition intertwined with those involved in excitation? What is the nature of the signal output from the PFC to other neural regions? Is it a coherent burst of neural activity such as a gamma oscillation? These questions are only beginning to be addressed but promise great insights into how the PFC implements executive control.

References

Alexander, G. E., Newman, J. D., & Symmes, D. (1976). Convergence of prefrontal and acoustic inputs upon neurons in the superior temporal gyrus of the awake squirrel monkey. *Brain Research, 116,* 334–338.

Bahramali, H., Gordon, E., Lim, C. L., Li, W., Lagapoulus, J., Rennie, C., & Meares, R. A. (1997). Evoked related potentials with and without an orienting reflex. *Neurore-port*, 8, 2665–2669.

Barcelo, F., & Knight, R. T. (2000). Prefrontal lesions alter context dependent value of novel stimuli during visual attention. *Society of Neuroscience Abstracts*, 26, 2233.

Barcelo, F., & Knight, R. T. (2002). Both random and perseverative errors underlie WCST deficits in prefrontal patients. *Neuropsychologia*, 40, 349–356.

Barcelo, F., Suwazono, S., & Knight, R. T. (2000). Prefrontal modulation of visual processing in humans. *Nature Neuroscience*, 3, 399–403.

Bartus, R. T., & Levere, T. E. (1977). Frontal decortication in Rhesus monkeys: A test of the interference hypothesis. *Brain Research*, 119, 233–248.

Bauer, R. H., & Fuster, J. M. (1976). Delayed-matching and delayed-response deficit from cooling dorsolateral prefrontal cortex in monkeys. *Journal of Comparative and Physiological Psychology*, 90, 293–302.

Bechera, A., Damasio, H., Tranel, D., & Anderson, S. W. (1998). Dissociation of working memory from decision making within the human prefrontal cortex. *Journal of Neuroscience*, 18, 428–437.

Brodmann, K. (1909). Vergleichende lokalisationlehre der grosshirnrinde in ihren prinzipoen dargestellt auf grund des zellenbaues (p. 324). Leipsig: J. A. Barth.

Brutkowski, S. (1965). Functions of prefrontal cortex in animals. *Physiolological Review*, 45, 721–746.

Büchel, C., & Friston, K. J. (1997). Modulation of connectivity in visual pathways by attention: Cortical interactions evaluated with structural equation modeling and fMRI. *Cerebral Cortex*, 7, 768–778.

Carr, D. B., & Sesack, S. R. (1998). Callosal terminals in the rat prefrontal cortex: Synaptic targets and association with GABA-immunoreactive structures. *Synapse*, 29, 193–205.

Chao, L. L., & Knight, R. T. (1995). Human prefrontal lesions increase distractibility to irrelevant sensory. *Neuro-Report*, 6, 1605–1610.

Chao, L. L., & Knight, R. T. (1998). Contribution of human prefrontal cortex to delay performance. *Journal of Cognitive Neuroscience*, 10, 167–177.

Chawla, D., Rees, G., & Friston, K. J. (1999). The physiological basis of attentional modulation in extrastriate visual areas. *Nature Neuroscience*, 2, 671–676.

Comerchero, M. D., & Polich, J. (1998). P3a, perceptual distinctiveness, and stimulus modality. *Cognitive Brain Research*, 7, 41–48.

Comerchero, M. D., & Polich, J. (1999). P3a and P3b from typical auditory and visual stimuli. *Clinical Neurophysiology*, 110, 24–30.

Corbetta, M. (1998). Frontoparietal cortical networks for directing attention and the eye to visual locations: Identical, independent, or overlapping neural systems? *Proceedings of the National Academy of Sciences U.S.A.*, 95, 831–838.

Courchesne, E., Hillyard, S. A., & Galambos, R. (1975). Stimulus novelty, task relevance, and the visual evoked potential in man. *Electroencephalography and Clinical Neurophysiology*, 39, 131–143.

Daffner, K. R., Mesulam, M. M., Holcomb, P. J., Calvo, V., Acar, D., Chabrerie, A., Kikinis, R., Jolesz, F. A., Rentz, D. M., & Scinto, L. F. (2000a). Disruption of attention to novel events after frontal lobe injury in humans. *Journal of Neurology, Neurosurgery and Psychiatry*, 68, 18–24.

Daffner, K. R., Mesulam, M. M., Scinto, L. F., Acar, D., Calvo, V., Faust, R., Chabrerie, A., Kennedy, B., & Holcomb, P. (2000b). The central role of the prefrontal cortex in directing attention to novel events. *Brain*, 123, 927–939.

Daffner, K. R., Mesulam, M. M., Scinto, L. F., Calvo, V., West, W. C., & Holcomb, P. (2000c). The influence of stimulus deviance on electrophysiologic and behavioral response to novel events. *Journal of Cognitive Neuroscience*, 12, 393–406.

Damasio, A. S., & Anderson, S. W. (1993). The frontal lobes. In K. M. Heilman, & E. Valenstein (Eds.), *Clinical neuropsychology* 3rd ed. pp. 409–460. New York: Oxford University Press.

Desimone, R. (1998). Visual attention mediated by biased competition in extrastriate cortex. *Philosophical Transactions of the Royal Society of London, Ser. B*, 353, 1245–1255.

D'Esposito, M., Aguirre, G. K., Zarahn, E., & Ballard, D. (1998). Functional MRI studies of spatial and non-spatial working memory. *Cognitive Brain Research*, 7, 1–13.

D'Esposito, M., Detre, J. A., Alsop, D. C., Shin, R. K., Atlas, S., & Grossman, M. (1995). The neural basis of the central executive system of working memory. *Nature*, 378, 279–281.

D'Esposito, M., & Postle, B. R. (1999). The dependence of span and delayed-response performance on prefrontal cortex. *Neuropsychologia*, 37, 1303–1315.

D'Esposito, M., Postle, B. R., Ballard, D., & Lease, J. (1999). Maintenance versus manipulation of information held in working memory: An event-related fMRI study. *Brain & Cognition, 41*, 66–86.

D'Esposito, M., Postle, B. R., Jonides, J., & Smith, E. E. (1999). The neural substrate and temporal dynamics of interference effects in working memory as revealed by event-related functional MRI. *Proceedings of the National Academy of Sciences U.S.A., 96*, 7514–7519.

Diamond, A. (1988). Differences betweeen adult and infant cognition: Is the crucial variable presence or absence of language? In L. Weiskrantz (Ed.), *Thought without language* (pp. 337–370). Oxford: Oxford University Press.

Dias, R., Robbins, T. W., & Roberts, A. C. (1997). Dissociable forms of inhibitory control within prefrontal cortex with an analog of the Wisconsin Card Sort Test: Restriction to novel situations and independence from "on-line" processing. *Journal of Neuroscience, 17*, 9285–9297.

Duncan, J., & Owen, A. M. (2000). Common regions of the human frontal lobe recruited by diverse cognitive demands. *Trends in Neuroscience, 10*, 475–483.

Edinger, H. M., Siegel, A., & Troiano, R. (1975). Effect of stimulation of prefrontal cortex and amygdala on diencephalic neurons. *Brain Research, 97*, 17–31.

Escera, C., Alho, K., Winkler, I., & Naatanen, R. (1998). Neural mechanisms of involuntary attention to acoustic novelty and change. *Journal of Cognitive Neuroscience, 10*, 590–604.

Eslinger, P. J., & Damasio, A. R. (1985). Severe disturbance of higher cognition after bilateral frontal lobe ablation: Patient EVR. *Neurology, 35*, 1731–1741.

Funahashi, S., Bruce, C. J., & Goldman-Rakic, P. S. (1989). Mnemonic coding of visual space in the monkey's dorsolateral prefrontal cortex. *Journal of Neurophysiology, 61*, 331–349.

Funahashi, S., Bruce, C. J., & Goldman-Rakic, P. S. (1993). Dorsolateral prefrontal lesions and oculomotor delayed-response performance: Evidence for mnemonic "scotomas." *Journal of Neuroscience, 13*, 1479–1497.

Fuster, J. M. (1997). *The prefrontal cortex: Anatomy, physiology, and neuropsychology of the frontal lobes.* 3rd ed. New York: Raven Press.

Fuster, J. M., & Alexander, G. E. (1971). Neuron activity related to short-term memory. *Science, 173*, 652–654.

Fuster, J. M., Brodner, M., & Kroger, J. K. (2000). Cross-modal and cross-temporal associations in neurons of frontal cortex. *Nature, 405*, 37–351.

Galambos, R. (1956). Suppression of auditory nerve activity by stimulation of efferent fibers to the cochlea. *Journal of Neurophysiology, 19*, 424–437.

Garavan, H., Ross, T. J., & Stein, E. A. (1999). Right hemispheric dominance of inhibitory control: An event-related functional MRI study. *Proceedings of the Natural Academy of Sciences U.S.A., 96*, 8301–8306.

Godfrey, O., & Rousseaux, M. (1997). Novel decision making in patients with prefrontal or posterior brain damage. *Neurology, 49*, 695–701.

Goldberg, E., Podell, K., & Lovell, M. (1994). Lateralization of frontal lobe functions and cognitive novelty. *Journal of Neuropsychiatry and Clinical Neuroscience, 6*, 371–378.

Grady, C. L., Van Meter, J. W., Maisog, J. M., Pietrini, P., Krasuski, J., & Rauschecker, J. P. (1997). Attention-related modulation of activity in primary and secondary auditory cortex. *Neuroreport, 8*, 2511–2516.

Guillery, R. W., Feig, S. L., & Lozsadi, D. A. (1998). Paying attention to the thalamic reticular nucleus. *Trends in Neuroscience, 21*, 28–32.

Guitton, D., Buchtel, H. A., & Douglas, R. M. (1985). Frontal lobe lesions in man cause difficulties in suppressing reflexive glances and in generating goal-directed saccades. *Experimental Brain Research 58*, 455–472.

Hecaan, H., & Albert, M. L. (1975). *Human Neuropsychology.* New York: John Wiley and Sons.

Heinze, H. J., Mangun, G. R., Burchert, W., Hinrichs, H., Scholz, M., Munte, T. F., Gos, A., Scherg, M., Johannes, S., Hundeshagen, H., Gazzaniga, M. S., & Hillyard, S. A. (1994). Combined spatial and temporal imaging of brain activity during visual selective attention in humans. *Nature, 372*, 543–546.

Hillyard, S. A., & Anllo-Vento, L. (1998). Event-related brain potentials in the study of visual selective attention. *Proceedings of the National Academy of Sciences U.S.A., 95*, 781–787.

Hillyard, S. A., Hink, R. F., Schwent, U. L., & Picton, T. W. (1973). Electrical signs of selective attention in the human brain. *Science, 182*, 177–180.

Hopfinger, J. P., Buonocore, M. H., & Mangun, G. R. (2000). The neural mechanisms of top-down attentional control. *Nature Neuroscience, 3*, 284–291.

Janowsky, J. S., Shimamura, A. P., Kritchevsky, M., & Squire, L. R. (1989a). Cognitive impairment following frontal lobe damage and its relevance to human amnesia. *Behavioral Neuroscience, 103,* 548–560.

Janowsky, J. S., Shimamura, A. P., & Squire, L. R. (1989b). Memory and metamemory: Comparisons between patients with frontal lobe lesions and amnesic patients. *Psychobiology, 17,* 3–11.

Johnson, M. K. (1992). MEM: Mechanisms of recollection. *Journal of Cognitive Neuroscience, 4,* 268–280.

Johnson, M. K., & Raye, C. L. (1981). Reality monitoring. *Psychological Review, 88,* 67–85.

Kahneman, D., & Miller, D. T. (1986). Norm theory: Comparing reality to its alternatives. *Psychological Review, 93,* 136–153.

Karis, D., Fabiani, M., & Donchin, E. (1984). "P300" and memory: Individual differences in the Von Restorff effect. *Cognitive Psychology, 16,* 177–216.

Kastner, S., Pinsk, M. A., de Weerd, P., Desimone, R., & Ungerleider, L. G. (1999). Increased activity in human visual cortex during directed attention in the absence of visual stimulation. *Neuron, 22,* 751–761.

Katayama, J., & Polich, J. (1998). Stimulus context determines P3a and P3b. *Psychophysiology, 35,* 23–33.

Knight, R. T. (1984). Decreased response to novel stimuli after prefrontal lesions in man. *Electroencephalography. Clinical Neurophysiology, 59,* 9–20.

Knight, R. T. (1997). Distributed cortical network for visual attention. *Journal of Cognitive Neuroscience, 9,* 75–91.

Knight, R. T., & Grabowecky, M. (2000). Prefrontal cortex, time and consciousness. In M. Gazzaniga (Ed.), *The new cognitive neurosciences* (pp. 1319–1339). Cambridge, MA: MIT Press.

Knight, R. T., & Scabini, D. (1998). Anatomic bases of event-related potentials and their relationship to novelty detection in humans. *Journal of Clinical Neurophysiology, 15,* 3–13.

Knight, R. T., Scabini, D., & Woods, D. L. (1989). Prefrontal cortex gating of auditory transmission in humans. *Brain Research, 504,* 338–342.

Knight, R. T., Staines, W. R., Swick, D., & Chao, L. L. (1999). Prefrontal cortex regulates inhibition and excitation in distributed neural networks. *Acta Psychologia, 101,* 159–178.

Knight, R. T., Hillyard, S. A., Woods, D. L., & Neville, H. J. (1981). The effects of frontal cortex lesions on event-related potentials during auditory selective attention. *Electroencephalography Clinical Neurophysiology, 52,* 571–582.

Konishi, S., Nakajima, K., Uchida, I., Sekihara, K., & Miyashita, Y. (1998). No-go dominant brain activity in human inferior prefrontal cortex revealed by functional magnetic resonance imaging. *European Journal of Neuroscience, 10,* 1209–1213.

Kraus, N., Ozdamar, O., & Stein, L. (1982). Auditory middle latency responses (MLRs) in patients with cortical lesions. *Electroencephalography and Clinical Neurophysiology, 54,* 275–287.

Leuders, H., Leser, R. P., Harn, J., Dinner, D. S., & Klem, D. (1983). Cortical somatosensory evoked potentials in response to hand stimulation. *Journal of Neurosurgery, 58,* 885–894.

Lhermitte, F. (1986). Human autonomy and the frontal lobes. Part II: Patient behavior in complex and social situations: The "environmental dependency syndrome." *Annals of Neurology, 19,* 335–343.

Lhermitte, F., Pillon, B., & Serdarv, M. (1986). Human anatomy and the frontal lobes. Part I: Imitation and utilization behavior: A neuropsychological study of 75 patients. *Annals of Neurology, 19,* 326–334.

Luck, S. J., Chelazzi, L., Hillyard, S. A., & Desimone, R. (1997). Neural mechanisms of spatial selective attention in areas V1, V2, and V4 of macaque visual cortex. *Journal of Neurophysiology, 77,* 24–42.

Luria, A. R. (1966). *Higher cortical functions in man.* New York: Basic Books.

Malmo, R. R. (1942). Interference factors in delayed response in monkeys after removal of frontal lobes. *Journal of Neurophysiology, 5,* 295–308.

Mangels, J., Gershberg, F. B., Shimamura, A., & Knight, R. T. (1996). Impaired retrieval from remote memory in patients with frontal lobe damage. *Neuropsychology, 10,* 32–41.

Mangun, G. R. (1995). Neural mechanisms of visual selective attention. *Psychophysiology, 32,* 4–18.

Martinez, A., Anllo-Vento, L., Sereno, M. I., Frank, L. R., Buxton, R. B., Dubowitz, D. J., Wong, E. C., Hinrichs, H., Heinze, H. J., & Hillyard, S. A. (1999). Involvement of striate and extrastriate visual cortical areas in spatial attention. *Nature Neuroscience, 2,* 364–369.

McIntosh, A. R., Grady, C. L., Ungerleider, L. G., Haxby, J. U., Rapoport, S. I., & Horwitz, B. (1994). Network analysis of cortical visual pathways mapped with PET. *Journal of Neuroscience*, *14*, 655–666.

Mesulam, M. M. (1998). From sensation to cognition. *Brain*, *121*, 1013–1052.

Miller, E. K. (1999). The prefrontal cortex: Complex neural properties for complex behavior. *Neuron*, *22*, 15–17.

Milner, B. (1963). Effects of different brain regions on card sorting. *Archives of Neurology*, *9*, 90–100.

Muller, N. G., Machado, L., & Knight, R. T. (2002). Contributions of subregions of prefrontal cortex to working memory: Evidence from brain lesions in humans. *Journal of Cognitive Neuroscience*.

Nielsen-Bohlman, L., & Knight, R. T. (1999). Prefrontal cortical involvement in visual working memory. *Cognitive Brain Research*, 8, 299–310.

Perret, E. (1974). The left frontal lobe of man and the suppression of habitual responses in verbal categorical behaviour. *Neuropsychologia*, *12*, 323–330.

Rainer, G., Asaad, W. F., & Miller, E. K. (1998a). Memory fields of neurons in the primate prefrontal cortex. *Proceedings of the National Academy of Sciences U.S.A.*, *95*, 15008–15013.

Rainer, G., Asaad, W. F., & Miller, E. K. (1998b). Selective representation of relevant information by neurons in the primate prefrontal cortex. *Nature*, *393*, 577–579.

Rainer, G., & Miller, E. K. (2000). Effects of visual experience on the representation of objects in the prefrontal cortex. *Neuron*, *27*, 179–189.

Rajkowska, G., & Goldman-Rakic, P. S. (1995a). Cytoarchitechtonic definition of prefrontal areas in the normal human cortex: I. Remapping of areas 9 and 46 using quantitative criteria. *Cerebral Cortex*, *5*, 307–322.

Rajkowska, G., & Goldman-Rakic, P. S. (1995b). Cytoarchitechtonic definition of prefrontal areas in the normal human cortex: II. Variability in locations of areas 9 and 46 and relationship to the Talairach coordinate system. *Cerebral Cortex*, *5*, 323–337.

Rees, G., Frackowiak, R., & Frith, C. (1997). Two modulatory effects of attention that mediate object categorization in human cortex. *Science*, *275*, 835–838.

Richer, F., Decary, A., Lapierre, M., Rouleau, I., Bouvier, G., & Saint-Hilaire, J. (1993). Target detection deficits in frontal lobectomy. *Brain and Cognition*, *21*, 203–211.

Rogers, R. D., & Monsell, S. (1995). Costs of a predictable switch between simple cognitive tasks. *Journal of Experimental Psychology: General*, *124*, 207–231.

Rossi, A. F., Rotter, P. S., Desimone, R., & Ungerleider, L. G. (1999). Prefrontal lesions produce impairments in feature-cued attention. *Society for Neuroscience Abstracts*, 29:2.

Saver, J. L., & Damasio, A. R. (1991). Preserved access and processing of social knowledge in a patient with acquired sociopathy due to ventromedial frontal damage. *Neuropsychologia*, *29*, 1241–1249.

Shallice, T., & Burgess, P. W. (1991). Deficits in strategy application following frontal lobe damage in man. *Brain*, *114*, 727–741.

Shimamura, A. P., Gershberg, F. B., Jurica, P. J., Mangels, J. A., & Knight, R. T. (1992). Intact implicit memory in patients with focal frontal lobe lesions. *Neuropsychologia*, *30*, 931–937.

Shimamura, A. P., Janowsky, J. S., & Squire, L. R. (1990). Memory for the temporal order of events in patients with frontal lobe lesions and amnesic patients. *Neuropsychologia*, *28*, 803–813.

Shimamura, A. P., Janowsky, J. S., & Squire, L. S. (1991). What is the role of frontal lobe damage in memory disorders? In H. Levin, H. Eisenberg, & A. Benton (Eds.), *Frontal lobe function and dysfunction*. New York: Oxford University Press.

Shimamura, A. P., Jurica, P. J., Mangels, J. A., Gershberg, F. B., & Knight, R. T. (1995). Susceptibility to memory interference effects following frontal lobe damage: Findings from tests of paired-associate learning. *Journal of Cognitive Neuroscience*, *7*, 144–152.

Skinner, J. E., & Yingling, C. D. (1977). Central gating mechanisms that regulate event-related potentials and behavior. In J. E. Desmedt (Ed.), *Progress in clinical neurophysiology* (Vol. 1, pp. 30–69). Basel: S. Karger.

Sokolov, E. N. (1963). Higher nervous functions: The orienting reflex. *Annual Review of Physiology*, *25*, 545–580.

Somers, D. C., Dale, A. M., Seiffert, A. E., & Tootell, R. B. (1999). Functional MRI reveals spatially specific attentional modulation in human primary visual cortex. *Proceedings of the National Academy of Sciences U.S.A.*, *96*, 1663–1668.

Steinmetz, P. N., Roy, A., Fitzgerald, P. J., Hsiao, S. S., Johnson, K. O., & Niebur, E. (2000). Attention modulates synchronized neuronal firing in primate somatosensory cortex. *Nature*, *404*, 187–189.

Stone, V. E., Baron-Cohen, S., & Knight, R. T. (1998). Does frontal lobe damage produce theory of mind impairment? *Journal of Cognitive Neuroscience, 10*, 640–656.

Stroop, J. R. (1935). Studies of interference in serial verbal reactions. *Journal of Experimental Psychology, 18*, 643–662.

Stuss, D. T., Alexander, M. P., Palumbo, C. L., Buckle, L., Sayer, L., & Pogue, J. (1994). Organizational strategies of patients with unilateral or bilateral frontal lobe injury in word list learning tasks. *Neuropsychology, 8*, 355–373.

Stuss, D. T., & Benson, D. F. (1984). Neuropsychological studies of the frontal lobes. *Psychological Bulletin, 95*, 3–28.

Stuss, D. T., & Benson, D. F. (1986). *The frontal lobes.* New York: Raven Press.

Suwazono, S., Machado, L., & Knight, R. T. (2000). Predictive value of novel stimuli modifies visual event-related potentials and behavior. *Clinical Neurophysiology, 111*, 29–39.

Swick, D. (1998). Effects of prefrontal lesions on lexical processing and repetition priming: An ERP study. *Cognitive Brain Research, 7*(2), 143–157.

Swick, D., & Knight, R. T. (1998). Lesion studies of prefrontal cortex and attention. In R. Parasuraman (Ed.), *The attentive brain.* Cambridge, MA: MIT Press.

Thompson-Schill, S. L., D'Esposito, M., Aguirre, G. K., & Farah, M. J. (1997). Role of left inferior prefrontal cortex in retrieval of semantic knowledge: a reevaluation. *Proceedings of the Natural Academy of Sciences U.S.A., 94*, 14792–14797.

Tomita, H., Ohbayashi, M., Nakahara, K., Hasegawa, I., & Miyashita, Y. (1999). Top-down signal from prefrontal cortex in executive control of memory retrieval. *Nature, 401*, 699–703.

Tversky, A., & Kahneman, D. (1983). Extensional versus intuitive reasoning: The conjunction fallacy in probability judgement. *Psychological Review, 90*, 293–315.

Von Restorff, H. (1933). Uber die wirkung von bereischsbildungen im spurenfeld. *Psychlogische Forschung, 18*, 299–342.

Webster, M. J., Bachevalier, J., & Ungerleider, L. G. (1994). Connections of inferior temporal areas TEO and TE with parietal and frontal cortex in macaque monkeys. *Cerebral Cortex, 5*, 470–483.

Woldorff, M. G., Gallen, C. C., Hampson, S. A., Hillyard, S. A., Pantev, C., Soble, D., & Bloom, E. F. (1993). Modulation of early sensory processing in human auditory cortex during auditory selective attention. *Proceedings of the National Academy of Sciences U.S.A., 90*, 8722–8726.

Woldorff, M. G., & Hillyard, S. A. (1991). Modulation of early auditory processing during selective listening to rapidly presented tones. *Electroencephalography and Clinical Neurophysiology, 79*, 170–191.

Woldorff, M. G., Fox, P. T., Matzke, M., Lancaster, J. L., Veeraswamy, S., Zamarripa, F., Seabolt, M., Glass, T., Gao, J. H., Martin, C. C., Jerabek, P. (1997). Retinotopic organization of early visual spatial attention: Effects as revealed by PET and ERP data. *Human Brain Mapping, 5*, 280–286.

Woods, D. L. (1990). The physiological basis of selective attention: Implications of event-related potential studies. In J. Rohrbaugh, J. R. Johnson, & R. Parasurman (Eds.), *Event-related brain potentials* (pp. 178–210). New York: Oxford University Press.

Woods, D. L., & Hillyard, S. A. (1978). Attention at the cocktail party: Brainstem evoked responses reveal no peripheral gating. In D. A. Otto (Ed.), *Multidisciplinary perspectives in event-related brain potential research* (pp. 230–233). Washington, DC: U. S. Government Printing Office.

Woods, D. L., & Knight, R. T. (1986). Electrophysiological evidence of increased distractibility after dorsolateral prefrontal lesions. *Neurology, 36*, 212–216.

Yago, E., & Knight, R. T. (2000). Tonic and phasic prefrontal modulation of extrastriate processing during visual attention. *Society for Neuroscience Abstracts, 26*, 2232.

Yamaguchi, S., & Knight, R. T. (1990). Gating of somatosensory inputs by human prefrontal cortex. *Brain Research, 521*, 281–288.

Yamaguchi, S., & Knight, R. T. (1991). Anterior and posterior association cortex contributions to the somatosensory P300. *Journal of Neuroscience, 11*, 2039–2054.

Yamaguchi, S., & Knight, R. T. (1992). Effects of temporal-parietal lesions on the somatosensory P3 to lower limb stimulation. *Electroencephalography and Clinical Neurophysiology, 84*, 139–148.

Yingling, C. D., & Skinner, J. E. (1977). Gating of thalamic input to cerebral cortex by nucleus reticularis thalami. In J. E. Desmedt (Ed.), *Progress in Clinical Neurophysiology* (Vol. I, pp. 70–96). Basel: S. Kargar.

Contributors

Geoffrey K. Aguirre, M.D. Ph.D.
Department of Neurology and
Center for Cognitive Neuroscience
University of Pennsylvania
Philadelphia, Pennsylvania

Michael P. Alexander, M.D.
Department of Neurology
Beth Israel Medical Center
Harvard University
Boston, Massachusetts

Jeffrey R. Binder, M.D.
Department of Neurology
Medical College of Wisconsin
Milwaukee, Wisconsin

Anjan Chatterjee, M.D.
Department of Neurology and
Center for Cognitive Neuroscience
University of Pennsylvania
Philadelphia, Pennsylvania

H. Branch Coslett, M.D.
Department of Neurology and
Center for Cognitive Neuroscience
University of Pennsylvania
Philadelphia, Pennsylvania

Mark D'Esposito, M.D.
Helen Wills Neuroscience Institute and
Department of Psychology
University of California, Berkeley
Berkeley, California

Darren R. Gitelman, M.D.
Department of Neurology and Cognitive Neurology
and Alzhelmer's Disease Center
Northwestern University Medical School
Chicago, Illinois

Scott Grafton, M.D.
Center for Cognitive Neuroscience and
Department of Psychological and Brain Sciences
Dartmouth College
Hanover, New Hampshire

John R. Hodges, M.D.
MRC Cognition and Brain Sciences Unit and
University Department of Neurology
Addenbrooke's Hospital
Cambridge, UK

Robert T. Knight, M.D.
Helen Wills Neuroscience Institute and
Department of Psychology
University of California, Berkeley
Berkeley, California

Michael S. Mega, M.D. Ph.D.
Department of Neurology
University of California, Los Angeles
School of Medicine
Los Angeles, California

Robert Rafal, M.D.
Centre for Cognitive Neuroscience and
School of Psychology
University of Wales
Bangor, Wales, UK

Index